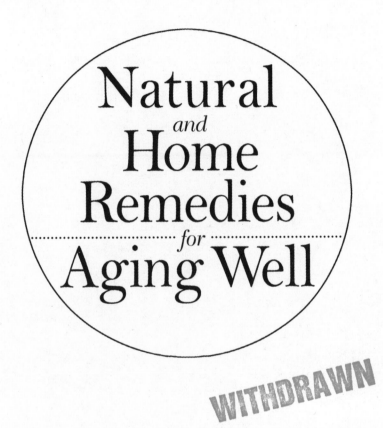

Natural
and
Home
Remedies
for
Aging Well

Also by Bottom Line Inc.

52 Ways to Beat Diabetes
Aging Well with Diabetes

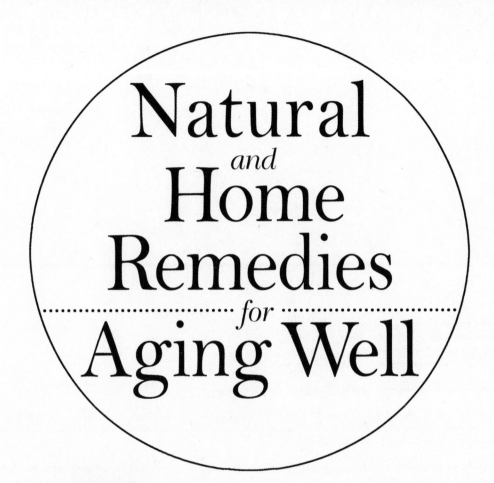

Natural *and* Home Remedies *for* Aging Well

196 Alternative Health and Wellness Secrets That Will Change Your Life

BottomLineInc

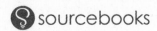

sourcebooks

Copyright © 2018 by Bottom Line Inc.
Cover and internal design © 2018 by Sourcebooks, Inc.
Cover design by The Book Designers
Cover images © kurhan/Shutterstock Images, Feelkoy/Shutterstock Images

Published by Sourcebooks, Inc.
P.O. Box 4410, Naperville, Illinois 60567-4410
(630) 961-3900
Fax: (630) 961-2168
sourcebooks.com

Library of Congress Cataloging-in-Publication data is on file with the publisher.

Printed and bound in the United States of America.
VP 10 9 8 7 6 5 4 3 2 1

Table of Contents

Preface

Medication can be effective and even lifesaving, but Americans might be too quick to seek a quick fix without exploring less risky options. Whatever the ailment, there's supposed to be a pill to save the day. Well, it's time to step back and consider a different approach.

You see, these quick fixes can come with a lot of risk. If age has already left you a bit unsteady, side effects of drugs may easily worsen balance and cause a fall.[*] Adverse effects from medications are the fourth-leading cause of death in the United States (after heart disease, cancer, and stroke). About 6 percent of patients who take two medications daily will experience a drug interaction.[†] If you're taking five medications a day (and a survey of older adults by researchers at the University of Illinois at Chicago found that nearly 36 percent used five or more prescription medications), the risk of having drug interactions rises to 50 percent.[‡]

The other problem with medication is that it's generally prescribed to control the condition, not treat the reasons you have it. Natural therapies, on the other hand, are more likely to target the root causes of illness, increasing the likelihood of a cure. But even when just treating

....

[*]   Ihsan M. Salloum, MD, MPH, "Accidental Addicts—5% of Seniors Abuse Drugs," Bottom Line Inc., May 4, 2010, https://bottomlineinc.com/health/drugs/accidental-addicts-5-seniors-abuse-drugs.

[†]   Armon B. Neel Jr., PharmD, "Are Your Prescriptions Killing You?" Bottom Line Inc., January 1, 2013, https://bottomlineinc.com/health/drug-interactions/are-your-prescriptions-killing-you.

[‡]   D. M. Qato et al., "Changes in Prescription and Over-the-Counter Medication and Dietary Supplement Use Among Older Adults in the United States, 2005 vs. 2011," *Journal of the American Medical Association* 174, no. 4 (April 2016): 473–482.

symptoms, a natural approach can have the same—or better—effect with little to no risk of dangerous side effects. Nondrug approaches also can be a powerful complement to necessary medications, enabling you lower to your doses, improve your quality of life, or even slow the progression of a chronic disease.

While it's true that many nondrug approaches have been based primarily on their thousands of years of use by Asian, Indian, and other traditional cultures, there is now an impressive body of scientific evidence that makes natural medicine a smarter choice than ever before for many health conditions.

The editors at Bottom Line Inc. are proud to bring you *Natural and Home Remedies for Aging Well*, the first book published to gather trustworthy and actionable health and wellness information specifically for mature readers and their families. In the pages of this collection, you'll find what you need to live a fuller, happier life over the age of fifty, from natural foods and supplements to other nondrug approaches for the complications brought on by arthritis, sleep trouble, cancer, or incontinence.

How do we find all these top-notch medical professionals? Over the past four decades, we at Bottom Line have built a network of thousands of leading physicians in both alternative and conventional medicine. They are affiliated with the premier medical institutions and the best universities throughout the world. We read the important medical journals and follow the latest research that is reported at health conferences worldwide. We regularly talk to our advisors in major teaching hospitals, private practices, and government health agencies for their insider perspectives.

Natural and Home Remedies for Aging Well is a result of our ongoing research and connection with these experts and is a distillation of their latest findings and most important advice. We have worked with top experts in natural and complementary medicine and from leading research centers, such as Tufts University, New York University School of Medicine, Rush University Medical Center, University of Tokyo School of Medicine, and University of Washington School of Medicine, to compile the information you need to know. We trust that you will glean new, helpful, and affordable information about living a healthy life!

As a reader, please be assured that you are receiving well-researched information from a trusted source. But please use prudence in health matters. Natural medicine is not do-it-yourself medicine… and just because something is "natural" or "drug free" doesn't mean that it's safe for you. Always work with a knowledgeable health-care provider before starting any new regimen, be it taking vitamins or supplements, stopping a prescribed medication, changing your diet, or beginning an exercise program. If you experience side effects from any regimen, contact your doctor immediately.

Be well,

The Editors, Bottom Line Inc., Stamford, Connecticut

1

Arthritis

Key to Beating Arthritis: The Right Foods and Supplements

Osteoarthritis has long been considered a "wear-and-tear" disease associated with age-related changes that occur within cartilage and bone.

Now: A growing body of evidence shows that osteoarthritis may have a metabolic basis. Poor diet results in inflammatory changes and damage in cartilage cells, which in turn lead to cartilage breakdown and the development of osteoarthritis.

The increase in osteoarthritis cases corresponds to similar increases in diabetes and obesity, other conditions that can be fueled by poor nutrition. Dietary approaches can help prevent—or manage—all three of these conditions.

Key scientific evidence: A number of large studies, including many conducted in Europe as well as the United States, suggest that a diet emphasizing plant foods and fish can support cartilage growth and impede its breakdown. People who combine an improved diet with certain supplements can reduce osteoarthritis symptoms and possibly stop progression of the disease.

A SMARTER DIET

By choosing your foods carefully, you can significantly improve the pain and stiffness caused by osteoarthritis. Here's how to get started.

Avoid acidic foods. The typical American diet, with its processed foods, red meat, and harmful trans fatty acids, increases acidity in the body. A high-acid environment within the joints increases free radicals, corrosive molecules that both accelerate cartilage damage and inhibit the activity of cartilage-producing cells known as chondrocytes.

A Mediterranean diet, which includes generous amounts of fruits, vegetables, whole grains, olive oil, and fish, is more alkaline. (The body requires a balance of acidity and alkalinity, as measured on the pH scale.) A predominantly alkaline body chemistry inhibits free radicals and reduces inflammation.

What to do: Eat a Mediterranean-style diet, including six servings daily of vegetables, three servings of fruit, and two tablespoons of olive oil. (The acids in fruits and vegetables included in this diet are easily neutralized in the body.) Other sources of healthful fats include olives, nuts (such as walnuts), canola oil, and flaxseed oil or ground flaxseed.

Important: It can take twelve weeks or more to flush out acidic toxins and reduce arthritis symptoms after switching to an alkaline diet.

Limit your intake of sugary and processed foods. Most Americans consume a lot of refined carbohydrates as well as sugar-sweetened foods and soft drinks, all of which damage joints in several ways. For example, sugar causes an increase in advanced glycation end products (AGEs), protein molecules that bind to collagen (the connective tissue of cartilage and other tissues) and make it stiff and brittle. AGEs also appear to stimulate the production of cartilage-degrading enzymes.

What to do: Avoid processed foods, such as white flour (including cakes, cookies, and crackers), white pasta, and white rice, as well as soft drinks and fast food. Studies have shown that people who mainly eat foods in their whole, natural forms tend to have lower levels of AGEs and healthier cartilage.

Important: Small amounts of sugar—used to sweeten coffee or cereal, for example—will not significantly increase AGE levels.

Get more vitamin C. More than ten years ago, the Framingham Heart Study found that people who took large doses of vitamin C had a *threefold* reduction in the risk for osteoarthritis progression.

Vitamin C is an alkalinizing agent due to its anti-inflammatory and antioxidant properties. It blocks the inflammatory effects of free radicals. Vitamin C also decreases the formation of AGEs and reduces the chemical changes that cause cartilage breakdown.

What to do: Take a vitamin C supplement (1,000 mg daily for the prevention of osteoarthritis, 2,000 mg daily if you have osteoarthritis).* Also increase your intake of vitamin C–rich foods, such as sweet red peppers, strawberries, and broccoli.

Drink green tea. Green tea alone won't relieve osteoarthritis pain, but people who drink green tea and switch to a healthier diet may notice an additional improvement in symptoms. That's because green tea is among the most potent sources of antioxidants, including catechins, substances that inhibit the activity of cartilage-degrading enzymes.

What to do: For osteoarthritis, drink one to two cups of green tea daily. (Check with your doctor first if you take any prescription drugs.)

Eat fish. Eat five to six three-ounce servings of omega-3-rich fish (such as salmon, sardines, and mackerel) weekly. Omega-3s in such fish help maintain the health of joint cartilage and curb inflammation. If you would prefer to take a fish oil supplement rather than eat fish, see the recommendation below.

SUPPLEMENTS THAT HELP

Dietary changes are a first step to reducing osteoarthritis symptoms. However, the use of certain supplements also can be helpful.

Fish oil. The two omega-3s in fish, docosahexaenoic acid (DHA) and eicosapentaenoic acid (EPA), block chemical reactions in our cells that convert dietary fats into chemical messengers (such as prostaglandins), which affect the inflammatory status of our bodies. This is the same process that's inhibited by nonsteroidal anti-inflammatory drugs (NSAIDs), such as ibuprofen.

What to do: If you find it difficult to eat the amount of omega-3-rich fish mentioned above, ask your doctor about taking fish oil supplements that supply a total of 1,600 mg of EPA and 800 mg of DHA daily. Look for a pharmaceutical grade fish oil product, such as Sealogix or Natural Factors RxOmega-3.

If, after twelve weeks, you need more pain relief or have a strong family history of osteoarthritis, add:

Glucosamine, chondroitin, and MSM. The most widely used supplements for osteoarthritis are glucosamine and chondroitin, taken singly or in combination. Most studies show that they work.

Better: A *triple* combination that contains methylsulfonylmethane (MSM) as well as glucosamine and chondroitin. MSM is a sulfur-containing compound that provides the raw material for cartilage

---

* Check with your doctor before taking any dietary supplements.

regrowth. Glucosamine and chondroitin reduce osteoarthritis pain and have anti-inflammatory properties.

What to do: Take daily supplements of glucosamine (1,500 mg), chondroitin (1,200 mg), and MSM (1,500 mg).

Instead of—or in addition to—the fish oil and the triple combination, you may want to take **SAMe.** Like MSM, S-adenosylmethionine (SAMe) is a sulfur-containing compound. It reduces the body's production of TNF-alpha, a substance that's involved in cartilage destruction. It also seems to increase cartilage production.

In one study, researchers compared SAMe to the prescription anti-inflammatory drug celecoxib. The study was double-blind (neither the patients nor the doctors knew who was getting which drug or supplement), and it continued for four months. Initially, patients taking the celecoxib reported fewer symptoms, but by the second month, there was *no* difference between the two groups.

Other studies have found similar results. SAMe seems to work as well as over-the-counter and/or prescription drugs for osteoarthritis, but it works more slowly. I advise patients to take it for at least three months to see effects.

What to do: Start with 200 mg of SAMe daily and increase to 400 mg daily if necessary after a few weeks.

> Peter Bales, MD, board-certified orthopedic surgeon at Columbia Memorial Hospital in Astoria, Oregon. A research advocate for the Arthritis Foundation (www.arthritis.org), he is author of *Osteoarthritis: Preventing and Healing Without Drugs.*

Green Tea Recipes That Heal

G reen tea can be healing for arthritis sufferers. Buy dried tea leaves (fresh are rare) online or at a health-food store, Asian market, or large grocery store. If you shop for tea leaves in person, whenever possible, check their aroma. If it's weak, the flavor will be weak too, so buy only tea leaves that smell robust. Most types cost around two dollars an ounce, although some less common types, such as premium green tea, can run seventeen dollars an ounce or more. If you have tea bags, you also can just cut the bags open and use those tea leaves.

Here are two easy, delicious ways to use tea in your cooking:

+ **Use tea leaves in a rub.** Grind one tablespoon of tea leaves in an electric coffee grinder or spice mill until they become a fine powder. (Make sure it's not a grinder that has been used to grind coffee, because the aroma and flavor of the coffee will linger and overwhelm the tea aroma and flavor.) Add the powder to one tablespoon of another type of flavoring, then rub it onto one serving of raw fish or poultry with your hands. Let stand for ten minutes before cooking. For example, try green tea with roasted sesame seeds.

+ **Use tea leaves in a marinade.** Add one tablespoon of tea leaves, ground as above, to eight ounces of a marinade. Marinate one serving of fish or poultry in the mixture for thirty minutes before grilling or sautéing. Try green tea with chive-honey-ginger-garlic.

> Robert Wemischner, pastry chef and culinary educator, Los Angeles. He is coauthor of *Cooking with Tea* and author of *The Dessert Architect.* RobertWemischner.com.

Arthritis-Fighting Curry Dry Rub

+ ½ cup mild curry powder
+ 2 tablespoons kosher salt
+ 2 teaspoons crushed red pepper flakes
+ 2 teaspoons ground coriander
+ 1 teaspoon ground turmeric
+ 1 teaspoon ground ginger

1. Combine spices, then sprinkle or pat onto food. Don't rub hard into the food. You can damage the meat's fibers and texture. If seasoning the food overnight, leave out the salt. It will dehydrate the food. But be sure to sprinkle on salt about 15 minutes before you start to cook.

2. Makes 12 tablespoons. Generally, about ¾ to 1 tablespoon of this rub will cover 3 pounds of meat. Great on chicken breast and tofu.

> Linda Gassenheimer, award-winning author of several cookbooks, including *Fast and Flavorful: Great Diabetes Meals from Market to Table.* Her free webinar, "Delicious Diabetes Dinners Everyone Will Love," is available at BottomLineExpertsLive.com.

Relieve Arthritis Pain with Ayurvedic Herbs

Your poor joints are stiff, inflamed, and achy from osteoarthritis, but the medications that reduce your pain also can have serious side effects, such as gastrointestinal bleeding, liver and kidney damage, and increased risk for heart attack and stroke.

Safer solution: Consider the Ayurvedic approach to osteoarthritis treatment, which relies on natural herbs and spices to bring relief.

The following four Ayurvedic arthritis remedies have been used in ancient Indian medicines and in cooking for more than five thousand years. And they really work. A study presented at a meeting of the American College of Rheumatology showed a combination herbal Ayurvedic therapy to be as effective in treating knee osteoarthritis as the commonly prescribed medication celecoxib.

Boswellia (Indian frankincense). This comes from the resin of the *Boswellia serrata* plant. It works by blocking an enzyme involved in the formation of leukotrienes, chemicals that trigger inflammation.

Note: Boswellia may cause a reaction in people who are allergic to ragweed, and it can irritate the gastrointestinal tract (especially if taken alone rather than in a balanced combination formula as traditionally used).

Turmeric. The active ingredient in this spice, curcumin, interferes with three important inflammation-producing enzymes, so it disrupts the inflammatory process at three different stages. Turmeric also may provide some protection against the damage that pain-relieving medications can do to the gastrointestinal tract.

Ginger. Various studies have demonstrated ginger's ability to reduce pain and inflammation by interfering with inflammatory enzymes.

Bonus: Ginger also aids digestion. Why should that matter? Because according to Ayurvedic principals, poor digestion is a primary trigger for arthritis. When we eat improper foods or our digestion is weak, food is not broken down into small molecules, so larger-than-normal molecules get absorbed into the bloodstream. These biochemical impurities circulate, eventually getting localized in a tissue and initiating swelling. When the affected tissue is a joint, the result is arthritis.

Ashwagandha. This herb is also known as winter cherry or Indian ginseng. Studies suggest that it has anti-inflammatory properties that protect against cartilage damage. In addition, animal studies provide evidence that the herb combats stress. When we are stressed, the hormones cortisol and epinephrine cause a breakdown of various body tissues. Ashwagandha helps alleviate the damaging effects of stress by restoring the proper hormonal balance to the nervous system, which in turn strengthens the immune system and further reduces inflammation.

Caution: Since ashwagandha makes your immune system more active, it is not appropriate for people who have an autoimmune disorder, including rheumatoid arthritis. Rarely, ashwagandha can irritate the gastrointestinal tract.

USING AYURVEDIC HERBS

Ayurvedic herbal products are available in health-food stores and online. For maximum convenience and effect, osteoarthritis patients should take an herbal supplement that combines several of the herbs and spices listed above, such as Maharishi Ayurveda's Flexcel, which contains boswellia, ashwagandha, and ginger as well as other natural ingredients that further support joint and bone health. This product does not contain turmeric, so you can use the spice liberally in the kitchen. Turmeric added to food is more important than in a formula because you can get a much greater quantity that way. Add turmeric to every meal and cook it into each dish, even if only in small amounts, for its cumulative anti-inflammatory and antioxidant protection.

Important: According to a Boston University study, some commercial Ayurvedic herbal remedies contain lead, mercury, and/or arsenic in amounts exceeding regulatory standards. I endorse Maharishi Ayurveda (www.mapi.com), a company that has been in business for nearly thirty years. If you are interested in a different brand, to guard against contamination, contact the seller to make sure the company tests every batch in the United States for heavy metals, as well as for parasites and fungus.

To make sure that the specific ingredients are safe and appropriate for you and to get dosage recommendations, consult a physician who is knowledgeable about Ayurvedic medicine. To find such a practitioner, visit the website of the Light on Ayurveda Education Foundation (www .loaj.com).

Try this Ayurvedic approach for eight weeks to see whether these remedies relieve your osteoarthritis symptoms. If they do, continue to take them indefinitely, reducing to the lowest dose that maintains your improvement.

> Nancy Lonsdorf, MD, in private practice in Fairfield, Iowa. Dr. Lonsdorf is author of *The Ageless Woman: Natural Health and Beauty After Forty with Maharishi Ayurveda* and coauthor of *A Woman's Best Medicine: Health, Happiness and Long Life through Maharishi Ayur-Veda.* Ayurveda-ayurvedic.org.

Natural Soothers for Joint Pain

Many arthritis patients find these supplements and natural therapies helpful.

Red seaweed extract. Red seaweed extract (*Lithothamnion calcareum*) can help people with osteoarthritis. One study reported in *Nutrition Journal* and funded by Marigot, the company that makes Aquamin (a patented red seaweed extract), found that taking the extract for one month was associated with a 20 percent reduction in arthritis pain. Patients also reported less stiffness and better range of motion and were able to walk farther than those taking a placebo. A typical dose would be 2,400 mg of seaweed extract in capsule form each day. (Note: Seaweed contains iodine in amounts that may be dangerous to thyroid patients.)

Vitamin D. Research indicates that vitamin D may play a key role in slowing the development and progression of both osteoarthritis and rheumatoid arthritis. If you have either, it's a good idea to get your blood level of vitamin D checked. If you are deficient, take at least 1,000 IU of vitamin D-3 (cholecalciferol) each day.

Peat/peloid packs (also called balneotherapy). Commonly used in Europe, this is a form of thermal mud therapy that holds heat particularly well. Peat (or peloid packs that are sheets of peat mud on fabric) is applied to the aching area for about twenty minutes. The treatment can be done at home, but it is far better to work with a physical therapist or doctor who is knowledgeable in the technique, as the packs are cumbersome and must be carefully applied to protect the skin

from burning. Peat therapy treatments are typically administered over the course of several visits, declining in frequency as the patient's pain begins to ease. The results are long-lasting, and you can resume treatment if and when the pain returns.

Methylsulfonylmethane (MSM). MSM is a sulfur derivative that is beneficial for some people with osteoarthritis. It may help prevent cartilage degeneration, and it's also known to decrease pain and improve physical function. It's thought that MSM works better when combined with glucosamine—take one gram of MSM twice daily with meals.

Massage and acupuncture. Many people, including those with rheumatoid arthritis or osteoarthritis, find these treatments to be soothing. This makes sense, since both techniques increase blood flow to the muscles and ligaments around the joints (particularly the knees and hips), which are stressed by arthritis.

Exercise. This often is the last thing people in pain feel like doing, but exercise is still essential for both osteoarthritis and rheumatoid arthritis patients. The primary benefit is that exercise delivers fresh blood cells to the affected areas, bringing in nutrients and removing waste, including acidic waste products in the muscles that may provoke inflammation. Try swimming, walking, or perhaps working with a trainer who is knowledge-able about arthritis.

Weight control. Keeping your weight down reduces the pressure on painful joints for both osteoarthritis and rheuma-toid arthritis patients. An NIH study found twice as much arthritis in obese people as in people of healthy weight. One study showed that losing just eleven pounds reduced risk for knee osteoarthri-tis by half and significantly reduced pain in the knees of those already afflicted.

› Kimberly Beauchamp, ND, licensed naturopathic doctor and health and nutrition writer, North Kingstown, Rhode Island. KimberlyBeauchamp.com.

Joint Pain: Four Surprising Cures

Exercise has so many health benefits that it's hard to understand why everyone isn't doing it on a regular basis. But what if it hurts to exercise? If you have joint pain, you may wonder whether exercise is good for you or even possible to do. In conventional medicine, joint pain is treated with synthetic medication, typically nonsteroidal anti-inflammatory drugs (NSAIDs), such as naproxen or ibuprofen. These medicines usually are effective for short-term use, but they do not cure the problem, and they can harm your stomach. For these reasons, I prefer to start with natural methods, which usually do a terrific job at reducing—and sometimes even eliminating—joint pain. These are my favorite remedies for joint pain, roughly in order of importance.

Get serious about stress reduction. An increasing body of evidence now shows that stress reduction really does reduce pain. You may have noticed this through your own experiences—for example, your pain lessens while you're on vacation or during a relaxed weekend. Three stress-reducing methods that I highly recom-mend are yoga, meditation, and massage. I advise patients to engage in one or more of these practices on a regular basis. An ideal stress-reducing regimen might include daily meditation, yoga three times a week, and/or massage once a week.

Investigate food allergies. Eating food to which you are allergic can significantly increase pain. Wheat, soy, and peanuts are common food aller-gens. To start, eliminate suspected foods to see if your symptoms improve and then reappear when the foods are reintroduced. Or ask a naturopathic physician to test you for food allergies using a blood test for immunoglobu-lin G (IgG), an antibody that reaches high levels with food allergies. If food allergies don't seem to be contributing to your pain, you may want to consider giving up animal-based foods, including meat. Animal-based foods are generally inflammatory, which means that they contain a high percentage of arachidonic acids that can promote and aggravate pain. Keep in mind that you can often get more inflammation-fighting omega-3s from plant sources, such as flaxseed and walnuts, than from fish.

Try boswellia. This herbal remedy contains nutrients that reduce inflammation and improve both acute and chronic joint pain.

Typical dose: 300 mg three times a day for four weeks, then 300 mg one to three times a day if needed for pain. It's generally safe, but check with your doctor before trying this remedy.

Get some mild exercise. Many people mistakenly assume that exercise will damage joints and increase pain, but studies show that regular mild exercise, such as swimming, yoga, or Pilates, promotes circulation within joints and will reduce inflammation and pain. Work out up to the point of pain, then stop and repeat the exercise the next day, ideally until you can do the activity for an hour a day, six days a week. If you have joint degeneration or severe pain, check with your doctor first.

› Jamison Starbuck, ND, naturopathic physician in family practice and a guest lecturer at the University of Montana, both in Missoula. She is past president of the American Association of Naturopathic Physicians. Starbuck is a columnist for the *Bottom Line Health Insider* and hosts *Dr. Starbuck's Health Tips for Kids* on Montana Public Radio. DrJamisonStarbuck.com.

Foods That Worsen Arthritis Symptoms

The only way to know which of the foods below affect your joint pain is to eliminate each one for at least two weeks and assess your symptoms. That way, you'll know which type of food increases your inflammation and pain.

Avoid foods that increase inflammation. There are a variety of foods that trigger the body to produce cytokines—naturally occurring proteins that can promote inflammation, leading to pain and deterioration of cartilage in the joints.

These include beef and other red meat, foods cooked at high temperatures, particularly fried foods, and any foods containing man-made trans fats (often called partially hydrogenated fats or oils on food labels), including junk food and commercial baked goods. Eat these types of foods sparingly.

Reduce intake of foods from animal products. I tell my patients to eat turkey and chicken in moderation. But the fact is that all animal products—including poultry, some farm-raised fish, egg yolks, and other dairy products—contain arachidonic acid, a fatty acid that is converted by the body into prostaglandins and leukotrienes, two other types of inflammation-causing chemicals. I've had many patients tell me that they reduced arthritis symptoms by adopting a modified vegetarian diet.

Key: Decrease your intake of animal protein and increase the amount of protein you get from fish and plant sources, such as beans, nuts, soy, portobello mushrooms (a common meat substitute), and whole grains. Start by substituting one-fourth of the animal protein you normally eat with plant-based foods, cold-water fish, and low-fat dairy. After two or three months, increase the substitution to half, adding more vegetables, fruits, lentils, beans, fish, whole grains, and low-fat dairy. After a while, many of my patients choose to give up all animal protein because they enjoy the benefit of reduced pain and inflammation.

Note: A small percentage of people find that certain vegetables—including tomatoes, white potatoes, peppers, and eggplant—make their arthritis worse. These nightshade family plants contain solanine, a substance that can be toxic if not sufficiently digested in the intestines. Eliminate all these foods, then add them back one at a time, as long as you do not have pain or inflammation.

Stay away from foods with a high glycemic index. While high-glycemic foods (foods that quickly raise your blood sugar) should be avoided by people with diabetes or prediabetes, they pose problems for people with arthritis as well.

Reason: They increase insulin production, which promotes accumulation of body fat and causes a rebound sensation of hunger a few hours after eating, making it harder to maintain a healthy weight, which is important for reducing arthritis symptoms. High-glycemic foods include table sugar, baked white potatoes, French fries, pretzels, white bread and rolls, white and brown rice, potato and corn chips, waffles, doughnuts, and corn flakes.

....

› Harris McIlwain, MD, board-certified specialist in rheumatology and geriatric medicine, McIlwain Medical Group, Tampa, Florida. He is coauthor of *Pain-Free Arthritis—A 7-Step Program for Feeling Better Again.* MmgHealth.com.

....

The Best Pain-Fighting Foods for Osteoarthritis, Rheumatoid Arthritis, and Gout

Many of us turn to medications to relieve pain. But research has shown that you can help reduce specific types of pain—and avoid the side effects of drugs—just by choosing the right foods (unless otherwise noted, aim to eat the recommended foods daily). Here are some common causes of pain and the foods that can help.

OSTEOARTHRITIS

Osteoarthritis causes pain and inflammation in the joints.

Best foods: Bing cherries, ginger, avocado oil, and soybean oil.

A study in the *Journal of Nutrition* found that men and women who supplemented their diets with Bing cherries (about two cups of cherries throughout the day) had an 18 to 25 percent drop in C-reactive protein, a sign of inflammation. Bing cherries contain flavonoids, plant-based compounds with antioxidant properties that lower inflammation.

Ginger also contains potent anti-inflammatory agents that can reduce joint pain. A double-blind, placebo-controlled study found that 63 percent of people who

consumed ginger daily had less knee pain when walking or standing. I recommend one to two teaspoons of ground fresh ginger every day.

Avocado oil and soybean oil contain avocado soybean unsaponifiables (ASUs), which reduce inflammation and cartilage damage in arthritis patients.

RHEUMATOID ARTHRITIS

This autoimmune disease causes systemic inflammation—your joints, your heart, and even your lungs may be affected.

Best foods: Fish and vitamin C–rich foods.

The omega-3 fatty acids in fish increase the body's production of inhibitory prostaglandins, substances with anti-inflammatory effects. A recent study found that some patients who consumed fish oil supplements improved so much that they were able to discontinue their use of aspirin, ibuprofen, and similar medications.

Ideally, it's best to eat two to three servings of fish a week. Or take a daily fish oil supplement. The usual dose is 1,000 to 3,000 mg. Be sure to work with a qualified health professional to determine what supplement regimen is right for you.

Foods rich in vitamin C (citrus fruits, berries, red bell peppers) are effective analgesics because they help decrease joint inflammation. These foods also help protect and repair joint cartilage. A study in the *American Journal of Nutrition* found that patients who ate the most vitamin C–rich fruits had 25 percent lower risk for inflammation.

GOUT

Gout is a form of arthritis that causes severe joint pain that can last for days and that flares up at unpredictable intervals.

Weight loss and avoiding refined carbohydrates, such as white bread, commercially prepared baked goods, and other processed foods can help minimize flare-ups. You also should eat foods that reduce uric acid, a metabolic by-product that causes gout.

Best foods: Celery and cherries.

Celery contains the chemical compound 3-n-butylphthalide, which reduces the body's production of uric acid. Celery also reduces inflammation.

Both sweet (Bing) and tart (Montmorency) pie cherries contain flavonoids, although the bulk of science supporting the anti-inflammatory and pain-relieving properties of cherries has been done using tart cherries. (An exception is the study that found that Bing cherries relieve osteoarthritis.) It is hard to find fresh tart cherries, so I recommend dried tart cherries or tart cherry juice.

› David Grotto, RD, registered dietitian and founder and president of Nutrition Housecall, LLC, a Chicago-based nutrition consulting firm that provides nutrition communications, lecturing, and consulting services as well as personalized, at-home dietary services. He is an adviser to *Fitness* magazine and blogs for the Real Life Nutrition community featured on WebMD. He is author of *The Best Things You Can Eat: For Everything from Aches to Zzzz*. DavidGrotto.com.

Arthritis Relief That's Safer Than NSAIDs

What can you do about unremitting osteoarthritis pain after you've tried it all—conventional specialists, assorted prescriptive and over-the-counter pharmaceutical medications, and even the much talked about natural substance glucosamine? More drugs may not be the answer. But an alternate natural remedy could be.

As a nurse, sixty-one-year-old Betsy knew better than most people about the risks inherent in taking many OTC drugs, including the painkilling NSAIDs—nonsteroidal anti-inflammatory drugs. Betsy ached constantly from the arthritis in her knees and hips, especially since her job kept her on her feet all day. The hours she spent in bed at night had become painful as well, making it difficult for her to sleep. Painkilling drugs seemed to offer the only option for obtaining some measure of pain-free time, and for several years, they did help, but now they had ceased to be effective, so Betsy made an appointment with me at a friend's recommendation.

A STEP IN THE RIGHT DIRECTION

In our first meeting, I discovered that along with the painkilling NSAID pills, Betsy had already started to use natural substances in hopes of combating her arthritis. Several years previously, she had read that glucosamine sulfate would ease arthritis pain. Consequently, in addition to the multivitamin and vitamin C she'd been taking daily for years, she had added 1,500 mg of glucosamine to her daily regimen. She continued to take the glucosamine faithfully, but she admitted it hadn't really helped. In fact, her joints were aching worse than ever. Betsy was also thirty pounds overweight, which exacerbated her joint pain. I immediately put her on a weight loss program, but now I also had to find a natural substance that would address Betsy's joint stiffness and pain since the glucosamine, which is helpful for many people, was not working for her.

The substance I determined would likely help Betsy was an oral collagen-containing hyaluronic acid supplement. Collagen-containing hyaluronic acid is less well known than glucosamine for treating osteoarthritis. Many of my patients have found it to be extremely effective, since hyaluronic acid exists in all tissues and fluids in the body with the highest concentrations of it in connective tissues, including the collagen between bones that cushions the joints. Hyaluronic acid supplements made from animal cartilage can help with connective tissue formation and especially with production of synovial fluid in the joints, another way the body protects the joints from stiffness and pain. I prescribed 500 mg of collagen-containing hyaluronic acid twice a day for Betsy.

OTHER PROBLEMS CAUSED BY NSAIDS

With an aging population, osteoarthritis has become more widespread than ever. Many people reach for NSAIDs to ease their pain, but overuse of these drugs—as is frequently the case in treating a chronic problem such as arthritis—can be, as Betsy discovered, ineffective. For some patients, they're even dangerous. The drugs can be hard on the digestive system, the stomach in particular, causing bleeding and ulceration. There is also evidence that NSAIDs are associated with kidney and liver problems and possibly increased cardiovascular risk. The problems they can cause may be far worse than those people started with.

While many people find that glucosamine (the original supplement Betsy took) helps soothe their arthritis pain, it's not always successful, and even when it is, it sometimes stops working after a while. This is one reason it's so important to have a physician trained in natural medicine oversee your use of supplements. My prescription of collagen-containing hyaluronic acid, much less well known than glucosamine, offers relief for many who aren't finding success with glucosamine. It should be used until symptoms subside. One product I use often is BioCell Collagen II, which is a patented form with research showing it to be well tolerated.

THE PATIENT'S PROGRESS

After just three weeks, Betsy was feeling much better, and after eight weeks of treatment, her improvement was considerable. Betsy was also helped by losing her excess weight. I recommended a daily calorie intake of 1,500 calories—moderate protein, high fiber, balanced fats, and avoiding most refined carbs. She was taking a weekly aqua aerobics class and biking several days a week as well. At a follow-up visit one year later, Betsy reported she was 80 percent better and that although she continues to take collagen-containing

hyaluronic acid, she no longer has any need for painkilling drugs.

....

› Mark A. Stengler, NMD, naturopathic doctor and founder of the Stengler Center for Integrative Medicine in Encinitas, California. He is author and coauthor of numerous books, including *The Natural Physician's Healing Therapies* and *Bottom Line's Prescription for Natural Cures*, and is the author of the newsletter *Health Revelations*. MarkStengler.com.

....

How to Use Marijuana to Fight Arthritis

T*he U.S. government classifies marijuana* (cannabis) as a Schedule I controlled substance—a dangerous drug with no medical value. Yet the Institute of Medicine, an elite group of scientists and physicians, has concluded that the chemical compounds in marijuana do have therapeutic properties.

The wrangling between scientists and policy makers won't stop anytime soon. Neither will the wrangling between the federal government and the states, as more and more allow the use of medical marijuana—some even legalized marijuana for recreational use for people over age twenty-one. But marijuana can be an effective medicine for some patients and can be very helpful in reducing pain.

Caution: Always use medical marijuana under a doctor's supervision.

The anti-inflammatory and pain-relieving substances in cannabis appear to make it a good choice for different forms of arthritis, including rheumatoid arthritis and osteoarthritis.

In the past, cannabis often was recommended for nausea, even in the absence of weight loss. It was clearly more effective than the early generation antinausea medication dronabinol, which is synthesized from cannabis-based compounds. However, newer drugs for nausea, such as ondansetron, are probably more effective than cannabis.

HOW TO USE IT

I don't recommend that my patients who use cannabis smoke it. Smoking can increase the risk for bronchitis or other respiratory problems. Here are some better methods.

Vaporization. When patients use a vaporizer, the active compounds in cannabis "boil" and turn into vapor—the plant material doesn't get hot enough to burn. This eliminates the harsh compounds in the smoke. It also causes less intoxication, because the lower temperatures don't activate tetrahydrocannabinol (THC), the compound that causes most of the "high" associated with smoking marijuana.

Sublingual tincture. With a prescription, you can buy this form of cannabis at some dispensaries. You also can make it at home by steeping one ounce of cannabis flowers (available at dispensaries) in six ounces of glycerin for about a week. You put three or four drops under your tongue when you need a dose. It works almost as quickly as vaporized cannabis.

Juicing. You can put a small amount of cannabis in a blender, add your choice of liquids such as milk or juice, and drink it as a beverage. The intoxicating effects are reduced because the THC isn't heated.

Some people eat cannabis by adding it to brownies or other prepared foods. Don't do it. The intoxicating effects can be very strong. And because it can take an hour or longer to work, patients may think that they're not getting enough. They consume even more—and wind up getting too much.

HOW MUCH TO TAKE

Some cannabis dispensaries (and growers) use devices called gas chromatographs to measure the amounts of THC and other compounds in their products. This makes it easier to achieve batch-to-batch consistency. Typically, the cannabis sold by dispensaries has a THC concentration of about 15 to 20 percent.

Doctors who recommend cannabis

usually rely on patient-titrated dosing. This simply means taking a small amount when you need a dose, waiting for about twenty to thirty minutes to see how you feel, and then increasing or decreasing subsequent doses as needed. Effects typically last one to two hours.

WHAT AND WHERE TO BUY

Different types of cannabis have markedly different effects. Cannabis that is rich in cannabidiol (CBD) has fewer psychoactive effects than cannabis with a lot of THC. Patients who want to minimize the intoxicating effects can choose a strain with a higher percentage of CBD.

You can buy marijuana at dispensaries in the states where it is legal. Describe your symptoms to the clerk so that he/she can help you choose the right type of cannabis. If, for example, you have pain that mainly bothers you at night, you probably will want a cannabis that's high in CBD—it will help you fall asleep. Patients with certain conditions where fatigue is a symptom and who need a lift might do better with a higher-THC product.

SIDE EFFECTS

Recreational users of marijuana want to get high. For medical patients, this often is the main drawback.

I recommend to my patients that they "start low, go slow." Take the lowest possible dose at first. Later, you can increase the dose if you need more relief. If you find that you're getting intoxicated, use less.

Obviously, you shouldn't drive, operate tools or machinery, or perform tasks that require a lot of concentration up to three hours after using cannabis, though residual effects have been reported up to twenty-four hours after using any medication that impairs mental functions.

Caution: If you have a serious psychiatric illness, such as bipolar disorder or schizophrenia, don't use cannabis without the supervision of a psychiatrist. I don't recommend cannabis for patients with a history of drug and/or alcohol abuse unless they've been referred by an addiction specialist.

> Gregory T. Carter, MD, physiatrist, medical director at St. Luke's Rehabilitation Institute in Spokane, Washington. His research interests include the use of cannabis and other treatments for amyotrophic lateral sclerosis (ALS). He is senior associate editor for *Muscle & Nerve* and coauthor of *Medical Marijuana 101.* St-Lukes.org.

How Meditation Can Help Arthritis

*S*tress is bad for everybody but particularly for people who suffer from a chronic inflammatory condition such as asthma, rheumatoid arthritis, or inflammatory bowel disease. That's because stress contributes to inflammation, so it makes sense to take steps to reduce stress.

A particular type of stress-reducing technique appears to be uniquely beneficial when it comes to quelling inflammation, according to a recent study. Best of all, this technique requires no drugs (or any foreign substance, for that matter), it's easy to do, and it can be done anywhere.

How the study was done: Healthy volunteers were divided into two groups. One group was instructed in mindfulness-based stress reduction (MBSR), a technique in which a person meditates by focusing attention on his breathing and bodily sensations while sitting still, walking, or doing yoga. The thing to notice is that this sort of meditation emphasizes mindfulness, which means to foster an awareness of each sensation, emotion, or thought as it unfolds in the moment, catching and then releasing it without judgment. The other group participated in a program that combined physical activity, music therapy, and instruction

in improved nutrition, all of which are known to improve well-being but do not include the idea of mindfulness. Both groups received the same amount of training and did the same amount of at-home practice for eight weeks.

Before starting and again after the end of the eight-week programs, the researchers provoked stress in the participants by asking them to give short impromptu speeches and to do some mental arithmetic problems. Next, a cream with an irritant was placed on the participants' forearms to induce inflammation, then a sucking device was applied to raise blisters. This allowed the researchers to collect some fluid from the irritated skin so that levels of two cytokines (proteins released by the immune system) could be measured. Researchers also measured the size of the resulting inflamed areas of skin and the amount of the stress hormone cortisol secreted in the participants' saliva at various times throughout the day.

Results: It was not surprising that the stress caused by giving speeches and doing mental math caused increases in markers for stress, and the levels of the cytokines and cortisol were about the same in both groups. But participants who had practiced mindfulness meditation showed significantly less stress-induced inflammation (as measured by the area of inflamed skin) than those in the other group, and their cortisol levels on a normal day showed a healthier circadian rhythm.

In other words, the meditators had reduced their bodies' inflammatory response—something that would be good for anyone but that could provide an especially profound health benefit for a person with an inflammatory condition!

Bottom line: If you have a chronic inflammatory health problem, or if you want an extra measure of protection against the harmful effects of inflammation, consider taking a class in mindfulness meditation. It's a very popular sort of meditation, and you shouldn't have trouble finding a class in your area. Or visit the website of the University of Massachusetts Center for Mindfulness in Medicine, Health Care, and Society (www.umassmed.edu/cfm) to search for an MBSR-trained practitioner near you.

> Melissa A. Rosenkranz, PhD, associate scientist, Waisman Laboratory for Brain Imaging and Behavior and Center for Investigating Healthy Minds, University of Wisconsin, Madison. Her study was published in *Brain, Behavior, and Immunity.*

Get Fit in the Water! If You Have Arthritis, It's the Workout of Choice

Many people avoid exercise because they assume that they are too out of shape to get started or fear that they will get injured or their muscles will ache after workouts. Sound familiar?

If so, water exercise could be your solution. It involves much more than swimming. A good water workout may include jogging, pushing, and pulling—all in the water.*

Key advantage: The buoyancy of water reduces your "weight" by 90 to 100 percent (depending on the depth of the water), so there's far less stress on your joints and muscles.

This makes water exercise an excellent option for people with osteoarthritis, rheumatoid arthritis, or back problems. It's also ideal for those with peripheral arterial disease (reduced blood flow to the extremities) or other circulatory problems—the force of water against your body stimulates blood circulation.

Don't assume that you can't get a good workout from water exercises. When done

---

* Water exercise may not be recommended if you have a skin condition, such as psoriasis, or have recently undergone surgery.

properly, this form of exercise can boost your cardiovascular fitness.

Water exercise also improves muscular strength, endurance, and flexibility—all of which help with daily activities ranging from grocery shopping to gardening.

A TOUGH WORKOUT THAT DOESN'T HURT

Water exercise is safe and comfortable. Water's natural buoyancy—it resists downward movement and assists upward movement—allows you to virtually eliminate any jarring physical impact on your lower body, especially your hips, knees, and ankles.

The gravity-defying effects of water also eliminate any risk of falling during your workout. In addition, water's natural resistance—currents push and pull against the body—strengthen your core muscles (the abdominals and back) to improve your posture, promote better balance, and reduce lower back pain.

BEST WATER WORKOUTS

The following workout, which is a good introduction to water exercises, is best performed in a water depth slightly above the navel. Perform the workout at least twice weekly—ideally, in addition to exercises on land, such as walking.

Jog and scull boosts heart health.

What to do: Begin by moving your hands across the water's surface as if smoothing sand. This movement, called *sculling*, helps promote balance. While keeping your ears, shoulders, and hips in a straight line, jog up and down with your knees raised high, as if marching, and continue to scull with your hands just beneath the water's surface.

Jog up and down the lanes of a lap pool. (If the pool ranges from shallow to deep, run side to side across the shallow end.) Continue for three to five minutes, increasing to ten minutes or more as you build stamina. In addition, aim to gradually increase your speed and the height of your knees as you jog.

Tandem stand promotes balance and reduces your risk of falling on land.

What to do: Stand with one foot in front of the other as if walking on a line. Move your arms so that you alternate with one arm in front and the other one behind the hips. As you move your arms, the water currents will challenge your balance and strengthen your core. Continue for thirty seconds to one minute, then switch feet front to back. Repeat three to four times.

Rock forward, rock back improves posture and back strength.

What to do: While standing on one leg, tilt your upper body forward with your other leg bent at the knee and your hands held flat in front of you for balance.

Then rock back and pull your arms slightly back, while squeezing your shoulder blades together and keeping your hands turned so that your thumbs are pointed upward. Switch legs and repeat. Perform one to three sets (eight to fifteen repetitions each).

DON'T HAVE A POOL?

You don't need your own backyard swimming pool to perform water exercise. Nonprofit organizations, such as the YMCA/YWCA and Jewish Community Centers, operate approximately four thousand swimming pools across the United States. Memberships, which range from thirty to ninety dollars monthly depending on location, are often less expensive than those at for-profit health clubs. Municipal pools also are common in the United States. Many do not charge admission, and some offer water exercise classes.

....
> Mary E. Sanders, PhD, adjunct professor of health education, University of Nevada School of Medicine, Reno. A research fellow of the American College of Sports Medicine, she serves as an advisory board member for the International Council on Active Aging and has developed water exercise programs based on research that she has conducted for more than fifteen years.
....

Pain-Free Knees without Surgery

M*ost people over age fifty* can expect to live longer than their parents or grandparents, but many are doing so without their original knees.

What's happening: Knee-replacement procedures, known as total knee arthroplasty, have become one of the most commonly performed surgeries in the United States.

Each year, more than six hundred thousand Americans undergo knee replacement to help relieve the pain associated with knee osteoarthritis, rheumatoid arthritis, or other forms of degenerative joint disease—and the numbers just keep rising. This trend is due largely to an aging population and obesity, a leading cause of joint damage.

But is surgery really the right solution for all these people? Not necessarily.

Here's the catch: Many people who receive knee replacements could have avoided surgery—along with the risk for infection and the painful weeks of postsurgical rehabilitation—with simple exercises that strengthen the knee and help prevent deterioration of the tendons, ligaments, and bones.

A HEALTHY-KNEE PROGRAM

In addition to exercise, normal body weight is critical for long-term knee health. If you're overweight or obese, your knees are subjected to unnecessary force. Research has shown that losing as little as eleven pounds can cut the risk of developing knee arthritis by 50 percent.

But if you're overweight, losing *any* amount of weight can help. One study, published in the journal *Arthritis & Rheumatism,* found that every pound of lost weight translates into a four-pound reduction in knee stress—with each and every step.

Why exercise helps: Patients who stretch and strengthen the muscles around the knees have better joint support. There is also an increase in synovial fluid, a gel-like substance that keeps the joints moving smoothly.

What's more, exercise increases bone density in these patients and results in better range of motion.

FOUR MUST-DO EXERCISES

Everyone can benefit from knee exercises. Even if you don't suffer from knee pain now, the following exercises may help prevent problems from developing. People who have received surgery to replace or repair a knee also can benefit by strengthening their muscles to help guard against future knee injuries.

The goal of knee exercises is to work the muscles *around* the joint. These include the quadriceps (on the front of the thigh), the hamstrings (back of the thigh), and the muscles in the calves. Strength and flexibility in these areas support the knees and help keep them aligned. Alignment is critical, because asymmetry increases pressure and joint damage.

Perform the following regimen daily—it can be completed in about fifteen to thirty minutes. If you have an advanced knee problem due to a condition such as rheumatoid arthritis, your doctor may also prescribe additional exercises that are targeted to address your specific issues.

Important: All the exercises described in this article should be performed within a range of motion that does not cause pain. If a slight strain occurs with the first repetition, that is acceptable, as long as the pain diminishes with subsequent repetitions. If the pain worsens with subsequent repetitions, stop the exercise.

1. **Knee-to-chest stretch.** This exercise improves flexibility in the lower back, hips, and hamstrings. People who do this stretch will notice an opening of their hips, allowing them to stand taller. This improvement in posture is important for reducing knee stress.

   Bonus: You can use this movement

to diagnose knee problems. If the knee you're bending doesn't come straight toward your shoulder and stay in line with your foot, you'll know that you have an alignment problem that needs to be corrected.

This knee exercise can be performed in bed if that is more comfortable than doing it on a carpeted floor or on a padded surface. Here's what to do.

- *Lie on your back with your knees bent and your feet flat on the floor (or bed).*
- *Using both hands, slowly pull one knee toward your chest. (To avoid straining the knee, grip behind it, not on the front.) Go as far as you can without discomfort—you should feel a stretch in your lower back but no pain.*
- *Hold the position for fifteen to thirty seconds, then slowly lower the leg. Perform the movement eight to twelve times. Repeat with the other leg.*

2. **Knee-to-chest stretch with resistance.** This is similar to the exercise described above, except that you use a latex exercise band to increase resistance and strengthen muscles.

   - *Lie on your back with your legs straight. Loop the latex band around the bottom of one foot. Grip the loose ends of the band with both hands.*

   - *Use the band to pull your knee toward your chest.*
   - *Hold the position for fifteen to thirty seconds, then straighten the leg while pushing against the band. Hold the band taut to increase resistance. Do this eight to twelve times, then repeat with the other leg.*

3. **Standing one-leg balance.** This move is more challenging than it looks, because you're using the weight of your body to strengthen your legs as well as the core muscles in the abdomen. These muscles, which connect the torso and pelvis, help control motions in your whole body. Core weakness is a common cause of asymmetric motion, which often leads to knee problems.

   - *Stand next to a wall, with your right shoulder just touching the wall.*
   - *Lift your left knee until the foot is off the floor. If you can, keep raising it until the thigh is about parallel to the floor. Make sure that your posture is upright at all times.*
   - *Hold the position for about fifteen seconds, then lower your foot. Repeat eight to twelve times, then turn around and do the same thing with the other leg.*

Important: If you can't balance for fifteen seconds, or if you find yourself using the wall for support or moving your arms or dancing around to balance on one foot, your legs are weaker than they should be. This means you should definitely also do the next exercise.

Note: Even if you can easily perform the one-leg balance above, it's a good idea to do the one below to maintain your strength.

4. **Standing one-leg balance with resistance.** This is similar to the exercise that's described above, except that you use a latex band to strengthen muscles in the thighs and hamstrings.

- *Stand with your right shoulder barely touching a wall. Loop a latex band under your left foot. Hold the loose ends of the band in each hand.*
- *With your hands at waist level, raise your left foot until your thigh is about parallel to the floor. Shorten the band by wrapping it around your hands to keep some tension on the band.*
- *While holding the band taut and your knee elevated, slowly press your foot forward, as though you're taking a big step. Keep the band taut to increase resistance. Maintain your balance!*
- *Now, pull on the band to return to*

the bent-knee position. Repeat eight to twelve times, then turn around and repeat with the other leg.

> Steven P. Weiniger, DC, a postgraduate instructor at Logan College of Chiropractic, outside of St. Louis, Missouri, and a managing partner of BodyZone.com, a national online health information resource and referral directory to chiropractors, physical therapists, and certified posture exercise professionals (CPEPs). He is author of *Stand Taller, Live Longer: An Anti-Aging Strategy.* StandTallerLiveLonger.com.

Keep Your Hands Young and Strong: Seven Simple Exercises to Reduce Pain and Stiffness

If you have been diagnosed with arthritis, it's wise to protect your hands *right away.* Approximately 40 percent of arthritis patients must eventually restrict their daily activities because of joint pain or stiffness—and the hands often get the worst of it.

Both osteoarthritis (known as "wear-and-tear" arthritis) and rheumatoid arthritis (an autoimmune disease) can damage cartilage and sometimes the bones themselves.

What's missing from the typical arthritis prescription: Unfortunately, most patients with either type of arthritis do not recognize the importance of simple daily hand exercises, which can improve joint lubrication, increase your range of motion and hand strength, and maintain or restore function. These exercises also are helpful for people who have a hand injury or who heavily use their hands.

SAVE YOUR HANDS WITH EXERCISE

Most hand and wrist exercises can be done at home without equipment. But don't exercise during flare-ups, particularly if you have rheumatoid arthritis. Patients who ignore the pain and overuse their hands and wrists are more likely to suffer long-term damage, including joint deformity.

Important: Warm the joints before doing these exercises. This helps prevent microtears that can occur when stretching cold tissue. Simply run warm water over your hands in the sink for a few minutes right before the exercises, or you can warm them with a heating pad.

Before doing the hand exercises here, it also helps to use the fingers of the other hand to rub and knead the area you'll be exercising. This self-massage improves circulation to the area and reduces swelling.

If you have osteoarthritis or rheumatoid arthritis, do the following exercises five times on each hand and work up to ten times, if possible. The entire sequence should take no more than five minutes. Perform the sequence two to three times a day.*

1. **Tendon glides.** *Purpose:* Keeps the tendons functioning well to help move all the finger joints through their full range of motion.

   What to do: Rest your elbow on a table with your forearm and hand raised (fingertips pointed to the ceiling). Bend the fingers at the middle joint (form a hook with your fingers), and hold this position for a moment. Then bend the fingers into a fist, hiding your nails. Don't clench—just fold your fingers gently while keeping the wrist in a neutral position. Now make a modified fist with your nails showing. Next, raise your fingers so that they are bent at a ninety-degree angle and your thumb is resting against your index finger (your hand will look similar to a bird's beak). Hold each position for three seconds.

2. **Thumb active range of motion.** *Purpose:* Improves your ability to move your thumb in all directions.

---

* For more exercises, see an occupational therapist. To find one, consult the American Occupational Therapy Association at aota.org.

Do the movements gently so that you don't feel any pain.

What to do: Rest your elbow on a table with your forearm and hand in the air. Touch the tip of the thumb to the tip of each finger (or get as close as you can). Then flex the tip of your thumb toward the palm. Hold each of these positions for three seconds.

3. **Web-space massage.** *Purpose:* Strengthens muscles in the active hand while increasing circulation in the passive hand by using one hand to massage the other.

   What to do: Clasp your left hand with your right hand as if you are shaking hands. With firm but gentle pressure, use the length of your left thumb to massage the web (space between the thumb and the index finger) next to your right thumb. Then reverse the position and massage the web next to your left thumb. Massage each web for thirty seconds.

4. **Wrist active range of motion.** *Purpose:* Maintains proper positioning of the wrist, which helps keep the fingers in correct alignment.

   What to do: Rest your right forearm on a table with your wrist hanging off the edge and your palm pointing downward—you'll be moving only your wrist. Then place your left hand on top of your right forearm to keep it stable. With the fingers on your right hand held together gently, raise the wrist as high as it will comfortably go. Hold for three seconds.

   Next, make a fist and raise it so the knuckles point upward. Lower the fist toward the floor. Hold each position for three seconds.

5. **Digit extension.** *Purpose:* Strengthens the muscles that pull the fingers straight—the movement prevents chronic contractions that can lead to joint deformity.

   What to do: Warm up by placing the palms and fingers of both hands together and pressing the hands gently for five seconds. Then place your palms flat on a table. One at a time, raise each finger. Then lift all the fingers on one hand simultaneously while keeping your palm flat on the table. Hold each movement for five seconds.

6. **Wrist flexion/extension.** *Purpose:* Stretches and promotes muscle length in the forearm. Forearm muscles move the wrist and fingers. Flexion (bending your wrist so that your palm approaches the forearm) and extension (bending your wrist in the opposite direction) help maintain wrist strength and range of motion.

   What to do: Hold your right hand

in the air, palm down. Bend the wrist upward so that the tips of your fingers are pointed toward the ceiling. Place your left hand against the fingers (on the palm side) and gently push so that the back of your right hand moves toward the top of your right forearm. Hold for fifteen seconds. Switch hands and repeat.

Next, bend your right wrist downward so that the fingers are pointed at the floor. Place your left hand against the back of your right hand and gently push so your palm moves toward the bottom of the forearm. Hold for fifteen seconds. Switch and repeat.

7. **Finger-walking exercises.** *Purpose:* Strengthens fingers in the opposite direction of a deformity. This exercise is particularly helpful for rheumatoid arthritis patients.

What to do: Put one hand on a flat surface. Lift the index finger up and move it toward the thumb, then place the finger down. Next, lift the middle finger and move it toward the index finger. Lift the ring finger and move it toward the middle finger. Finally, lift the little finger and move it toward the ring finger. Repeat on your other hand.

› Anjum Lone, OTR/L, CHT, occupational and certified hand therapist and chief, department of occupational therapy, Phelps Memorial Hospital Center, Sleepy Hollow, New York.

Quick Yoga Cure to Relieve Arthritis

Yoga *aficionados know that this* ancient practice can tone muscles and calm the mind. But few people are aware of yoga's ability to cure everyday ailments that can cause pain and sap our energy.

As a low-impact exercise that focuses on physical postures (*asanas*) and breathing techniques, yoga helps relieve a number of chronic conditions by increasing blood flow, for example, and improving range of motion.

And even though regular yoga practice offers the broadest range of health benefits, doing targeted yoga moves, as needed, can often help you feel better within minutes. Do not worry about doing the move perfectly. Simply breathe deeply while gently moving your body into position.

Consider trying the single, carefully chosen yoga pose described here. This can help other treatments, such as medication, work more effectively, or in some cases, the pose alone may alleviate the problem. Stay in the pose for five to ten deep, long breaths.

Hands and knees fist release. For many people, this pose helps the swelling, joint pain, stiffness, and limited range of motion that accompany rheumatoid arthritis and osteoarthritis, especially in the hands.

What to do: Gently, get on your hands and knees. Make tight fists with both hands. Bend your elbows out to your sides, and place the tops of your hands on the ground, with your knuckles facing each other. Begin to straighten your elbows, but keep your fists tight and only do as much as you can without causing pain. You should feel a stretch on the tops of your wrists.

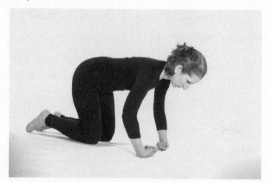

How it works: Whether you have arthritis or just sit at a desk all day, which dramatically limits your range of motion, this move increases flexibility in the wrists, hands, arms, and back—important in easing arthritis pain.

....

› Tara Stiles, founder and owner, Strala Yoga, New York City. She is author of two books, *Yoga Cures:* *Simple Routines to Conquer More Than 50 Common Ailments and Live Pain-Free* and *Slim Calm Sexy Yoga: 210 Proven Yoga Moves for Mind/Body Bliss.* Stiles has also created several yoga DVDs with Jane Fonda, Deepak Chopra, and others. TaraStiles.com.

....

Natural Remedies for Gout

*A*n attack of gout comes on quickly but can really take its time going away. This painful form of arthritis commonly affects the joint at the base of the big toe or other joints, such as the ankle, thumb, wrist, elbow, or knee. Inflammation leaves the joint red, swollen, and so tender that it hurts to have clothes or bedsheets touch it.

Gout can be treated very effectively with a natural approach that features detoxification, nutritional supplements, and diet changes. Here's what you need to know.

WHY IT OCCURS

Gout results from elevated blood levels of uric acid, a waste by-product created when your body breaks down purines, compounds found in foods such as organ meats, anchovies, asparagus, mushrooms, and beer. Gout traditionally was associated with the consumption of fatty foods and alcohol, which is why it was once known as a rich man's disease. Today, we know that gout is not always related to diet. With this condition, the kidneys are unable to filter high levels of uric acid out of the blood. Over time, excess uric acid forms crystals that accumulate in joint tissue, leading to attacks of joint pain. Men are more likely than women to get gout. Women are more susceptible after menopause.

Insulin resistance, obesity, fungal overgrowth, and hypothyroidism all have been linked to gout. Taking niacin for heart disease can exacerbate gout. Regular use of aspirin (any dose) and some blood pressure medications (thiazide diuretics) can cause gout.

Gout medications lower blood levels of uric acid, but these medications all have side effects, ranging from nausea and skin rash to disruptions in liver enzymes and blood-cell production. Fortunately, gout can be treated very effectively without these harsh drugs.

TREATING AN ACUTE GOUT ATTACK

I recommend starting the following regimen at the first sign of joint pain caused by gout.

Do first: The first two on the following list, then the others. These remedies, which all are available at health-food stores, are safe to take together. There are no side effects except as noted.

◆ **Juice detoxification.** In an acute gout attack, it's essential to quickly eliminate uric acid from your body. You can do this with a three-day juice fast, which flushes excess purines from the body. I usually recommend drinking eight to ten cups of juice daily, mainly from vegetables.

Good choices: Green drinks, such as those made from wheatgrass, chlorella, and spirulina, pure water, and herbal teas.

Another good choice: Unsweetened cherry juice. Just a few tablespoons give you the beneficial anthocyanins that can decrease blood uric acid levels. Dilute the juice with as much water as you like.

Don't fast for more than three days. Prolonged periods without food can raise uric acid levels. (Most middle-aged people with gout have no trouble going without solid food for a few days, but it is wise to consult your doctor before fasting.)

◆ **Celery seed extract.** This anti-inflammatory herb (not to be confused with the spice celery seed, which is much less concentrated) can ease joint pain. Celery seed extract contains compounds that inhibit the enzymes that produce uric acid. The extract comes in tablet and capsule form.

Dose: 400 mg to 500 mg three times daily during an acute attack. Do not use this herb if you have kidney disease (because of its diuretic effect) or if you are pregnant.

Other helpful remedies to take during an attack of gout:

+ **Homeopathic colchicum.** This remedy can relieve acute gout attacks in which pain worsens with movement.

    Dose: During waking hours, take a 30C-potency pellet every two hours for no more than two days.

+ **Nettle root (also known as stinging nettle root).** This herb, available in liquid or capsules, neutralizes uric acid.

    Dose: 250 mg of concentrated root extract three times daily during an attack.

LONG-TERM GOUT PROTECTION

When gout symptoms have eased, I have my patients implement the following preventive regimen.

+ **Celery seed extract.** I recommend taking this important antigout supplement at a reduced dose of 400 to 500 mg only once daily.

+ **Fish oil.** Omega-3 fatty acids can help prevent gout-related joint inflammation.

Dose: 2,000 mg of combined EPA and DHA daily.

+ **Vitamin C.** Studies have shown that vitamin C can reduce the risk for gout.

    Dose: 500 mg daily.

+ **Antigout diet.** You will want to avoid foods that increase uric acid production, including those with refined flour or sugar and those containing saturated, hydrogenated, and partially hydrogenated fats. Concentrate on consuming moderate amounts of protein (such as cold-water fish and soy products) and plenty of plant foods. And high-fiber foods, such as whole grains and nuts, can help your body eliminate uric acid. Drink eight to ten eight-ounce glasses of water throughout the day to keep uric acid flushed from your body.

+ **Antifungal diet.** Fungal overgrowth in the digestive tract may increase uric acid. You may want to try an antifungal diet, which involves eliminating sugar, grains, and yeast products and taking antifungal herbs.

› Mark A. Stengler, NMD, naturopathic doctor and founder of the Stengler Center for Integrative Medicine in Encinitas, California. He is author and coauthor of numerous books, including *The Natural Physician's Healing Therapies* and *Bottom Line's Prescription for Natural Cures,* and is the author of the newsletter *Health Revelations.* MarkStengler.com.

2

Back and Neck

Stop Hurting Your Back! Avoid These Common Mistakes

As many as 80 percent of Americans will suffer an episode of back pain at some time in their lives—the older you are, the more common it is. Back problems are among the main reasons for doctor visits, and they can be excruciatingly slow to heal.*

What people don't realize is that most back injuries are predictable, and how to avoid them might surprise you. Here are the six worst mistakes that people make that hurt their backs.

WEIGHT AND EFFORT MISMATCH

Suppose you lift a box that is heavier than you expected. You get it a few inches off the floor and then realize that it's really heavy. It's going to crash back down if you don't bring all your strength into play. The sudden contraction of unprepared back muscles can cause an instant strain.

Or maybe you're lifting a box that you think is heavy but turns out to be as light as a feather. All the muscle force that you generated causes a "snap" in the muscles (and the box goes flying).

Self-protection: Before you lift something, test the weight. Slide it a few inches or lift just a corner. You have to know what you're dealing with. If it's heavy, get your legs under you, and use the muscles in your legs more than the muscles in your back. If it's light, lift with a smooth motion—you won't need that initial hard jerk to get it moving.

---

* American Chiropractic Association, "Back Pain Facts and Statistics," accessed January 10, 2017, https://www.acatoday.org/Patients/Health-Wellness-Information/Back-Pain-Facts-and-Statistics.

OVERHEAD BIN REACH

If you think that the cramped, knees-to-chest seating in today's airplanes is hard on your back, wait until you use the overhead bins. You will pay in pain what you saved on checked luggage.

Travelers often overstuff their carry-ons. A twenty-pound bag that's easy to carry (or wheel) can feel like fifty pounds when you're off-balance and reaching overhead. Unloading also is a hazard. You probably had to angle, wedge, and stuff your bag to get it to fit. You will have to give it a hard yank to get it out, a motion that is very hard on the back.

Self-protection: Pack light. If you're in reasonable shape, you probably can manage, say, a ten-pound bag when your arms are extended and you're standing on tiptoe. Use both hands to place the bag in the bin; don't swing it up with one arm. Store it with the handle facing out. That way, you can grip the handle with one hand and use your other hand for support. For anything much heavier, put it in checked baggage—it's worth it even if you have to pay.

SUPERSOFT CHAIR RECLINE

It feels good to sink into a soft chair or sofa, but it is hard to extricate yourself from the pillowy depths.

Surprising fact: Sitting in a soft chair is hard work.

When you sit in a firm chair, your back is supported, so it relaxes. But a soft chair doesn't provide the same sensory input, so the muscles stay contracted. After an hour or so, you might notice that your back is hurting even though you haven't done anything more strenuous than read a book or work the TV remote.

Self-protection: When you're settling in, choose a chair that provides a decent amount of back support. It doesn't have to be hard, but it should be firm.

Also helpful: If you have a history of back problems, you probably will do better if you stand up for one to two minutes now and then, say, every fifteen or twenty minutes.

THE CAR TRUNK LEAN

How many times have you felt a pinch when you lift a suitcase or a sack of groceries from a car's trunk or cargo area? It's not so much the weight that causes problems but your position. When you bend over and lift, you are at a mechanical disadvantage. You are not using the big muscles in your legs. Your back muscles aren't very strong. Their job is to stabilize your spine, not help with heavy lifting.

Self-protection: Get as close to the vehicle as you can before pulling the item to the front of the trunk and taking it out. This allows you to bring your leg muscles into play. Most people stand back from the rear of the car because they don't want to get their clothes dirty. Step in closer. It's easier to clean your clothes than to deal with a month or two of back pain.

TWIST AND SHOUT

"Twist and shout" is what I call the stab of pain that occurs when people use a twisting motion to bend over. Suppose that you're picking something up off the floor that's a little bit off to your side. You might pivot at the hips and swing one hand down to snag it. Don't! This is an unnatural motion, because the spinal joints are designed to shift from front to back, not side to side. Twisting strains the soft tissues and can lead to sprains and spasms.

Self-protection: Before you pick something up, take a fraction of a second to move into a position of strength. With both feet facing the object, squat down and pick it up. Face it square, and use your legs more and your back less.

SHOVELING ANYTHING HEAVY

Back specialists see a lot of new patients in the spring after they have been working in the yard shoveling mulch, dirt, or gravel. The same is true after snowstorms. Even when snow looks light and fluffy, each shovelful packs a lot of weight, and you never move just one shovelful.

Self-protection: Warm up before picking up the shovel. Walk around the house for a few minutes. Stretch out the muscles in your back, legs, and arms.

Once you're outside, let your legs do the work. Bend your knees when you load the shovel, then straighten them when you lift. Don't bend your back any more than you have to. And don't take the heaviest shovelfuls that you can manage—if you're grunting, it's too much.

Also helpful: Home-supply stores stock a variety of ergonomic shovels that make it easier to stand upright when you're shoveling.

....

› David G. Borenstein, MD, clinical professor of medicine, George Washington University Medical Center, Washington, DC, and partner, Arthritis & Rheumatism Associates, the largest rheumatology practice in Washington/Maryland. He is host of *Speaking of Health with Dr. B*, a weekly radio program, and author of *Heal Your Back: Your Complete Prescription for Preventing, Treating, and Eliminating Back Pain*. DrBHealth.org.

....

Change Your Sleep Position to Relieve Back and Neck Pain

When you slip into bed at night, you probably go straight to your favorite sleep position, perhaps on your side or on your back. But sleep positions can sometimes be tricky. Certain positions can help—or worsen—back and neck pain.

BACK PAIN

Back sleeping is a good position for people with back pain. However, if you're lying flat on your back, you may feel more comfortable with a pillow under your knees. This will keep your back in a more natural position and eliminate an excessive arch between your lower back and the mattress.

Self-test: If you can easily slip your hand into an open space between your lower back and the mattress, raise your knees a little more. Your lower back should be flat against your hand.

For back pain, you may also find it comfortable to sleep on your side with a pillow between your legs.

NECK PAIN

If your neck is tight and/or painful, do not sleep on your stomach.

Reason: Unless you sleep with your face pressed into the mattress, you'll need to turn your head to the side. This puts a lot of stress on the neck joints as well as the muscles and soft tissues in the neck and upper back.

Better: Sleep on your side with a pillow

under your neck. The pillow should fill the distance between your neck and shoulder. You can use a special pillow for side sleeping with more support for your neck and a cutout for your head (available online or from home-goods stores). Alternately, you can use a rolled-up towel to give your neck more support. You also can sleep on your back as long as you don't prop up your head too high, which will strain your neck. (Usually, one pillow is enough.)

HOW TO CHANGE HOW YOU SLEEP

Suppose that you are a side sleeper, but you know that you should be sleeping on your back. Before you go to sleep, think about the position that you want to maintain and start in that position. Remind yourself of this whenever you happen to wake up and return to the desired position.

It may take a few weeks (or even months), but the mental reminders and time in the desired position will eventually change the way that you sleep most of the time.

IS IT TIME TO REPLACE YOUR MATTRESS?

If you can't remember when you bought your mattress, you're probably due for a new one. Mattresses start to sag and lose their support after about eight or ten years.

Choose a mattress that's on the firm

side or firm but with some cushioning on top, such as a plush-top mattress. About every three months, rotate the mattress. Flip it over if it has two sleep sides.

Also: Invest in more pillows. You can use them in different ways when you need more support or padding—for example, between your legs, for hugging, and under your knees. Depending on the size of the pillows, two to four will generally be enough to provide added support for your body.

› Mary Ann Wilmarth, PT, DPT, chief of physical therapy, Harvard University, Cambridge, Massachusetts, and former director, doctor of physical therapy (DPT) program, Northeastern University, where she was the assistant dean for the College of Professional Studies. She is also the founder and CEO of Back2Back Physical Therapy, a private practice based in Andover, Massachusetts. Back2BackPT.com.

Is Your Pillow Causing Your Pain?

Lots of people think that mattresses are more important than pillows when it comes to getting a good night's sleep. But that's a mistake. If you have occasional or frequent body aches, pillows are just as important as mattresses—or even more so.

NECK PAIN

If you randomly X-rayed one hundred people over age fifty-five, 70 to 80 percent would have arthritis of the neck.

If you have neck pain, don't sleep on your stomach. This position twists the neck. Instead, sleep on your side while hugging a second pillow. This offers the comforting sensation of something against your stomach but is far better for your neck.

My advice: If you have arthritis of the neck or neck pain due to another condition (such as muscle strain or injury) and find that it's comfortable to sleep on your side, choose a pillow that is just thick enough to fill the space between your downside ear and neck and the mattress.

To determine the proper pillow thickness for you: When lying on your side with your head on the pillow, your head should be parallel to the mattress. Ask someone to see whether your nose is aligned with the middle of your chest. If your nose is higher than your chest, you need a thinner pillow. If it's lower, you need a thicker pillow.

Before buying a pillow: At the store, compress the pillow with your head by lying down on it or lean your head on the pillow up against the store wall.

Smart idea: Call around before shopping to find stores that allow for pillow returns.

If you have neck pain and typically sleep on your back, choose a pillow that just fills the gap between your neck and the mattress. A pillow that is too thick will push your neck forward, placing stress on the muscles in the back of the neck.

Good choices: A fluffable down pillow, such as the Superior Goose Down Pillow.

Or try an easily shapeable buckwheat pillow, such as those from BuckwheatCo., which can also be heated in the microwave before bed. A heated buckwheat pillow smells like freshly baked bread.

LOWER BACK PAIN

For years, lower back pain sufferers were advised to sleep on their backs on very firm mattresses or even on the floor. We now know that these people should choose whatever sleeping position feels best—except on the stomach, which can increase the forward curve of the lower back and jam the spinal joints.

My advice: If you have back pain and like to sleep on your back, slip a pillow under your knees. This flattens your lower back against the mattress, discouraging the muscle spasms that can occur if the lower back is arched. The pillow can be made of any material as long as it's about three to four inches thick.

Good choice: The Duro-Med Elevating Leg Rest ($24).

If you're a side sleeper, you may straighten your bottom leg and bend your upper leg in front of you to avoid the discomfort of your knees rubbing together. But this position twists your body from the waist, placing strain on your lower back.

My advice: Place a pillow or a rolled-up towel between your knees to keep your top leg parallel with the bed.

Good choice: The Back Buddy Knee Pillow.

If you tend to switch back and forth in your sleep between your side and back, try a dual pillow, such as Therapeutica's Sleeping Pillow. It is designed to offer correct support and stability whether you're sleeping on your back or side.

ROUNDED SHOULDERS

Most people's shoulders are rounded to some degree, due, for example, to spinal arthritis or prolonged computer usage. If you typically sleep on your side, your top shoulder may sag forward, exacerbating poor posture.

My advice: Try a boomerang-shaped pillow that supports your head and neck while curving down the front of your torso to provide shoulder support.

Good choice: The Dr. Mary Side Sleeper Pillow.

› Bill Lauretti, DC, associate professor of chiropractic clinical sciences at the New York Chiropractic
College in Seneca Falls, New York. He is the author
of numerous journal articles and textbook chapters
on neck and back pain.

Three Simple Exercises to Improve Your Posture

Stop reading this for a minute and think about your shoulders. Where are they? Are they rounded or slumped? Are they causing a strain in your neck?

Many of us have little or no awareness of our posture, but poor posture can contribute to a host of problems, including muscle pain and injury when performing regular activities, such as getting dressed or carrying groceries. The good news is that it's easy to take control of our upper-body posture.

When our upper body is in alignment, we optimize the movement of our joints, have increased muscle strength, and are at decreased risk for injury. The exercises below borrow from Pilates, an exercise modality uniquely able to help improve posture. During Pilates, you perform controlled, mindful moves that improve the flexibility and strength of muscles required for good posture.

RETRAINING YOUR MUSCLES

You can align your head, neck, and back by retraining your muscles. These easy-to-do exercises are designed to help you with this by improving the range of motion and strength of the muscles of the back and neck so that it is easier to bring them into alignment. Repeat each exercise up to ten times daily. Do each repetition carefully, and you won't need to do more to benefit. Consult with a doctor before doing any new exercises.

1. **Rolldown.** Improves movement of the spine and increases postural awareness.

    What to do: Stand against a wall with the back of your head, rib cage, and buttocks touching the wall. Walk your feet about one foot away from the wall, and put your hands on your thighs. Slowly roll forward, sliding your hands gently down the fronts of your thighs. As you roll forward, feel each vertebra leave the wall. When you have gone as far as you can, roll back up, touching one vertebra at a time to the wall. People with osteoporosis should not do this exercise—bending the spine forward is not recommended for those with low bone density. The movement can result in microfractures of the spine.

2. **Paint the ceiling.** Increases range of motion in the neck.

   What to do: While seated, imagine a long artist's paintbrush extending up from the crown of your head. Remain seated as you position your head so that the crown of your head is as close to the ceiling as you can get it. With the "paintbrush," nod your head forward and backward, drawing a one- to two-inch line on the ceiling. Move just your head. Next, "paint" a short line on the ceiling from side to side. Finally, paint a small circle by rotating your head in both directions.

3. **The pre-swan.** Increases the strength and mobility of the muscles of the upper spine and helps correct a forward curve in the upper spine.

   What to do: Lie on your stomach on the floor on a mat or carpet. Bend your elbows so that your hands are under your shoulders. Inhale, and gently press your hands into the floor. Reach your elbows toward your heels, and peel your upper chest off the floor, keeping the lowest ribs in contact with the floor. This small movement should be felt only in the upper back and chest. (If you feel this in the lower back, you may have rolled up too high.) People with back problems should consult a doctor before doing this exercise.

To find a certified Pilates instructor to help you improve your posture, visit the Pilates Method Alliance, a nonprofit organization that provides a list of qualified instructors around the country.

› Brent Anderson, PhD, physical therapist, adjunct instructor, University of Miami, and president and CEO, Polestar Pilates, Coral Gables, Florida. PolestarPilates.com.

Most Back Pain Has Emotional Roots

As anyone who routinely gets migraine or tension headaches or upset stomachs will confirm, real pain can originate in the mind.

When tension mounts, any of a wide range of uncomfortable conditions can develop, from spastic colon to asthma to eczema. In fact, the mind can use practically any body organ or system as a defense mechanism to sidetrack itself from the awareness of undesirable, negative emotions.

Currently, the most popular distraction is pain in the back, neck, or shoulders. It has not always been so. Forty years ago, no one took these pains seriously. Now, they are costing Americans more than $90 billion a year.

Fifty years ago, ulcers, colitis, and tension headaches were the best distracters. But people knew they were caused by tension, and doctors learned to clear them up with medication, so the brain had to look around for a better hiding place.

The back was perfect, because no one suspected it, and it gradually took over the number-one spot.

What the brain created was something I call the tension myositis syndrome, or TMS, in which pain is caused simply by reducing the blood flow a little. I have found it to be the most common cause of back pain by far. Fortunately, understanding what's going on usually stops the pain.

WHO CAN GET TMS

It is fair to say that everybody is susceptible. I used to think that it was only the "nervous" types who got it, but we now realize that anyone who has pressure in his/her life can get TMS. And strangely, the greatest pressure comes from our own personalities, because we pressure ourselves to be perfect and to be good. Since the middle years of life (thirty to sixty) have the greatest pressures, TMS is most common during these years. This is why persistent pain in the back, neck, or shoulders is usually due to TMS.

Caution: Never assume you have TMS unless you have seen a doctor and ruled out serious disorders like tumors, cancer, bone disease, and the like.

Each person with TMS develops a pattern of what time of the day or night the pain will appear, what part of the body will be involved, what activities will make it better or worse, and how severe the pain will be.

One patient may say, "I'm fine when I get up, but as the day goes on, it gets worse. By late afternoon, I can't sit for more than five minutes at a time."

Another patient may have pain-racked nights followed by increasing relief through the day. They both have TMS.

SEEKING TREATMENT

People with back pain understandably want to know what is wrong and how to get better. They go from practitioner to practitioner, often getting a different diagnosis with each visit.

Surgery is commonly done, but since structural abnormalities are rarely responsible for the pain, in my experience, this does not solve the problem. The pain returns to the same or another place, or the problem switches to another organ or system.

A very common misconception is that recurrent back pain is due to an old injury.

Example: "I was ice skating ten years ago and fell on my tailbone, and my back has hurt on and off ever since." This makes no sense, for the body tends to heal itself, quickly and completely. Recurrent attacks are due to TMS.

Another mistaken idea is that if the pain is excruciating, there must be a structural abnormality. In fact, such severe pain is due to muscle spasm, a powerful contraction of muscle when it is suddenly deprived of its full complement of oxygen, as occurs with TMS.

Instead of attributing their pain to psychological factors, most people would rather believe it is the result of some structural abnormality that can be treated surgically or with medication or some other kind of therapy. It is my impression that eight out of ten people are unable to accept the diagnosis of TMS.

Unfortunate: People who would benefit most from a psychological diagnosis tend to be the least able to accept it.

Am I saying that people consciously induce their own pain? Of course not. It is the stress and pressures of life that bring on the pain, because they lead to internal bad feelings, like anger, which the brain then avoids by turning our attention to the pain.

Patients are often told in pain clinics that they are unconsciously making their pain worse in order to gain certain benefits like sympathy, attention, money, etc. I don't believe that is a significant factor in chronic pain.

Why don't more doctors diagnose TMS? Unfortunately, medical teaching still tends to view the body as a magnificent machine and the doctor as an engineer to that machine. There is still very little awareness in the ranks of medicine of the intimate connection of the mind and body. This is a tragedy for the average patient.

How can you prove that TMS exists? It doesn't show up on an X-ray or blood test, but if a large number of patients (thousands) get better when treated for that diagnosis, it must exist.

The cure: Repudiate the structural explanation for the pain and acknowledge that it is due to pressure and tension. This is accomplished through teaching and group meetings. In about 10 percent of cases, it is also necessary to work with a psychotherapist who is familiar with the disorder.

Through the years, many people have written to me and described how they were cured by carefully studying my book, *Healing Back Pain.* This is logical, because information is the primary therapeutic ingredient. It's what I give my patients.

> The late John E. Sarno, MD, who was professor of clinical rehabilitation medicine, New York University School of Medicine, and attending physician,

Howard A. Rusk Institute of Rehabilitation Medicine, NYU Medical Center, New York City. He was author of *Mind Over Back Pain: A Radically New Approach to the Diagnosis and Treatment of Back Pain* and *Healing Back Pain: The Mind-Body Connection.*

....

Five Do-It-Yourself Remedies for Back Pain

Argh!" If you've ever hurt your lower back, you're familiar with that microsecond of awareness that signals something is wrong, followed by a sudden jolt of pain. You know that you're in for days, weeks, or even months of painful back spasms and nagging backaches. After the initial injury, pain can be brought on even by simple tasks such as turning over in bed or getting in or out of the car.

Fortunately, there are natural back pain remedies that really work. If you follow these steps for run-of-the-mill back pain, you should feel much better within about a week.

Walking—on hills. Recent research tells us that walking regularly is as effective as physical therapy, chiropractic care, and medication for many types of lower back pain. That's because walking uses and strengthens muscles in the back and abdomen but doesn't overwork them. As these muscles are gently worked,

circulation improves, tissues repair, and spasms relax.

Secret that will make walking even more effective for lower back pain: If possible, do *hill* walking. Why is this better? Walking uphill requires you to lift your leg more than flat walking does. In doing this, the muscles along the spine are elongated, stretched, and strengthened more effectively than with flat walking. Downhill walking is less helpful than walking uphill, though it does generally help and strengthens thigh muscles.

Important: Hill walking does not mean climbing up mountains or steep hills. If you want to try hill walking for back pain, look for rolling hills and choose a route with more up than down if possible. Walk a minimum of twenty minutes per day, four times a week. If this is painful, start with five-minute walks, spread throughout the day, and work up to twenty or more minutes per walk when you are able.

Ice. Many people think that ice helps only right after you've injured your back. This isn't so. Ice reduces pain and inflammation as long as your back is still hurting.

What to do: Keep a gel pack or bag of frozen peas in your freezer. Wrap in a thin cloth, and apply to your lower back for ten minutes only, several times a day.

Stretching. Gentle stretching is great

for reducing back pain. Breathe deeply and stretch (reach overhead, bend forward, and lean from side to side), but only as far as you can without causing pain.

T-Relief. This ointment, which contains arnica, chamomile, and other herbs in homeopathic form, is anti-inflammatory, promotes circulation, and reduces pain. Apply a small amount to the painful area twice daily as needed for up to a month. T-Relief is available from naturopathic physicians' offices and over the counter at natural-food stores and pharmacies as well as online.

White willow bark. This herb, which reduces pain and inflammation, contains salicin, a chemical that is similar to aspirin. I often recommend 400 mg three times daily for lower back pain relief. Like aspirin, white willow can bother the stomach, so take it with a small amount of food. Check with your doctor first if you have a chronic medical condition or take medication (especially a blood thinner, beta blocker, or diuretic).

> › Jamison Starbuck, ND, naturopathic physician in family practice and a guest lecturer at the University of Montana, both in Missoula. She is past president of the American Association of Naturopathic Physicians. Starbuck is a columnist for the *Bottom Line Health Insider* and hosts *Dr. Starbuck's Health Tips for Kids* on Montana Public Radio. DrJamisonStarbuck.com.

How to "Untie" a Knot in Your Back

D*on't you hate it when* a muscle in the middle of your back cramps up, creating a knot of hot pain? You long to rub away the agony, but unless you're as flexible as an acrobat, the tender spot is impossible to reach.

Such cramps often are the result of muscles overreacting to try to protect you from whatever stress you are under, whether that stress is emotional or physical (for instance, the result of sitting too long in one position). The muscle fibers, which normally are stretchy, temporarily lose their pliability and clench up. This cuts off circulation, depriving the tissue of needed nutrients and oxygen and leading to pain.

Massage techniques and other tactics can help disperse tension from muscle fibers and promote healing by restoring circulation to the affected area. To release a hard-to-reach knot in your back, try the following:

+ **Tennis ball tip.** Place a tennis ball inside the toe end of a long sock. Grasping the open end of the sock, toss the ball over one shoulder and stand with your back close to a wall. Lean backward so the ball is pressed between you and the wall, positioned directly against the sore spot.

Maintain as much pressure as possible for as long as you can stand it, though that may be only a few seconds to start. Rest for a moment, then repeat several times. Use the technique as needed throughout the day.

- **Candy cane cure.** For more precise control, use the Thera Cane Deep Pressure Massager, which is shaped like a two-foot-long candy cane with several projections that allow for a firm grip and various self-massaging options. Experiment to determine the specific positions and degrees of pressure that bring the most relief.
- **Hot-and-cold healing.** Between your self-massage sessions, wrap an ice pack in a towel, and lie on top of it so that the sore spot is in contact with the ice pack (but don't let your skin get uncomfortably cold). Or try alternating the ice pack with a warm pack, such as a hot water bottle or heating pad, at intervals of fifteen minutes or less. The ice brings relief by numbing the area, while the heat relaxes the contracted muscle and improves circulation. Repeat the sequence three times throughout the day.
- **Get up and go.** You probably don't feel like moving much when your back is causing you pain, but staying stationary may only exacerbate the muscle

cramp. So rather than sitting (or lying) around for hours on end, get up at least every hour and walk around, shrug and roll your shoulders, and gently stretch your neck and arms.

If symptoms persist: See a professional massage therapist. Ask your doctor for a referral or check the website of the American Massage Therapy Association.

› Donald O. Miles, PhD, LMT, CNC, licensed massage therapist, Fitness Plus, Saint Francis Medical Center, Cape Girardeau, Missouri, and Caring Touch Center, Jackson, Missouri. FitnessPlus.sfmc.net.

Natural Painkillers You Haven't Heard Of

Move over *Tylenol and Advil.* There are natural pain relievers that work just as well as—or better than—over-the-counter pain relievers. And they are much gentler on your body. Drugs may be fine for temporarily relieving pain, but they have unhealthful side effects that you might not be aware of. These side effects are particularly noticeable when you use these pain medications and others over time for chronic conditions—they can irritate the stomach, cause stomach and intestinal ulcers, and increase heart disease risk. These three herbs can help with a variety of ailments, including lower back pain. Take the first natural painkiller on the list for four weeks. If you notice an improvement, stay with it. If not, try the next one. They are all available at health-food stores or online.

Caution: Women who are pregnant or breastfeeding should not take these remedies, because they have not been studied in these populations.

For lower back pain, take devil's claw, white willow bark, or curcumin.

For muscle aches and pains, take white willow bark or curcumin.

DEVIL'S CLAW

Devil's claw (Harpagophytum procumbens), a shrub found in southern Africa, works similarly to many pharmaceutical pain relievers—by blocking the action of pain-promoting compounds in the body—but without damaging the digestive tract. In studies involving people with chronic lower back pain, devil's claw extract proved as effective as prescription pain relievers.

Dose: Devil's claw extract is available in capsules. Look for 1.5 to 2 percent harpagoside, one of the active ingredients. Take 1,000 mg three times daily of a standardized extract.

Side effect: The only significant potential side effect is diarrhea.

WHITE WILLOW BARK

White willow bark is a pain reliever that has anti-inflammatory and blood-thinning benefits similar to those of aspirin, but unlike aspirin, it doesn't appear to damage the stomach lining. For centuries, the bark of the white willow (*Salix alba*), a tree found in Europe and Asia, was noted for its pain-relieving qualities. Its active ingredient is salicin, which the body converts to salicylic acid, a close cousin to aspirin (acetylsalicylic acid).

Dose: Take 120 mg daily of white willow bark extract capsules. If this amount does not reduce pain, try 240 mg.

Caution: Don't take this if you have an aspirin allergy and for one week before undergoing surgery. White willow bark is a blood thinner, so take it only while being monitored by a physician if you take blood-thinning medication.

CURCUMIN

Curcumin (diferuloylmethane), a constituent of turmeric, is the pigment compound that gives the spice its distinctive yellow coloring. In one study of rheumatoid arthritis patients, 1,200 mg daily of curcumin extract improved morning stiffness and joint swelling.

Dose: Take 500 mg of standardized turmeric extract (containing 90 to 95 percent curcumin) three times daily.

Caution: It has blood-thinning properties, so do not take curcumin if you take blood-thinning medication, such as warfarin, unless monitored by a physician. Do not take curcumin if you have gallstones, since it can cause gallstones to block bile ducts.

....

> Mark A. Stengler, NMD, naturopathic doctor and founder of the Stengler Center for Integrative Medicine in Encinitas, California. He is author and coauthor of numerous books, including *The Natural Physician's Healing Therapies* and *Bottom Line's Prescription for Natural Cures*, and is the author of the newsletter *Health Revelations*. MarkStengler.com.

....

The Underwear That Reduces Back Pain

S urgery for back pain can sometimes make the problem worse. Happily, we have some pill- and surgery-free solutions to back pain.

Example: Wearing wool underwear can relieve lower back pain. In a study, men with lower back pain who wore merino wool underwear for two months reported 89 percent less pain and needed less pain medication than men who wore cotton underwear.

Wool's heat-retaining properties help keep back muscles flexible, reducing pain.

Merino wool underwear is widely available online and in outdoors-oriented stores.

....

> Study by researchers at Atatürk University, Erzurum, Turkey, published in *Collegium Antropologicum*.

....

The Stretches That Get Rid of Back Pain in Just Seven Minutes a Day

O f the more than thirty million Americans who suffer from lower back pain, only about 10 percent of the cases are caused by conditions that require surgery, such as pinched nerves or a slipped disk.

For the overwhelming majority of back pain sufferers, the culprit is tight, inflamed muscles.

Surprising: This inflammation usually is not caused by strain on the back muscles themselves but rather a strain or injury to the spine—in particular, to one of five motion segments in the lower back.

Each segment, which is constructed to bend forward and back and side to side, consists of a disk (the spongy cushion between each pair of spinal vertebrae), the two vertebrae directly above and below it, and the facets (joints) connecting the vertebrae to the disk.

Unfortunately, the segments' disks or facets can be injured in a variety of ways—by lifting something the wrong way, twisting too far, sitting too long or even sneezing too hard—causing the surrounding muscles to contract in order to protect the spine from further damage.

This contraction and the muscle inflammation that it produces is what causes the intense lower back pain that so many Americans are familiar with.

WHEN BACK PAIN STRIKES

Lower back pain caused by inflammation usually subsides on its own within three to six weeks. However, the healing process can be accelerated significantly by taking over-the-counter ibuprofen for several days after injury to reduce inflammation, if you don't have an ulcer (follow label instructions), and getting massage therapy to help loosen knotted muscles and increase healing blood flow to them. (If you suffer from severe back pain or back pain accompanied by fever, incontinence, or weakness or numbness in your leg, see a doctor right away to rule out a condition that may require surgery, such as serious damage to disks, ligaments, or nerves in the back.)

Also important: Perform the simple stretching routine described in this section. In my more than sixteen years of practice as an orthopedic spine surgeon, it is the closest thing I've found to act as a "silver bullet" for back pain.

How it works: All the muscles stretched in this routine attach to the pelvis and work in concert to stabilize the spine. Stretching increases blood flow to these specific muscles, thereby reducing the inflammation that leads to painful, tightened back muscles.

GETTING STARTED

In preparation for the back stretch routine described here, it's important to learn a simple approach that systematically stimulates and strengthens your core (abdominal, back, and pelvic muscles). This is one of the best ways to protect your spine. Although there are many types of exercises that strengthen the core, abdominal contractions are the easiest to perform.

What to do: Pretend that you have to urinate and then stop the flow—a movement known as a Kegel exercise. Then while lying on your back, place your hands on your pelvis just above your genitals. Now imagine that someone is about to punch you in the stomach, and feel how your lower abdomen tightens protectively.

To do a full abdominal contraction, combine these two movements, holding the Kegel movement while tightening your lower abdomen. Continuously hold the full abdominal contraction during all the stretches described in this article.

SEVEN-MINUTE STRETCHING ROUTINE

Do the following routine daily until your back pain eases (start out slowly and gently if you're still in acute pain). Then continue doing it several times a week to prevent recurrences. Regularly stretching these muscles makes them stronger, leaving your lower spine less prone to painful, back-tightening strains.

1. **Hamstring wall stretch.** Lie faceup on a carpeted floor (or on a folded blanket for padding), positioning your body perpendicular inside a door-frame. Bend your right leg and place it through the door opening. Bring your buttocks as close to the wall as possible and place the heel of your left foot up against the wall until it is nearly straight. Next, slide your right leg forward on the floor until it's straight, feeling a stretch in the back of your left leg. Hold for thirty seconds. Repeat twice on each side.

2. **Knees-to-chest stretch.** Lie on your back with your feet flat on the floor and your knees bent. Use your hands to pull your right knee to your chest. Next, try to straighten your left leg on the floor. While keeping your right knee held to your chest, continue the stretch for twenty seconds, then switch sides and repeat. Finally, do the stretch by holding both knees to your chest for ten seconds.

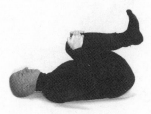

3. **Spinal stretch.** While on the floor with your left leg extended straight, pull your right knee to your chest (as in exercise 2), then put your right arm out to the side. Next, use your left hand to slowly pull your right knee toward your left side so that your right foot rests on the back of your left knee. Finally, turn your head toward your right side. Hold for twenty seconds, then reverse the movements and repeat.

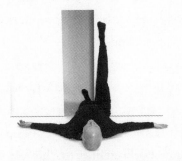

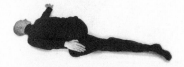

4. **Gluteal (buttocks) stretch.** Lie on your back with your feet flat on the floor and your knees bent. Cross your right leg over your left, resting your right ankle on your left knee. Next, grab your left thigh with both hands and bring both legs toward your body. Hold for thirty seconds, then switch sides and repeat.

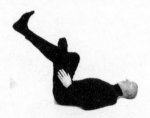

5. **Hip flexor stretch.** Kneel on your right knee (you can use a thin pillow for comfort) with your left leg bent ninety degrees in front of you and your foot flat on the floor. Place your right hand on your waist and your left hand on top of your left leg. Inhale and then, on the exhale, lean forward into your right hip, feeling a stretch in the front of your right hip. Hold for thirty seconds, then switch sides and repeat.

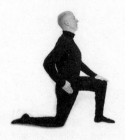

6. **Quadriceps stretch.** While standing, hold on to the back of a sturdy chair with your left hand for balance. Grasp your right foot with your right hand and gently pull your right leg back and up, with your toes pointing upward. Be sure to keep your right knee close to your left leg. Hold for thirty seconds, then switch sides and repeat.

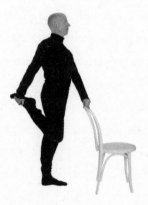

7. **Total back stretch.** Stand arm's length in front of a table or other sturdy object and lean forward with knees slightly bent so that you can grasp the table edge with both hands. Keep your arms straight and your head level with your shoulders. Hold for ten seconds.

Next, stand up straight with your left hand in front of you. Bring your right arm over your head with elbow bent, then bend your upper body gently to the left. Hold for ten seconds, then switch sides and repeat.

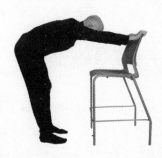

....

> Gerard Girasole, MD, orthopedic spine surgeon, the Orthopaedic & Sports Medicine Center, Trumbull, Connecticut. He is coauthor, with Cara Hartman, CPT, a Fairfield, Connecticut–based certified personal trainer, of *The 7-Minute Back Pain Solution—7 Simple Exercises to Heal Your Back Without Drugs or Surgery in Just Minutes a Day.*

....

Banish Back Pain with These Easy Yoga Poses

L ower back pain makes almost every-thing more difficult. But simple Iyengar-style yoga poses reduce pain and increase the ease of daily activities—without drugs.

Props: A mat, folding chair, blanket, towel, bolster (or two blankets rolled together), and strap. Breathe slowly and deeply; never push to the point of discomfort. Practice the poses below (which have been modified for people with back pain) in the order given three to seven days per week. Check with a health-care professional before beginning any new exercise routine.

◆ *Savasana* (corpse pose). Place the chair at the end of the mat, with a folded blanket on the seat. Lie on your back on the mat with your head on the folded towel. Rest your calves on the chair seat, knees comfortably bent and tailbone tucked under so your back is not arched. Let your arms rest at your sides, palms up. Relax completely. Hold for five minutes.

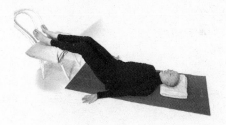

◆ *Supta tadasana* (reclining mountain pose). Place the short edge of the mat against a wall. Lie on your back with your head on the folded towel and your legs straight out in front of you, your feet hip-width apart, toes pointing up, soles pressed against the wall.

Hold the edges of the mat, elbows straight, outer arms pressed down. Hold for one minute.

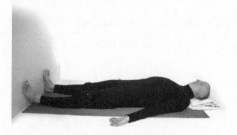

+ **Supta padangusthasana I** (supine big toe pose, bent knee). Start in supta tadasana pose (above). Keeping your left leg pressed to the floor and left sole against the wall, bend your right knee toward your chest, and clasp your shin with both hands. Hold for twenty seconds, then switch legs. Do three times per side.

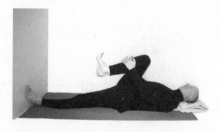

+ **Straight-leg variation:** Instead of clasping your shin, place the center of a strap across your right sole, and hold the ends of the strap. Straighten your leg and flex your foot so your sole faces the ceiling.

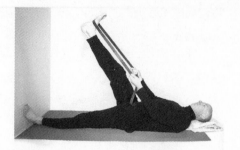

+ **Supta pavanmuktasana** (wind-releasing pose). Lie on your back with your head on a folded towel. Bending both knees, bring your knees toward your chest. Grasp your shins with your hands, keeping your knees hip-width apart. Hold for thirty seconds.

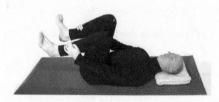

+ **Adho mukha svanasana** (downward-facing dog). Come to your hands and knees on the mat, hands shoulder-width apart, tips of your thumb and first two fingers touching the wall. Curl your toes under, and lift your knees off the floor, straightening your legs and raising your buttocks toward the ceiling. Pushing down and forward with your hands, stretch your shoulders back and away from the wall while stretching your heels toward the floor. Hold for thirty seconds.

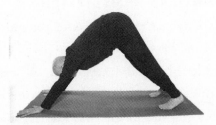

+ *Bharadvajasana* (seated twist on chair). Place the folded blanket on the chair seat, then sit backward with your hips close to the front edge of the seat. Spread your knees, and place your feet on the outside edges of the back chair legs. Place your right forearm on top of the chair back and grasp the front edge of the seat with your left hand. Keeping your chest lifted, turn your chest to the left, twisting gently. Hold for twenty seconds, then switch sides. Do three times per side.

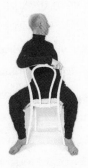

+ *Adho mukha virasana* (downward-facing hero). Place a bolster on the mat. Kneel at one end of the bolster,

knees apart and toes together. Sit back on your heels (tuck a folded blanket under your buttocks, if necessary). Place a rolled towel in your hip crease. Bending forward at the hips, place your hands on either side of the bolster for support while lowering your torso and forehead onto the bolster. Rest your forearms on the floor. Relax completely. Hold for five minutes.

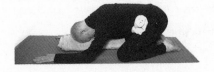

> Kimberly Williams, PhD, certified Iyengar yoga teacher at Inner Life Yoga Studio in Morgantown, West Virginia. IYogaPoses.com.

Simple Stretches to Ease a Stiff Neck

*L*et's say you're sitting *at* a computer for a while—it could be for an hour or more. You get up out of your chair, and ping, your neck aches and feels stiff. You can barely turn to look over your shoulder. Ouch! This type of pain can happen when we've been working at a desk, driving, even doing something relaxing such as working on a puzzle or craft.

Reason: Many of us sit with poor posture, and this affects the connecting muscles that control the position of the spine, including the neck. Stay in this position for a while and muscles become tight, resulting in pain and stiffness.

Stretching the neck muscles during and after you have been sitting for a while can help, so try the five stretches below. These five moves are easy to do and feel great. For all these exercises, sit up straight and comfortably in a hard-backed chair that has no armrests.

Note: If you have constant neck pain (that does not appear to be related to how much time you spend sitting), don't do these exercises for pain relief. While they might help you, it's much better to speak to a doctor or physical therapist, who can help determine the root cause of your pain.

HEAD STRETCH

This move stretches the large muscle that connects the base of the skull to the upper back, collarbones, and shoulder blades.

Place your right arm behind your back at waist level. Place your left hand over the top of your head and gently grasp the right side of your head. With your left hand, gently pull your head toward your left shoulder. Your left ear will be close to your left arm. Hold for one minute, or hold for thirty seconds, relax, and then repeat the move. Switch hands and repeat on the other side.

DOWNWARD HEAD STRETCH

This move eases tightness of the muscle that runs between the upper part of the shoulder blades and neck. You will really feel this stretch in the back of your neck.

As you did in the first exercise, place your right hand behind your back at waist level. Put your left hand on the top of your head. Turn your face toward your left armpit, and gently push your head toward the armpit (it's OK if your left hand slides back down your head to get a good stretch). Hold for thirty seconds and repeat. Or hold for one minute and only do one repetition. Repeat on the other side.

SHOULDER PINCH STRETCH

This move helps you maintain good posture. You will feel a stretch across your pectoral muscles in the upper chest.

Sit up tall. With your arms by your sides, bend your elbows at a ninety-degree angle, hands palm up. Position your arms so that the backs of your palms are a foot or so above your thighs. Pull your shoulder blades together, and as you do so, let your arms rotate out to your sides, keeping elbows bent. Repeat the rotating movement twenty times.

TORSO ROTATION

This move increases upper- and lower-back flexibility.

Cross your arms in front of you, and place your right hand on the front of your left shoulder and your left hand on the front of your right shoulder. Gentle rotate your torso and head to one side as far as you can go, then return to center. Rotate to the other side. Repeat ten times on each side.

SITTING KNEE PILLOW SQUEEZE

This move strengthens the hip flexors and solidifies your core muscles and the foundation upon which your neck depends. You will feel this move in your hips and inner thighs.

Sit straight up in your chair, and place a thick pillow between your knees. Roll your hips forward. Hold the pillow with your thighs, squeeze, and release. Repeat twenty times, and work up to three sets.

> Natalie Thomas, PT, DPT, doctor of physical therapy, managing director, In Motion O.C., Irvine, California. InMotionOC.com.

Myotherapy: Drug-Free Help for Back, Shoulder, and Hip Pain

*C*an you imagine living well into your nineties and being able to eliminate virtually all the aches and pains that you may develop from time to time?

Bonnie Prudden, a longtime physical fitness advocate, stayed pain free—even though she had arthritis that led to two hip replacements—by using a form of myotherapy ("myo" is Greek for muscle) that she developed more than thirty years ago. She died in 2011 at the age of ninety-seven.

Now: Tens of thousands of patients have successfully used this special form of myotherapy, which is designed to relieve trigger points (highly irritable spots in muscles) that develop throughout life due to a number of causes, such as falls, strains, or disease. By applying pressure to these sensitive areas and then slowly releasing it, it's possible to relax muscles that have gone into painful spasms, often in response to physical and/or emotional stress.

A simple process: Ask a partner (a spouse or friend, for example) to locate painful trigger points by applying his/her fingertips to parts of your body experiencing discomfort, or consult a practitioner trained in myotherapy.

If you're working with a partner, let

him know when a particular spot for each body area described in this article is tender.

Pressure should be applied for seven seconds (the optimal time determined by Prudden's research to release muscle tension) each time that your partner locates such a spot.

On a scale of one to ten, the pressure should be kept in the five- to seven-point range—uncomfortable but not intolerable.

The relaxed muscles are then gently stretched to help prevent new spasms.

If you prefer to treat yourself: Use a "bodo," a wooden dowel attached to a handle, and a lightweight, metal shepherd's crook.

For areas that are easy to reach, use the bodo to locate trigger points and then apply pressure to erase them. For spots that are difficult to reach, use the shepherd's crook to find and apply pressure to trigger points.

As an alternative to the specially designed tools, you can use your fingers, knuckles, or elbows on areas of the body that can be reached easily. If you are unable to find a practitioner near you, call local massage therapists and ask whether they are familiar with the techniques. Check with your doctor before trying this therapy if you have a chronic medical condition or have suffered a recent injury. Here are some common types of pain that can be relieved by this method.

LOWER BACK PAIN

Finding the trigger point: Lie facedown while your partner stands to your right and reaches across your body to place his elbow on your buttocks in the area where the left back pocket would appear on a pair of pants. For seven seconds, your partner should slowly apply pressure to each trigger point, not straight down but angled back toward himself.

Repeat on the other side. If the pressure causes slight discomfort, your partner has found the right spot! If not, your partner should move his elbow slightly and try the steps again. Two to three trigger points can typically be found on each buttock.

Pain-erasing stretch: Lie on your left side on a flat surface (such as a bed, table, or the floor). Bend your right knee, and pull it as close to your chest as possible. Next, extend your right leg, keeping it aligned with the left leg and about eight inches above it. Finally, lower the raised leg onto the resting one and relax for three seconds. Perform these steps four times on each leg.

SHOULDER PAIN

Finding the trigger point: Lie facedown while your partner uses his elbow to gently apply pressure to trigger points that can hide along the top of the shoulders and in the upper back. If you are very small or slender, your partner can use his fingers instead of his elbow.

Place one of your arms across your back at the waist while your partner slides his fingers under your shoulder blade to search for and apply pressure to additional trigger points. Repeat the process on the opposite side.

While still lying facedown, bend your elbows and rest your forehead on the backs of your hands. With his hands overlapped, your partner can gently move all ten of his fingers along the top of the shoulder to locate additional trigger points.

Pain-erasing stretch: The "shrug" is a sequence of shoulder exercises performed four times after myotherapy and whenever shoulder tension builds. From a standing or sitting position, round your back by dropping your head forward while bringing the backs of your arms together as close as possible in front of your body. Extend both arms back (with your thumbs leading) behind your body while tipping your head back and looking toward the ceiling. Next, with both arms at your sides, raise your shoulders up to your earlobes, then press your shoulders down hard.

HIP PAIN

Finding the trigger point: The trigger points for hip pain are often found in the gluteus medius, the muscles that run along either side of the pelvis.

Lie on your side with your knees slightly bent. Using one elbow, your partner should scan for trigger points along the gluteus medius (in the hip area, roughly between the waist and the bottom seam of your underpants) and apply pressure straight down at each sensitive spot for seven seconds.

The same process should be repeated on the opposite side of your body.

Pain-erasing stretch: Lie on your left side on a table with your right leg hanging off the side and positioned forward. Your partner should place one hand on top of your waist and the other hand on the knee of the dangling right leg. This knee should be gently pressed down eight times. The stretch should be repeated on the opposite side.

....

› The late Bonnie Prudden helped create the President's Council on Youth Fitness in 1956 and was one of the country's leading authorities on exercise therapy for more than five decades. In 2007, she received the Lifetime Achievement Award from the President's Council on Physical Fitness and Sports. She was author of numerous books, including *Pain Erasure*.

....

3

Brain

Four Surprising Ways to Prevent Alzheimer's

Every sixty-eight seconds, another American develops Alzheimer's disease, the fatal brain disease that steals memory and personality. It's the fifth-leading cause of death among people age sixty-five and older.

You can lower your likelihood of getting Alzheimer's disease by reducing controllable and well-known risk factors. But there are also little-known "secret" risk factors that you can address, too.

COPPER IN TAP WATER

A scientific paper published in the *Journal of Trace Elements in Medicine and Biology* theorizes that inorganic copper found in nutritional supplements and in drinking water is an important factor in today's Alzheimer's epidemic.

Science has established that beta-amyloid plaques—inflammation-causing cellular debris found in the brains of people with Alzheimer's—contain high levels of copper. Animal research shows that small amounts of inorganic copper in drinking water worsen Alzheimer's. Studies on people have linked the combination of copper and a high-fat diet to memory loss and mental decline. It may be that copper sparks beta-amyloid plaques to generate more oxidation and inflammation, further injuring brain cells.

What to do: There is plenty of copper in our diets—no one needs additional copper from a multivitamin/mineral supplement. Look for a supplement with no copper or a minimal amount (500 micrograms).

I also recommend filtering water. Water-filter pitchers, such as ones by Brita, can reduce the presence of copper.

I installed a reverse osmosis water filter in my home a few years ago when the evidence for the role of copper in Alzheimer's became compelling.

VITAMIN D DEFICIENCY

Mounting evidence shows that a low blood level of vitamin D may increase Alzheimer's risk.

A study in the *Journal of Alzheimer's Disease* analyzed ten studies exploring the link between vitamin D and Alzheimer's. Researchers found that low blood levels of vitamin D were linked to a 40 percent increased risk for Alzheimer's.

The researchers from UCLA, also writing in the *Journal of Alzheimer's Disease*, theorize that vitamin D may protect the brain by reducing beta-amyloid and inflammation.

What to do: The best way to make sure that your blood level of vitamin D is protective is to ask your doctor to test it and then, if needed, to help you correct your level to greater than 60 nanograms per milliliter (ng/mL). That correction may require 1,000 IU to 2,000 IU of vitamin D daily or another individualized supplementation strategy.

Important: When your level is tested, make sure that it is the 25-hydroxyvitamin D, or 25(OH)D, test and not the 1,25-dihydroxyvitamin D test. The latter test does not accurately measure blood levels of vitamin D but is sometimes incorrectly ordered. Also, ask for your exact numerical results. Levels above 30 ng/mL are considered normal, but in my view, the 60 ng/mL level is the minimum that is protective.

A CONCUSSION

A study published in Neurology showed that NFL football players had nearly four times higher risk for Alzheimer's than the general population, no doubt from repeated brain injuries incurred while playing football.

What most people don't realize: Your risk of developing Alzheimer's is doubled if you've ever had a serious concussion that resulted in loss of consciousness. This newer evidence shows that it is crucially important to prevent head injuries of any kind throughout your life.

What to do: Fall-proof your home, with commonsense measures such as adequate lighting, eliminating or securing throw rugs, and keeping stairways clear. Wear shoes with firm soles and low heels, which also helps prevent falls.

If you've ever had a concussion, it's important to implement the full range of Alzheimer's-prevention strategies in this article.

NOT HAVING A PURPOSE IN LIFE

In a seven-year study published in *Archives of General Psychiatry*, researchers at the Rush Alzheimer's Disease Center in Chicago found that people who had a purpose in life were 2.4 times less likely to develop Alzheimer's.

What to do: The researchers found that the people who agreed with the following statements were less likely to develop Alzheimer's and mild cognitive impairment: "I feel good when I think of what I have done in the past and what I hope to do in the future" and "I have a sense of direction and purpose in life."

If you cannot genuinely agree with the above statements, there are things you can do to change that. In fact, you even can change the way you feel about your past. It takes a bit of resolve, some action, and perhaps help from a qualified mental health counselor.

One way to start: Think about and make a list of some activities that would make your life more meaningful. Ask yourself, "Am I doing these?" and then write down small, realistic goals that will involve you more in those activities, such as volunteering one hour every week at a local hospital or signing up for a class at your community college next semester.

The following steps are crucial in the fight against Alzheimer's disease:

- Lose weight if you're overweight.
- Control high blood pressure.
- Exercise regularly.
- Engage in activities that challenge your mind.
- Eat a diet rich in colorful fruits and vegetables and low in saturated fat, such as the Mediterranean diet.
- Take a daily supplement containing 2,000 mg of omega-3 fatty acids.

> Marwan Sabbagh, MD, neurologist and director of the Alzheimer's disease and memory disorders division at Barrow Neurological Institute at Dignity Health St. Joseph's Hospital and Medical Center, Phoenix, Arizona. He is author of *The Alzheimer's Prevention Cookbook: 100 Recipes to Boost Brain Health.* MarwanSabbaghMD.com.

Alzheimer's Symptoms Reversed!

Can Alzheimer's symptoms be reversed? A breakthrough treatment suggests that they can. In a study published in the journal *Aging*, Dale Bredesen, MD, director of the Alzheimer's Disease Program at UCLA's David Geffen School of Medicine, presented an all-natural, multicomponent treatment program that reversed memory loss in four people with Alzheimer's and in five people with either subjective cognitive impairment or mild cognitive impairment (the stages of memory loss that typically precede Alzheimer's). Here, he describes the breakthrough.

RECENT THINKING

The current, widely accepted theory of Alzheimer's says that the protein beta-amyloid forms plaques outside neurons in the brain, somehow triggering the production of abnormal tau tangles inside neurons, thereby interfering with synapses, the information-laden connections between neurons that create memory and other mental activity.

Recent development: Normal mental function depends on a balance between synaptoblastic (synapse-making) and synaptoclastic (synapse-destroying) activity. If there is more synaptoclastic activity, memory loss may ensue. If there is chronic synaptoclastic activity, our research suggests that Alzheimer's occurs. My colleagues and I have identified thirty-six unique synapse-affecting factors (including beta-amyloid). Addressing only one or two of these factors—with a drug, for example— will not reverse Alzheimer's. But addressing many factors—ten, twenty or more—can effectively reverse the symptoms.

Here are several key factors in what we call the Metabolic Enhancement for Neuro Degeneration (MEND) program—factors anyone can use to prevent, slow, stop, or potentially even reverse memory loss.

RESTORING MEMORY

Synapse-making and synapse-destroying factors function in a loop that develops momentum, like a snowball rolling downhill. In the synapse-destroying momentum of Alzheimer's, you gradually lose memories, ultimately even basic ones such as the faces of loved ones. But because the synapse-making factors in the MEND program are so effective, they can reverse the momentum of Alzheimer's. The more of them that you incorporate into your daily life, the more momentum there is to protect and restore memory.

Optimize diet. Eliminate simple carbohydrates such as anything made from white flour and/or refined sugar. Don't eat processed foods with either trans fats or partially hydrogenated vegetable oil on the label. If you're sensitive to gluten, minimize your consumption of gluten-containing foods, such as wheat and rye (there are simple tests to determine whether you are indeed gluten-sensitive). Emphasize fruits and vegetables. Eat nonfarmed fish for neuron-protecting omega-3 fatty acids.

Why it works: This dietary approach reduces inflammation and high levels of insulin (the hormone that regulates blood sugar), both of which are synapse-destroying.

Important: Dietary changes have more impact than any other factor in preventing or reversing memory loss.

Helpful: Four books that have diets consistent with MEND are *Eat to Live: The Amazing Nutrient-Rich Program for Fast and Sustained Weight Loss* by Joel Fuhrman, MD, *The Blood Sugar Solution: The UltraHealthy Program for Losing Weight, Preventing Disease, and Feeling Great Now!* by Mark Hyman, MD, *The Spectrum: A Scientifically Proven Program to Feel Better, Live Longer, Lose Weight, and Gain Health* by Dean Ornish, MD, and *Grain Brain: The Surprising Truth about Wheat, Carbs, and Sugar—Your Brain's Silent Killers* by David Perlmutter, MD.

Have a nightly fast. Don't eat three hours before bedtime. Ideally, twelve hours should pass between the last time you eat at night and when you eat breakfast.

Example: Dinner ending at 8:00 p.m. and breakfast starting at 8:00 a.m.

Why it works: This eating pattern enhances autophagy (the body's ability to clean up dysfunctional cells, such as beta-amyloid) and ketosis (the generation of ketones, molecules that can help protect neurons). It also reduces insulin.

Reduce stress. Pick a relaxing, enjoyable activity—walking in the woods, yoga, meditation, playing the piano, etc.—and do it once a day or every other day for at least twenty to thirty minutes.

Why it works: Stress destroys neurons in the hippocampus, the part of the brain that helps create short- and long-term memory. Stress also boosts cortisol, a synapse-damaging hormone. And stress increases corticotropin-releasing hormone (CRH), which is linked to Alzheimer's.

Optimize sleep. Sleep seven to eight hours every night.

Why it works: Anatomical changes during sleep flush the brain of toxic, synapse-damaging compounds. If you have trouble sleeping, we have found that 0.5 mg of melatonin at bedtime is the best dose for restorative sleep.

Exercise regularly. I recommend thirty to sixty minutes per day, four to six days per week. Combining aerobic exercise (such as brisk walking) with weight-training is ideal.

Why it works: Among its many benefits, exercise produces brain-derived neurotrophic factor (BDNF), a powerfully synaptoblastic compound.

Stimulate your brain. Brain-training exercises and games stimulate and improve your ability to remember, pay attention, process information quickly, and creatively navigate daily life.

Why it works: Just as using muscle builds muscle, using synapses builds synapses. Scientists call this ability of the brain to change and grow plasticity.

Helpful: Brain HQ (BrainHQ.com) and Lumosity (Lumosity.com) are good, science-based online programs for stimulating your brain.

Take folate, vitamin B-6, and vitamin B-12. These three nutrients can reduce blood levels of the amino acid homocysteine, which is linked to an increase in tau protein, increased age-related shrinkage of the hippocampus, and double the risk for Alzheimer's disease.

However: To work, these supplements must undergo a biochemical process called methylation, and many older people don't methylate well, rendering the supplements nearly useless. To avoid the problem, take a form of the supplements that already is methylated (or activated)—folate as L-methylfolate, B-6 as pyridoxal-5-phosphate, and B-12 as methylcobalamin.

Take other targeted supplements. Along with the three B vitamins, there are many other supplements that target synaptoblastic and synaptoclastic factors. Check with your doctor about the right dosages. The supplements include vitamin D-3 (low levels double the risk for Alzheimer's); vitamin K-2; vitamin E (as mixed tocopherols and tocotrienols); the minerals selenium, magnesium, and zinc (zinc, for example, lowers copper, which is linked to Alzheimer's); DHA and EPA (anti-inflammatory omega-3 fatty acids); coenzyme Q10, N-acetylcysteine, and alpha-lipoic acid (they nourish mitochondria, energy-generating structures within cells); and probiotics (they improve the microbiome, helping to strengthen the lining of the gut, reducing body-wide inflammation). Also, certain herbs can be helpful. These include curcumin (1,000 mg per day), ashwagandha (500 mg once or twice per day), and bacopa (*Bacopa monnieri*) (200 to 300 mg per day). These have multiple effects, such as reducing inflammation and beta-amyloid peptide and enhancing neurotransmission.

› Dale Bredesen, MD, Augustus Rose Professor of Neurology and director of the Mary S. Easton Center for Alzheimer's Disease Research, Alzheimer's Disease Program and Neurodegenerative Disease Research in the David Geffen School of Medicine, UCLA. He is founding president of the Buck Institute for Research on Aging in Novato, California.

Berries and Your Brain

For more than a decade, scientists at the Jean Mayer USDA Human Nutrition Research Center on Aging at

Tufts University have been studying the effect of berries on the brain—in cells and in laboratory animals. They have found that regular ingestion of blueberries, strawberries, and/or blackberries can help improve plasticity, the ability of brain cells to form new connections with one another, generate new brain cells, stop inflammation and oxidation from damaging brain cells, ease the destructive effect of stress on the brain, prevent and reverse age-related memory loss, particularly short-term or working memory, and protect against beta-amyloid, the plaques in the brain that cause Alzheimer's disease. Now, research has shown that blueberries can help rejuvenate the aging *human* brain.

Startling findings: The researchers from Tufts studied thirty-seven people, ages sixty to seventy-five, dividing them into two groups. One group consumed one ounce of freeze-dried blueberries every day (the equivalent of one cup of fresh blueberries), and the other a blueberry placebo. At the beginning, middle, and end of the three-month study, the participants took tests measuring learning and memory. By the end of the study, those in the blueberry group had a 20 percent improvement in their scores on a memory test compared with those in the placebo group.

Strawberries are good too. The Tufts researchers gave participants either freeze-dried strawberry powder (the equivalent of two cups of fresh strawberries) or a placebo. After three months of daily intake, the strawberry group had much greater improvements in memory than the placebo group.

What to do: Eat one cup of blueberries or strawberries daily, either fresh or frozen. Choose organic. Every year, the Environmental Working Group announces its "Dirty Dozen," a list of the produce with the most pesticides. In 2017, strawberries topped the list, and blueberries ranked number 17.

› Bill Gottlieb, CHC, a certified health coach and health journalist. He is the author and coauthor of numerous books, including *Bottom Line's Speed Healing*. BillGottliebHealth.com.

Loneliness Doubles Alzheimer's Risk

For some time, we've known that social isolation is a risk factor for dementia. A recent study goes far deeper, with findings offering fascinating insight. Researchers at Rush University in Chicago and the University of Pennsylvania followed 823 people older than seventy for four years, using questionnaires administered by researchers to assess social isolation and conducting tests of cognitive functioning. They discovered that people who scored highest on the loneliness scale—regardless of whether or not they actually spent much time with people—were more than twice as likely to develop Alzheimer's during the follow-up period as people whose score was the lowest.

WHO GETS ALZHEIMER'S, AND WHO DOESN'T?

Loneliness is sometimes considered an early sign of Alzheimer's, but these findings show it is associated with increased risk and not an early symptom of its pathology.

Culturally, we've been inclined to regard problems of age to be inevitable with the passing of years. This study shows it's time to correct that assumption and more closely investigate ways to prevent the debilitation of old-age diseases including dementia. The kind of loneliness this study talks about is more like a trait than an emotional state. It's not the type of loneliness you might experience being away from home for an extended period, which is loneliness as a state, but rather the type that you feel all or most of the time, loneliness as a trait that follows you everywhere. Even so, there are still many ways to address and modify it. Medicine helps treat depression, which is usually part of loneliness,

but nondrug therapies including regular exercise, joining like-minded groups for activities, and expanding your circle of friends and acquaintances in general can be hugely beneficial—most especially when you've got strong networks already in place. If you live alone, you may want to consider moving to a retirement community, where even shy people can make connections, since most residents are looking to do so. Not only will being with others possibly help people avoid Alzheimer's in years to come, it will make for happier years right now.

› Robert S. Wilson, PhD, senior neuropsychologist of the Rush Alzheimer's Disease Center, Rush University Medical Center, Chicago.

Alzheimer's Could Really Be a B-12 Deficiency

*I*t *may seem like an* extreme form of wishful thinking to suggest that symptoms believed to signal the onset of Alzheimer's disease could instead be due to a lack of one particular vitamin, and yet studies over the years have been telling us just that. Some people fifty and older who are suffering from memory problems, confusion, irritability, depression, and/or paranoia could see those symptoms dramatically diminish simply by taking vitamin B-12.

Frighteningly, research shows that up to 30 percent of adults may be B-12 deficient, making them vulnerable to misdiagnosis of Alzheimer's. For years, doctors had believed that B-12 deficiency showed itself most significantly as the cause of anemia (pernicious anemia), but they now realize the lack of B-12 may even more dramatically be causing neurological symptoms, some of which are similar to Alzheimer's.

OTHERS AT RISK

Age is not the only risk factor for having a B-12 deficiency. Other at-risk groups include vegetarians (dietary B-12 comes predominantly from meat and dairy products) and people who have celiac disease, Crohn's disease, or other nutrient malabsorption problems. Evidence accumulating over the past few decades shows that regular use of certain medications also can contribute to vitamin B-12 deficiency. These include antacids, in particular proton pump inhibitors (PPIs) such as esomeprazole, lansoprazole, and many others that reduce stomach acid levels, making it difficult for B-12 to be fully absorbed. The diabetes drug metformin also can reduce B-12 levels.

MEASURING DEFICIENCY

A common symptom of vitamin B-12 deficiency is neuropathy, a tingly and prickly sensation, sometimes felt in the hands and feet and occasionally in the arms and legs as well. People with B-12 deficiency also tend to have problems maintaining proper gait and balance. I recommend testing B-12 levels for a few groups of people, including those on PPIs for more than a few months, people having memory problems and/or often feeling confused—and this can include people of any age, those with neuropathy in the feet and/or legs, and those who have unexplained anemia.

As mentioned above, deficiencies of B-12 in older adults are nearly always a direct result of too little stomach acid, which is essential for absorption of B-12. This explains why powerful antacids trigger B-12 deficiency. Another problem is that sometimes, especially in older people, the stomach isn't making enough of a protein called intrinsic factor (IF) that is needed to break down B-12 effectively. There is no way to increase IF, so the solution is to administer B-12 in large enough quantities to override the difficulty with absorption. Traditionally, this has been done with injections of B-12, but more recently, doctors have found that oral supplementation with high amounts of B-12 that dissolves under the tongue also is successful and certainly easier than regular injections. There is no reason to be concerned about balancing B vitamins as was once thought—B-12 is water soluble, and the body can excrete what it doesn't need.

WHAT YOU CAN DO

Adults can easily get the recommended daily amount of 2.4 micrograms (mcg) of B-12 from dietary sources, which include all animal products. For example, just three ounces of steamed clams supplies 34.2 mcg, and three ounces of salmon provides the necessary 2.4 mcg. However, this amount will not address the problems associated with aging and medications. Once again, the issue goes back to absorption—if you don't have enough stomach acid and/or IF to use the B-12 you ingest, it is almost irrelevant how much animal protein you eat. This is why the Institute of Medicine says that for people over age fifty and for vegetarians, the best way to ensure meeting your body's B-12 needs is to take a supplement or seek out foods fortified with it.

Reason: The body can more easily absorb the form of B-12 used for supplementation and fortification, even in people who have low levels of stomach acid.

Caution: B-12 tests are sometimes insufficiently sensitive, especially for vegans. If your test indicates levels are fine in spite of symptoms, have your doctor order a different test that will evaluate whether your B-12 system is intact. There is no need to suffer from any kind of B-12 deficiency symptoms, let alone risk misdiagnosis of Alzheimer's, when the solution is so close at hand!

> Irwin Rosenberg, MD, senior scientist and former director, Nutrition and Neurocognition Laboratory, Tufts University, Boston.

Four Supplements That Can Impair Your Brain

It is hardly news that supplements—just like drugs—can often cause physical side effects and reactions with prescribed medicines. Researchers are now learning more and more about unwanted mental changes that can occur when taking popular supplements (such as herbs and hormones).

These supplements can be a hidden cause of depression, anxiety, mania, and other mental changes because patients—and their doctors—often don't realize how these products can affect the brain.

MELATONIN

Melatonin is among the most popular supplements for treating insomnia, jet lag, and other sleep disorders. Melatonin is a natural hormone that's released by the pineal gland at night and readily enters the brain. Unlike many sleep aids, it doesn't render you unconscious or put you to sleep. It causes subtle brain changes that make you ready for sleep.

Studies have shown that people who take melatonin in the late afternoon or early evening tend to fall asleep more quickly when they go to bed. The amount of melatonin used in scientific studies ranges from 0.1 to 0.5 mg. However, the products in health-food stores typically contain much higher doses—usually 1 to 5 mg. Supplemental melatonin also may become less effective over time, which encourages people to increase the doses even more.

Effects on the brain: In people with depression, melatonin may improve sleep, but it may worsen their depression symptoms, according to the National Institutes of Health.

What to do: Melatonin can help when used short term for such problems as jet lag. It is not particularly effective as a long-term solution for other causes of insomnia.

ST. JOHN'S WORT

St. John's wort is probably the most studied herb for treating depression. Researchers who analyzed data from twenty-nine international studies concluded that St. John's wort was as effective as prescription antidepressants for treating minor to moderate depression.

St. John's wort appears to be safe, particularly when it's used under the supervision of a physician. However, it can cause unwanted mental changes.

Effects on the brain: St. John's wort may increase brain levels of "feel good" neurotransmitters, including serotonin and dopamine. But unwanted mental changes that may occur in anyone taking St. John's wort include anxiety, irritability, and vivid dreams. It may also lead to mania (a condition characterized by periods of overactivity, excessive excitement, and lack of inhibitions), especially in individuals who are also using antipsychotic drugs.

Caution: This supplement should never be combined with a prescription selective serotonin reuptake inhibitor (SSRI) antidepressant, such as sertraline or paroxetine. Taking St. John's wort with an SSRI can cause serotonin syndrome, excessive brain levels of serotonin that can increase body temperature, heart rate, and blood pressure—conditions that are all potentially fatal. It also can interact with certain drugs such as oral contraceptives and immunosuppressant medications.

What to do: If you have depression, do not self-medicate with St. John's wort. Always talk to your doctor first if you are interested in trying this supplement.

TESTOSTERONE

Older men whose testosterone levels are declining (as is normal with aging) are often tempted to get a prescription for supplemental "T," which is advertised (but not proven) to improve their ability to get erections. Some women also use testosterone patches or gels (in much lower doses than men) to increase sexual desire and arousal.

Effects on the brain: If your testosterone is low, taking supplemental doses may cause a pleasant—but slight—increase in energy. However, with very high doses, such as those taken by bodybuilders, side effects may include aggression and mood swings. Men and women may experience withdrawal symptoms, such as depression and loss of appetite, when they stop taking it.

Testosterone replacement for men is FDA approved only for those with a clinical deficiency, defined as blood levels under 300 nanograms per deciliter (ng/dL).

What to do: Testosterone has been shown to increase sexual desire in women.

It is not FDA approved for women but may be prescribed "off-label." The evidence supporting testosterone's ability to improve sexual function and well-being in normally aging men is weaker, unless they have been proven on more than one occasion to have low testosterone and related symptoms. Both men and women should take testosterone only under the supervision of a doctor.

WEIGHT-LOSS SUPPLEMENTS

Two ingredients that are commonly used in weight-loss supplements, beta-phenylethylamine (β-PEA) and p-synephrine, are said to increase energy and metabolism and burn extra calories.

Effects on the brain: Both β-PEA and p-synephrine (a compound made from bitter orange) can make you feel jittery and anxious, particularly when they are combined with stimulants such as caffeine.

Many weight-loss and energy products are complicated cocktails of active ingredients that haven't been adequately studied, nor have they been approved by the FDA. They're risky because they've been linked to dangerous increases in blood pressure.

Important: There is little evidence that any of these products is particularly effective as a weight-loss aid.

What to do: Don't rely on weight-loss supplements. To lose weight, you need to decrease your food intake and increase your exercise levels. No supplement can accomplish that!

> Cynthia Kuhn, PhD, professor of pharmacology, cancer biology, psychiatry, and behavioral sciences at Duke University School of Medicine in Durham, North Carolina. Dr. Kuhn is also coauthor of *Buzzed: The Straight Facts About the Most Used and Abused Drugs from Alcohol to Ecstasy.*

Best Nondrug Approaches for Parkinson's

The telltale tremors, *muscle stiffness*, and other movement problems that plague people with Parkinson's disease make even the mundane activities of daily living—such as brushing teeth, cooking, and dressing—more difficult.

Even though medications, such as levodopa (L-dopa) and newer drugs including pramipexole and selegiline, have long been the main treatment to control Parkinson's symptoms, researchers are discovering more and more nondrug therapies that can help.

Here are some of the best nondrug approaches (each can be used with Parkinson's medication).

EXERCISE

For people with Parkinson's, exercise is like a drug. It raises neurotrophic factors, proteins that promote the growth and health of neurons. Research consistently shows that exercise can improve motor symptoms (such as walking speed and stability) and quality of life.

For the best results: Exercise thirty to sixty minutes every single day. Aim to work hard enough to break a sweat, but back off if you get too fatigued—especially the following day (this indicates the body is not recovering properly). Parkinson's symptoms can worsen with too much exercise. Keep the following smart exercise habits in mind.

For better gait speed: Choose a lower-intensity exercise, such as walking on a treadmill (but hold on to the balance bars), rather than high-intensity exercise (such as running), which has a higher risk for falls and other injuries. A recent study showed that a walking group of Parkinson's patients performed better than a group of patients who ran.

Important safety tip: Parkinson's patients should exercise with a partner and take precautions to prevent falls—for example, minimizing distractions, such as ringing cell phones.

For aerobic exercise: Use a recumbent bicycle or rowing machine and other exercises that don't rely on balance.

For strength and flexibility: Do stretching and progressive resistance training.

Excellent resource: For a wide variety of exercises, including aerobic workouts, standing and sitting stretches, strengthening moves, balance exercises, and fall-prevention tips, the National Parkinson Foundation's Fitness Counts book is available as a free download at Parkinson.org/pd-library/books/fitness-counts.

For balance: Researchers are now discovering that yoga postures, tai chi (with its slow, controlled movements), and certain types of dancing (such as the tango, which involves rhythmic forward and backward steps) are excellent ways to improve balance.

COFFEE AND TEA

Could drinking coffee or tea help with Parkinson's? According to research, it can, when consumed in the correct amounts.

Here's why: Caffeine blocks certain receptors in the brain that regulate the neurotransmitter dopamine, which becomes depleted and leads to the impaired motor coordination that characterizes Parkinson's. In carefully controlled studies, Parkinson's patients who ingested low doses of caffeine—about 100 mg twice daily—had improved motor symptoms, such as tremors and stiffness, compared with people who had no caffeine or higher doses of caffeine.

My advice: Have 100 mg of caffeine (about the amount in one six-ounce cup of home-brewed coffee or two cups of black or green tea) twice a day—once in the morning and once in the midafternoon.

Note: Even decaffeinated coffee has about 10 to 25 mg of caffeine per cup.

SUPPLEMENTS

Researchers have studied various supplements for years to identify ones that could help manage Parkinson's symptoms and/or boost the effects of levodopa, but large studies have failed to prove that these supplements provide such benefits.

However, because Parkinson's is a complex disease that can cause about twenty different motor and nonmotor symptoms that evolve over time, the existing research may not apply to everyone. Some people with Parkinson's may benefit from the following:

+ **Coenzyme Q10 (CoQ10).** This supplement promotes the health of the body's mitochondria (energy generators in the cells), which are believed to play a role in Parkinson's. In a large study, people with Parkinson's who took 1,200 mg per day showed some improvement in symptoms over a sixteen-month study period. However, follow-up studies found no beneficial effects.

- **Riboflavin and alpha-lipoic acid.** These are among the other supplements that are continuing to be studied.

Important: If you wish to try these or other supplements, be sure to consult your doctor to ensure that there are no possible interactions with your other medications.

MARIJUANA

A few small studies have concluded that marijuana can improve some neurological symptoms, but larger studies are needed to show benefits for Parkinson's patients, especially for symptoms such as depression and anxiety.

However: Marijuana is challenging for several reasons. First, it is illegal in most states. If you do live in a state that allows medical marijuana use, it has possible side effects. For example, it can impair balance and driving; it is difficult to know the exact dosage, even if it's purchased from a dispensary; and with marijuana edibles (such as cookies and candies), the effects may take longer to appear, and you may accidentally ingest too much.

If you want to try marijuana: Work closely with your doctor to help you avoid such pitfalls.

SEEING THE RIGHT DOCTOR

For anyone with Parkinson's, it's crucial to see a neurologist and, if possible, one who has advanced training in Parkinson's disease and movement disorders.

Important finding: A large study showed that patients treated by a neurologist had a lower risk for hip fracture and were less likely to be placed in a nursing facility. They were also 22 percent less likely to die during the four-year study.

Neurologists are best equipped to treat the ever-changing symptoms of Parkinson's. For optimal care, see the neurologist every four to six months.

> Michael S. Okun, MD, professor and chair of the department of neurology and codirector of the Center for Movement Disorders and Neurorestoration at the University of Florida College of Medicine in Gainesville. He is also the medical director at the National Parkinson Foundation and has written more than four hundred medical journal articles. Dr. Okun is author of *10 Breakthrough Therapies for Parkinson's Disease.*

Natural Ways to Quiet Tremors

Natural therapies can help calm tremors by easing the stress and altering the brain chemicals and emotional responses that exacerbate the condition.

Important: Before trying natural remedies, be sure to avoid caffeine, smoking, and/or excess alcohol, all of which can worsen tremors. Also, make regular exercise (especially strength training) a priority. Tremors are more common when muscles become fatigued. Here are some natural treatments to tame any type of tremor.*

AROMATHERAPY

Breathing in the aroma of certain flowers and herbs can reduce tremors by enhancing brain levels of gamma-aminobutyric acid (GABA), a widely circulated neurotransmitter with proven stress-fighting effects. Raising GABA levels helps calm the overexcited neurons that can worsen tremors. What to try for tremors:

+ **Lavender.** This fragrant blue-violet flower has been shown in a number of small studies to produce calming, soothing, and sedative effects when its scent is inhaled. Lavender essential oil is widely available and can be inhaled in the bath (add five to eight drops to bath water for a long soak) or by dabbing a drop on your neck or temples.

SUPPLEMENTS

Certain supplements can ease tremors by enhancing muscle relaxation and/or reducing the body's overall stress levels or load of inflammatory chemicals, which can play a role in tremors caused by neuro-degenerative diseases. Check with your doctor to make sure these supplements don't interact with any medication you may be taking and won't affect any chronic condition you may have.†

+ **Magnesium.** This mineral helps to regulate nerve impulses and muscle contraction. Magnesium-rich foods include sesame seeds, beans, nuts,

---

*   Consult your doctor before trying these therapies to determine the cause of your tremors and for advice on the approaches best suited to your situation.

†   Because supplements aren't regulated by the FDA for purity, Giroux advises looking for products that bear the "USP-verified" stamp on the label. This means they have met rigorous testing standards to ensure quality by the scientific nonprofit U.S. Pharmacopeial Convention.

avocados, and leafy greens. To ensure that you're getting enough magnesium, consider taking a supplement.

Typical dose to ease tremors: 200 to 400 mg daily.

- **Fish oil.** The omega-3 fatty acids in fish oil offer proven anti-inflammatory effects. Systemic inflammation is implicated in neurodegenerative diseases such as MS and Parkinson's disease. Fish oil is abundant in fatty fish such as salmon, albacore tuna, mackerel, and herring. Aim for two servings per week. If you don't like fish, consider trying a supplement.

Typical dose to ease tremors: 1,000 to 1,500 mg daily.

- **Valerian, skullcap, and passionflower.** These calming herbs have been successfully used as part of a regimen to ease tremors. The supplements can be found in combination products, including capsules, teas, and tinctures. Follow instructions on the label.

BEAT TREMORS WITH YOUR MIND

If you suffer from tremors, it's common to think, *Oh no! My arm (or other body part) is shaking again. This is so embarrassing! I hate this!* While such thoughts are perfectly natural when tremors emerge, they are potentially destructive when trying to calm your condition.

What helps: Mindfulness can reset this negative thought pattern so that you stop viewing tremors as a problem, which only leads to distress that often worsens the condition.

Mindfulness is more than just relaxation. Often done in conjunction with deep-breathing exercises, mindfulness helps you simply observe your thoughts, feelings, and sensations and let them pass without judging them, labeling them, or trying to control them. By reducing the distress you feel about the tremors, you are no longer fueling the condition.

You can learn mindfulness from CDs or books.

My recommendations: Consult your local hospital to see if it offers mindfulness-based stress-reduction classes. Also consider trying other mind-body therapies that may help, such as hypnosis, biofeedback, and breath work.

....

› Monique Giroux, MD, neurologist and medical director and cofounder of the Movement & Neuroperformance Center of Colorado in Englewood, Colorado. Dr. Giroux was formerly a clinical fellow in integrative medicine at the University of Arizona and movement disorders at Emory University. She is the author of *Optimal Health with Parkinson's Disease.* CenterforMovement.org.

....

Cinnamon for Parkinson's

The Bible makes several references to it. The ancient Egyptians used it to preserve their mummies. The ancient Greeks and Romans used it to help them digest their feasts of lamb and wine. We know it's great for diabetes and glycemic control.

And now we find out that this substance fights Parkinson's disease. What is it? Cinnamon.

Besides being a commonly used spice, cinnamon has a long history as a medicine. Medieval physicians used it to treat arthritis, coughing, hoarseness, and sore throats. In fact, it was once so valuable, wars were fought over it.

Cinnamon can prevent symptoms of Parkinson's disease that include tremors; slow, jerky movement; stiffness; and loss of balance. My research has shown that cinnamon has this effect in mice acting as experimental models of Parkinson's disease.

Mouse studies often translate to humans when further research is done. Given how devastating Parkinson's disease can be and how familiar and safe cinnamon is, these cinnamon studies merit our attention right now. If these results are repeatable in Parkinson's disease patients, it would represent a remarkable advance in the treatment of this neurodegenerative disease.

The first thing to know is that we are not talking about just any kind of cinnamon but a specific, authentic kind.

Two types of cinnamon are sold in the United States—Chinese cinnamon (sometimes sold as Saigon cinnamon) and Ceylon cinnamon. Chinese cinnamon, or cassia, is the more common, less expensive type of cinnamon and is what you generally find in supermarkets. You know it—the usual cinnamon powder or that hard, aromatic curl of wood that you plunk into hot apple cider or cocoa. But this is not really "true" cinnamon and does not have its health benefits. Ceylon cinnamon is true cinnamon, and its sticks are softer and flakier than those of Chinese cinnamon. The powder is also lighter and sweeter smelling. There is virtually no way of knowing whether the powdered cinnamon you buy is true cinnamon or cassia or a mix unless it is specifically marked. Ceylon cinnamon is the spice of choice in medicinal research. So even just for general health, keep that in mind the next time you head out to the grocery store to replenish your spice rack—you may need to go to a higher-end market or even order online to get Ceylon cinnamon.

HOW DOES IT WORK?

As you may know, cinnamon is loaded with antioxidants. It may be therapeutic in Parkinson's disease, because its antioxidant effects counteract nitric oxide, a free radical that attacks proteins essential to supporting adequate levels of dopamine. Dopamine is the chemical in our brains that not only makes us feel happy and motivated, but also controls many of our muscle and limb movements.

It's known that the amount of proteins like DJ-1 and parkin decrease in the brains of patients with Parkinson's disease. We have found that these proteins also decrease in the brains of mice with Parkinson's disease because of nitric oxide production. After the mice ate ground cinnamon, their livers turned the cinnamon into an element, or metabolite, that cinnamon breaks down into during digestion, called sodium benzoate. Once the sodium benzoate got to the brain, it decreased the production of nitric oxide, which stopped the loss of parkin and DJ-1, protected brain cells, and allowed the mice to move around more normally, with steadier legs and less need for rest and downtime. It's possible that cinnamon could also prevent or lessen the symptoms of other diseases, such as types of palsy and Lewy body dementia, which are also caused by dopamine dysfunction.

HOW TO USE CINNAMON

These findings are potentially great news for people with Parkinson's disease and those who worry that they carry the potential for it in their genes. As it stands, Parkinson's disease patients must rely on drugs, such as levodopa, to replace dopamine, but these drugs neither cure nor change the course of the disease. They only provide temporary relief. Over time, symptoms become increasingly harder to control, and the drugs often have a wide range of serious side effects.

Cinnamon, however, and its metabolite sodium benzoate could potentially be among the safest approaches to stop the progression of Parkinson's disease once it's diagnosed.

Sodium benzoate is a common food preservative found in salad dressings, juices, condiments, and cosmetics. The National Institutes of Health's National Center for Complementary and Integrative Health has concluded that sodium benzoate and true cinnamon are safe and that true cinnamon is safe even in large amounts, but this is not true for cassia (Chinese cinnamon) because it contains coumarin, which, besides being a blood thinner, can damage the liver.

Unless you're allergic to cinnamon, take one teaspoon a day. But don't attempt to just swallow a teaspoon of dry cinnamon powder straight! It will make you gag and could cause you to cough and inhale the powder into your lungs, which is dangerous. Instead, mix cinnamon into food or drink.

You can bet there's much more research coming on cinnamon and Parkinson's. Meanwhile, generous helpings of this richly antioxidant spice could be well worth trying.

> Kalipada Pahan, PhD, professor of neurological sciences, Floyd A. Davis Professor of Neurology, Rush University Medical Center, Chicago. His study appeared in the *Journal of Neuroimmune Pharmacology*.

CoQ10 for Parkinson's

V itamin-like coenzyme Q10 (CoQ10) aids energy production in cells. In a study of eighty Parkinson's patients, those who took 1,200 mg of CoQ10 daily for sixteen months showed significantly less decline in motor function than other patients. A larger study is now testing an even higher dose.

> Katie Kompoliti, MD, neurologist, Rush University Medical Center, Chicago, and researcher in an ongoing multicenter clinical trial of six hundred Parkinson's patients.

Exercise Slows Parkinson's Disease

R *egular exercise has long been* known to improve symptoms and general quality of life for people with Parkinson's disease.

Now: Evidence shows that it may even slow progression of the disease.

Walking on a treadmill, riding a stationary bike, and strength training have been shown to improve general walking speed, strength, and overall fitness in Parkinson's patients. Picking up the pace may add even more benefit— one study found that symptoms and brain function improved more in Parkinson's patients the faster they pedaled on a stationary bike. Tai chi and even ballroom dancing have been shown to be especially effective at improving balance in Parkinson's patients.

Always talk to your doctor before starting a new exercise program. If you have a chronic illness, it may be useful to consult a physical therapist for advice on exercise dos and don'ts for your particular situation.

> John P. Porcari, PhD, program director of the Clinical Exercise Physiology (CEP) program at the University of Wisconsin–La Crosse. A past president of the American Association of Cardiovascular

and Pulmonary Rehabilitation, he has authored or coauthored more than 350 abstracts and 150 papers on exercise physiology.

....

Tai Chi: The Gentle Treatment for Parkinson's

I*magine feeling so unstable that* you are afraid of falling from the minute you get out of bed in the morning. That's what life can be like for many patients who are suffering from Parkinson's disease.

And while medications can help with the tremors and stiffness caused by Parkinson's, there is no pill to help with feeling unstable and unbalanced.

But research shows that there is a natural treatment that might help—tai chi. Past studies have shown that tai chi, an ancient Chinese exercise known for its slow and graceful movements (think yoga meets martial arts), can improve balance and stability in people with Parkinson's. But no studies comparing tai chi with other types of physical activity had been done before. So researchers set out to see how tai chi fared against resistance training (using weighted vests and ankle weights) and stretching and to find out, in particular, which might help Parkinson's patients improve their balance.

YOGA MEETS MARTIAL ARTS

The study participants included 195 men and women with Parkinson's between the ages of forty and eighty-five. They all had either mild or moderate Parkinson's but not severe, because those with severe Parkinson's are unable to stand unassisted, so they wouldn't have been able to do the exercises. The participants were randomly assigned to one of three different exercise programs—tai chi, resistance training, or stretching. All groups participated in a twice weekly, sixty-minute class for six months.

The tai chi program emphasized slow, continuous movements with multiple body parts moving at the same time, such as hand movements, trunk rotation, and weight shifting from foot to foot. The resistance-training program focused on strengthening muscles of the hips, knees, and ankles. The stretching program included light walking, arm, leg, and neck circles, and deep abdominal breathing.

At the end of the six-month study, the participants' balance was measured by looking at maximum excursion (which measured how far the person could lean over while standing without stumbling or falling), directional control while walking (which measured the amount of intentional movement toward a target compared with uncontrolled movement), and length of walking stride. Here are the findings:

* Tai chi participants increased their maximum excursion by 13 percent, while the resistance training group improved by only 6 percent, and the stretching group saw no improvement.
* The tai chi group increased their directional control by 11 percent, but neither the resistance-training group nor the stretching group saw any improvement.
* Those in the tai chi group had 67 percent fewer falls than those in the stretching group and marginally fewer falls than those in the resistance-training group.
* Length of stride improved for the tai chi participants by 10 centimeters (cm), compared with 4 cm for the resistance-training group and no improvement for the stretching group.

In other words, doing tai chi really helped these people with their balance and mobility! The research was published in the *New England Journal of Medicine*.

NATURAL HEALING
It's powerful, simple, and safe. If you have Parkinson's and you're interested in trying tai chi, mention it to your doctor (who will almost certainly say "by all means"), and then simply enroll in a class near you. Many gyms, YMCAs, and community centers offer tai chi. Or you can rent or buy a tai chi DVD. Tai chi doesn't require special equipment or fancy gym clothes, and it can be done indoors or outside. If you are unable to devote sixty full minutes to it twice a week, just remember that any amount is better than no amount.

> Fuzhong Li, PhD, senior research scientist, Oregon Research Institute, Eugene.

Best Workouts to Keep Your Brain "Buff"

We *all want to keep* our brains in top shape. But are crossword puzzles, online classes, and the other such activities that we've been hearing about for years the best ways to do that? Not really.

To improve memory and preserve overall cognitive function, the latest research reveals that it takes more than quiet puzzle solving and streaming lectures.

Even more intriguing: Some activities that we once thought were time wasters may actually help build intellectual capacity and other cognitive functions.

A HEALTHY BRAIN

The most important steps to keep your brain performing at optimal levels are lifestyle choices:

+ **Getting aerobic exercise (at least 150 minutes per week).**
+ **Maintaining a healthy body weight.**
+ **Not smoking.**
+ **Eating a diet that emphasizes fruits and vegetables and is low in refined sugar and white flour.**

Additional benefits are possible with regular brain workouts. In the past, experts thought that nearly any game or activity that challenges you to think would improve your general brain functioning.

What research now tells us: An increasing body of evidence shows that improved memory requires something more—you need to work against a clock. Games with a time limit force you to think quickly and with agility. These are the factors that lead to improved memory and mental focus. The following are among Dr. Green's favorite brain workouts. Aim for at least thirty minutes daily of any combination of the activities below.

BRAINY COMPUTER GAMES

Specialized brain-training computer programs (such as Lumosity, Fit Brains, and CogniFit) are no longer the darlings of the health community. Formerly marketed as a fun way to reduce one's risk for dementia, recent evidence has not supported that claim.

However, these programs do provide a variety of activities that may help improve intellectual performance, attention, memory, and mental flexibility. Lumosity and other programs are a good option for people who enjoy a regimented brain workout, including such activities as remembering sequences and ignoring distractions. Monthly prices range from $4.99 to $19.95.

Other options to consider trying:

+ **Action video games.** These games were once considered brain-numbing activities that kept players from developing intellectual and social skills. Yet research shows that action video games can promote mental focus, flexible thinking, and decision-making and problem-solving skills. Because these games are timed, they also require quick responses from the players.

    Good choices: World of Warcraft, The Elder Scrolls, and *Guild Wars,* all of which involve role-playing by assuming the identity of various characters to battle foes and complete quests, often with other virtual players. These games are available in DVD format for Mac or PC and with an online subscription for virtual play.

Caveat: An hour or two can be a brain booster, but don't overdo it. Too much role-playing takes you away from real-life interactions.

+ **Free brain-boosting computer game for a cause.** At Freerice.com, you can answer fun and challenging questions in such subjects as English vocabulary, foreign languages, math, and humanities. With each correct answer, enough money is generated to allow the United Nations World Food Programme to buy ten grains of rice and distribute it in a Third World country. To date, players have "earned" a total of nearly one hundred billion grains of rice—enough to create more than ten million meals.

To increase the challenge: Set a timer so that you must work against the clock.

APPS FOR YOUR BRAIN

If you'd prefer to use an app—a software application that you can use on a smartphone or similar electronic device—there are several good options. These are among the best fun/challenging apps (free on Android and Apple):

+ **Words with Friends.** This ever-popular game allows you to play a Scrabble-like game against your friends who have also downloaded the app on an electronic device. The game provides even more benefits if it's used with the time-clock feature.

+ **Word Streak with Friends** (formerly Scramble with Friends) is a timed find-a-word game. You can play on your own or with friends.

+ **Elevate** was named Apple's best app of 2014. It provides a structured game environment that feels more like a test, focusing on reading, writing, and math skills, than a game. Still, this timed app will give Apple users a good brain challenge.

TECH-FREE OPTIONS

If you'd rather not stare at the screen of a computer or some other electronic device for your brain workout, here are some good options:

+ **Tech-free games.** SET is a fast-paced card game that tests your visual perception skills. Players race to find a set of three matching cards (based on color, shape, number, or shading) from an array of cards placed on a table.

Bonus: This game can be played by one player or as many people as can fit around the table. The winner of dozens of "Best Game" awards, including the high-IQ group Mensa's Select award, SET is fun for kids and adults alike.

Another good choice: Boggle, which challenges you to create words from a given set of letter cubes within a three-minute period. It can be played by two or more people.

- **Drumming.** Playing any musical instrument requires attention and a keen sense of timing. Basic drumming is a great activity for beginner musicians (especially if you don't have the finger dexterity for piano or guitar).

  Even better: Join a drumming circle, which provides the extra challenge of matching your timing and rhythm to the rest of the drummers, along with opportunities for socialization.

  Bonus: Research has demonstrated that some forms, such as African djembe drumming, count as a low- to moderate-intensity activity that may reduce blood pressure, which helps protect the brain from blood vessel damage.

- **Meditation.** This practice improves cognitive function and sensory processing and promotes mental focus. Meditating for about thirty minutes daily also has been linked to greater blood flow to the brain and increased gray matter (associated with positive emotions, memory, and decision-making). The benefits have even been seen among some people with early-stage neurodegenerative diseases, such as Alzheimer's disease.

  A good way to get started: Begin with a simple "mindful eating" exercise—spend the first five minutes of each meal really focusing on what you're eating. Don't talk, read the paper, or watch TV; just savor the food. Eventually, you'll want to expand this level of attention to other parts of your day. Such mindfulness habits are a good complement to a regular meditation practice.

- **Coloring.** If you have kids or grandkids, don't just send them off with their crayons. Color with them.

  Even better: Get one of the new breed of coloring books with complex designs for adults. While there hasn't been specific research addressing the brain benefits of coloring, this form of play has been shown to reduce stress in children, and it is thought to boost creativity and have a meditative quality. You can find coloring books made for adults at bookstores and art-supply stores.

> Cynthia R. Green, PhD, practicing clinical psychologist and founder and president of Memory Arts, LLC, a brain-health and memory fitness consulting service in Montclair, New Jersey. She is also founding director of the Memory Enhancement Program at the Icahn School of Medicine at Mount Sinai in New York City. She is author of *Your Best Brain Ever: A Complete Guide & Workout.* TotalBrainHealth.com.

Meditate for a Bigger Brain

Compared with nonmeditators, *people who* had meditated between ten and ninety minutes a day for five to forty-six years had significantly greater brain volume in some regions linked to emotion, according to brain scans.

Theory: Meditation may promote better nerve connections or larger cells in certain brain regions, which may explain many meditators' emotional stability and mental focus.

> Eileen Luders, PhD, associate professor, department of neurology, Brain Mapping Center, University of California, Los Angeles, and lead author of a study of forty-four people.

Learn a Word a Day and Other Fun Ways to Add Healthy Years to Your Life

We all know that eating right and exercising can boost our chances of a long, healthy life. But sometimes it seems as if the changes we have to make to live a healthier life are simply too overwhelming. Just a few little changes can have a significant impact on our health. Here are some little changes that can make a big difference.

Learn a word a day. Pick a word out of the paper or dictionary every day. Or have a word emailed to you daily (Dictionary.Reference.com/wordoftheday). Put it on an index card, and drill yourself. This type of cognitive calisthenic keeps your brain sharp.

The brain continues to regenerate nerve cells throughout life. This process, known as neurogenesis, helps older adults to improve memory and other cognitive functions as they age.

Example: A 2006 study published in *JAMA: The Journal of the American Medical Association* compared two groups of older adults. Those in one group were given training in memory, reasoning, and mental processing. After just ten sessions of sixty to seventy-five minutes each, the participants had immediate and long-lasting improvements, compared with those who didn't get the training.

If learning a word a day doesn't appeal to you, pick an activity that you enjoy and find mentally challenging.

Examples: Reading history books, learning chess, or memorizing poems. When the activity starts getting easier, move on to harder challenges.

People who do this can regain as much as two decades of memory power. In other words, someone who starts at age seventy could achieve the memory of the average fifty-year-old.

Make social connections. Go on a cruise. Take a bus tour. Go to a reunion. All of these are great ways to connect with people. Why bother? Because emotional connections add years to your life.

Example: Studies published in the last ten years show that people in happy marriages have less heart disease and live longer than those in unhappy relationships or who are divorced or widowed. Being happily married at age fifty is a better predictor of good health at age eighty than having low cholesterol.

The same benefits occur when people maintain any close relationship—with friends, children, or even pets. People who are emotionally bonded with others suffer less depression. They also tend to have less stress and lower levels of disease-causing stress hormones. And inviting new people into your life can help you cope with the dislocations—due to death, divorce, retirement, etc.—that occur over time.

Emotional connections don't just happen—people have to work at them. Think of the friendships that are important to you. If you are like most people, maybe a few of these relationships are active, but others have gone dormant for a variety of reasons. Ask yourself why some relationships have lapsed and what you can do to revive them. If you have lost touch with someone special, send an email or pick up the phone.

We all have "relationship opportunities" that we can take advantage of. Talk to the stranger next to you at a concert or a sports event. If you volunteer, invite one of your coworkers for coffee.

Take a nap. It's a myth that older people need less sleep than younger adults. They often do sleep less, but this is mainly because they're more likely to have physical issues, such as arthritis or the need to use the bathroom at night, that interfere with restful sleep.

People who don't get enough sleep often have declines in immune function, which can increase the risk for cancer as well as infections. They also have a higher risk for hypertension and possibly prediabetes.

A short nap—no more than twenty

to thirty minutes—can make up for a bad night's sleep. But beware of excessive napping. A long nap or more than one short nap per day can ruin a good night's sleep. Napping late in the day, say, after 3:00, also can interfere with a night's sleep.

Climb the stairs. It takes very little time but is a great way to get your heart and lungs working. Most exercise guidelines recommend at least twenty to thirty minutes of exercise most days of the week. That much exercise—or more—is clearly beneficial, but short amounts of activity can have a significant impact.

In a study of five thousand people over age seventy, all the participants had some physical limitations, but those who got even minimal exercise (defined as the equivalent of walking a mile at least once a week) were 55 percent less likely to develop more serious physical limitations (defined as severe joint pain or muscle weakness) that could compromise independence.

Watch the birds. For many people, contact with the natural world has a restorative effect. A few minutes observing birds at a feeder or watching a sunset can restore our equilibrium.

The natural world has a pace that reminds us that life does not have to be lived in a rush. Taking a few moments to de-stress is worth doing, because an estimated 60 percent of all doctor visits are for stress-related disorders.

Connecting with nature also can boost our performance. A study at Kansas State University gave ninety women a five-minute typing assignment. The researchers found that those who worked with a bouquet of flowers nearby outperformed those with no flowers.

See a funny movie. A good guffaw is more complicated than most people imagine. Laughter involves fifteen facial muscles, along with the lungs, larynx, and epiglottis. It even seems to protect against heart disease.

A study at Loma Linda University School of Medicine found that volunteers who watched a humorous video had reduced levels of the stress hormones cortisol and epinephrine. These and other stress-related chemicals have been linked with increased inflammation and an elevated risk for heart disease and many other conditions.

> The late Robert N. Butler, MD, president and chief executive officer of the International Longevity Center-USA. He also was professor of geriatrics at Brookdale Department of Geriatrics and Adult Development at Mount Sinai Medical Center in New York City. He wrote *The Longevity Prescription: The 8 Proven Keys to a Long, Healthy Life* and won the 1976 Pulitzer Prize for his book *Why Survive? Being Old in America.*

Seven Foods That Make You Smarter

We *all know that we* need to eat right to keep our minds sharp. But some foods really pack a punch when it comes to memory, learning, and other cognitive abilities. Here, one of America's top brain specialists reveals the seven super brain boosters.

1. **Coconut water.** It's high in potassium, a mineral that is critical for brain health. Potassium causes nerve cells to fire at the right speed. People who don't get enough potassium tend to have a slower rate of brain activity and may experience confusion and slower reaction times.

   Potassium is particularly important if you eat a lot of salt. The body needs to maintain a proper sodium-potassium balance. You should consume roughly twice as much potassium as sodium.

   A medium-sized banana has more potassium (about 450 mg) than coconut water (about 250 mg per eight-ounce serving), but bananas also are higher on the glycemic index, a measure of how quickly the food is converted into glucose. The brain works more efficiently when sugars

enter the bloodstream gradually rather than spiking. Coconut water achieves this more readily than bananas.

   Recommended: About one cup of coconut water daily. It has a light taste and is low in calories. If you want, you can add it to smoothies or mix it with milk and pour it over breakfast cereals.

2. **Blueberries.** Sure, blueberries are good for you, but you may not realize just how super rich in inflammation-fighting antioxidants they are. Their oxygen radical absorbance capacity (ORAC, a measure of a food's antioxidant ability) is 2,400, compared with 670 for cherries and 483 for pink grapefruit.

   Studies at Tufts University showed that animals that had blueberries added to their diet performed better on cognitive tests than those given a standard diet. They also had increased cell growth in the hippocampus, the part of the brain associated with memory.

   Recommended: One-half cup daily. If you don't like blueberries, opt for strawberries or acai berries (a purple, slightly tart berry available in many health-food stores). Or try Concord grape juice. Researchers from the University of Cincinnati tested Concord grape juice versus a placebo beverage on twenty-one volunteers, average age seventy-six, suffering from mild cognitive impairment. After sixteen weeks, those in the grape-juice group scored better on tests of memory than those drinking the placebo. Also, MRI testing showed greater activation in key parts of the brain, suggesting increased blood flow.

3. **Sardines.** Salmon often is touted as a healthy fish that is high in omega-3 fatty acids, fats that protect the brain as well as the heart and arteries. Sardines are even better. They also contain generous amounts of omega-3s, but because of their small size, they accumulate lower levels of mercury and other toxins than larger fish.

    The membranes that surround brain cells require omega-3s for the efficient transmission of signals. A Danish study that looked at the diets of more than five thousand adults found that those who ate the most fish were more likely to maintain their memory than those who ate the least. Other research has shown that people who eat fish as little as once a week can lower their risk for dementia.

    Recommended: At least two to three servings of fish a week. If you prefer salmon to sardines, be sure to buy wild salmon. It contains more omega-3s than farm-raised fish.

    Also helpful: Avocados. They're among the best plant sources of omega-3s.

4. **Walnuts.** All nuts are good for the brain (as long as they're not roasted in oil and covered with salt). Like fish, nuts are rich in omega-3 fatty acids. They're also loaded with vitamin E, which, in some studies, has been shown to slow the progression of Alzheimer's disease.

    In addition, nuts reduce LDL "bad" cholesterol (important for preventing stroke). Walnuts are particularly good because they have very high levels of omega-3s. Macadamia nuts are another good choice.

    Bonus: The Adventist Health Study, conducted by researchers at Loma Linda University, found that people who ate nuts five or more times a week were about half as likely to have a heart attack as those who rarely ate nuts.

    Recommended: About one-quarter cup daily. Nuts are higher in calories than most plant foods, so you don't want to eat too many.

5. **Sweet potatoes.** They are another low-glycemic food that causes only small fluctuations in blood sugar.

This can help you maintain energy and concentration throughout the day. We routinely advise patients to eat sweet potatoes because they satisfy a craving for carbohydrates, and they're also high in beta-carotene and other important antioxidants that keep the brain sharp.

One sweet potato (when you eat the skin) provides more fiber than a bowl of oatmeal. Dietary fiber lowers cholesterol and improves brain circulation.

Recommended: Eat sweet potatoes two to three times a week. If you don't like sweet potatoes, eat yellow squash or spaghetti squash.

6. **Green tea.** It contains the potent antioxidant epigallocatechin gallate that protects brain cells from free radicals caused by air pollution, toxins, a high-fat diet, etc. Green tea also contains compounds that increase levels of dopamine in the brain. Dopamine is a neurotransmitter that stimulates the brain's reward and pleasure centers and makes you more motivated to make positive lifestyle choices.

Bonus: A double-blind study that looked at patients with mild cognitive impairment found that an amino acid in green tea, L-theanine, improved concentration and energy and reduced anxiety.

Recommended: Two cups daily.

7. **Turmeric.** The bright yellow color indicates high levels of antioxidants. People who use this spice several times a week have significant reductions in C-reactive protein, a substance that indicates inflammation in the brain and/or other tissues. A study that looked at more than one thousand elderly people found that those who ate curry—which includes generous amounts of turmeric—regularly did better on mental-status evaluations than those who rarely or never ate it. All spices with bright, deep colors are high in neuroprotective antioxidants.

Examples: Both ginger and cinnamon appear to have brain-protective properties similar to those of turmeric. And sage improves memory.

Recommended: Add one-quarter teaspoon to one-half teaspoon of any of these spices to your food every day.

....

› Daniel G. Amen, MD, and Tana Amen, RN, BSN. Dr. Amen is medical director of Amen Clinics, Inc. He is a clinical neuroscientist, psychiatrist, brain-imaging specialist, and author of *Use Your Brain to Change Your Age.* His wife, Tana Amen, is a nutritional and fitness expert. AmenClinics.com.

....

Water Helps Your Brain

*D*rinking water is the easiest thing you can do for your brain, but most people don't drink anywhere near enough.

Fact: About 80 percent of the brain is comprised of water. If you don't drink enough—or if you drink a lot of dehydrating liquids, such as coffee or alcohol—you're going to struggle to think clearly, and you may have memory problems. That's because dehydration increases stress hormones, and stress hormones interfere with cognitive abilities.

Recommended: Drink half your weight in water ounces every day.

Example: If you weigh 150 pounds, you'll want to drink seventy-five ounces of water a day. Drink more during the warm months or if you exercise regularly and lose water in perspiration.

› Daniel G. Amen, MD, and Tana Amen, RN, BSN. Dr. Amen is medical director of Amen Clinics, Inc. He is a clinical neuroscientist, psychiatrist, brain-imaging specialist, and author of *Use Your Brain to Change Your Age*. His wife, Tana Amen, is a nutritional and fitness expert. AmenClinics.com.

Five Best Brain-Boosting Drinks

*S*ome of the easiest-to-prepare brain foods—meaning foods that can preserve and even improve your memory and other cognitive functions—are actually delicious drinks.

You probably already know about green tea, which is high in epigallocatechin-3-gallate (EGCG), a potent compound that appears to protect neurons from age-related damage. But the following five drinks are scientifically proven to help your brain too.

BEET JUICE

Beets are a nutritional powerhouse, and so is the juice. It increases levels of nitric oxide, a blood gas that improves blood flow. How does that help your brain? Your brain needs good blood flow to function optimally.

One study looked at brain scans of participants before and after they drank beet juice. The postbeverage scans showed an increase in circulation to the brain's white matter in the frontal lobes, a part of the brain that's often damaged in people with dementia.

You can buy ready-made beet juice at health-food stores, although it's much less expensive to make your own with fresh beets (include the root and greens, which are nutritious as well).

Beet juice has a naturally sweet taste, but you may want to add a little apple juice or another fruit juice, both for flavor and to make the mixture more pourable.

BERRY SMOOTHIES

Acai, a South American fruit that reduces inflammation, is ranked near the top of brain-healthy foods because it dilates blood vessels and increases blood flow. Its juice has a pleasant taste—something like a cross between raspberry and cocoa—but it's very expensive (typically about thirty dollars or more for a quart).

What I recommend: Blend a variety of everyday frozen berries that have been shown to boost brain health—raspberries, blueberries, and strawberries, for example—along with a little acai juice (and a bit of any other fruit juice, if you wish) to make an easy, delicious smoothie.

Why use frozen berries? They retain the nutritional benefit of fresh berries; they're easy to buy and last a long time in the freezer; they give your smoothie a nice texture, which you can vary by adding more or less juice; and they're less expensive than fresh berries if you buy large bags.

CARROT JUICE

The old adage is that carrots are good for the eyes (indeed they are), but we now know that carrot juice is absolutely great for the brain. Like other deeply colored vegetables (sweet potatoes, kale, red peppers, etc.), carrots are high in beta-carotene, an antioxidant that reduces inflammation, believed to be a factor in brain deterioration.

If you have tried carrot juice but didn't like the taste (it's surprisingly sweet), that's no problem. It is a very good base for multivegetable juices. Some choices that are good for covering up the carrot flavor include kale, spinach, and other dark greens.

COCOA

A Harvard/Brigham and Women's Hospital study found that adults who drank two daily cups of cocoa did better on memory tests than those who didn't drink it.

The flavanols (a class of antioxidants) in cocoa relax the endothelial linings of blood vessels and help reduce blood pressure. High blood pressure is a leading risk factor for dementia. The antioxidants in cocoa also reduce the cell-damaging effects of free radicals, and this may improve long-term brain health.

Important: Do not go overboard with

sugar though. Sugar is not good for your brain (and the jury is still out on artificial sweeteners).

Here's my advice: Buy a brand of unsweetened cocoa powder that is processed to remain high in flavanols. You don't have to buy an expensive specialty brand to get the brain-protecting effects. Most major brands of cocoa powder have respectable levels of cocoa flavanols. I advise against using milk chocolate or chocolate syrup. They typically have the least amount of flavanols and the most sugar.

At first, make your hot cocoa with your usual amount of sugar, then slowly cut back. You'll grow to appreciate the deep and pleasantly bitter true taste of the cocoa itself as less and less sugar stops masking it. As for using milk or water for your cocoa, that's your choice.

RED WINE

Everyone knows that red wine promotes cardiovascular health (easy does it). What you might not know is that red wine has been linked to a lower risk for dementia.

One reason is that people who drink moderate amounts of red wine—up to two glasses a day for men or one glass for women—have an increase in HDL "good" cholesterol. Research from Columbia University has found that people with the highest levels of HDL were less likely

to develop dementia than those with the lowest levels.

Want to supercharge the brain-boosting power of your red wine? Make delicious sangria! You'll get the wine's benefits and extra antioxidants and other nutrients from the fruit.

Sangria is typically made by steeping pieces of fresh fruit—lemon, orange, apple, and just about any other fruit you like—in a rich red wine such as merlot or cabernet sauvignon (or a Spanish red if you want to be *autentico*) and adding sugar and another liquor, such as brandy or rum.

My advice: Skip the sugar and extra liquor, but go ahead and add some orange juice to dilute the wine a bit and add some sweetness.

› David Grotto, RD, registered dietitian and founder and president of Nutrition Housecall, LLC, a Chicago-based nutrition consulting firm that provides nutrition communications, lecturing, and consulting services as well as personalized, at-home dietary services. He is an adviser to *Fitness* magazine and blogs for the Real Life Nutrition community featured on WebMD. He is author of *The Best Things You Can Eat: For Everything from Aches to Zzzz.* DavidGrotto.com.

Turmeric: The Spice That May Prevent Alzheimer's

*I*n India, *the smell of* turmeric, the bright yellow spice used in curries, fills almost every restaurant and home. Indians eat turmeric because they like it, but rapidly growing evidence indicates that the spice is giving them much more than flavor.

Thousands of years ago, Ayurvedic and traditional Chinese medicine recognized turmeric as a healing agent for everything from flatulence to liver disease. Modern research demonstrates that properties in this zesty spice may be useful for lowering rates of breast, prostate, lung, and colon cancers and also for treating breast cancer, inflammatory bowel disease, Crohn's disease, and possibly cystic fibrosis.

But especially exciting research concerns the relationship between turmeric and Alzheimer's disease. Nearly ten years ago, researchers in India became curious about the influence turmeric might have on rates of Alzheimer's. They looked to see how many people over age sixty-five in a town in India had signs of the disease, versus a similar group of people in a similar-sized Pennsylvania town, where most people eat little or no turmeric.

What they found: In India, just 4.7 per 1,000 person-years (a common measure of incidence rate) showed signs of

Alzheimer's, compared with a rate of 17.5 per 1,000 person-years in Pennsylvania. In fact, India has among the lowest rates of Alzheimer's disease in the world. Another study, from the National University of Singapore, involved 1,010 people over age sixty. Those who reported that they ate curry "often or very often" or even "occasionally" scored higher on mental performance tests than those who rarely or never consumed it.

WHAT IS TURMERIC?

Turmeric is a powder made from the root of the plant *Curcuma longa*, which grows in southern Asia. The part of the plant that is responsible for healing is the yellow pigment, called curcumin.

When it comes to health-giving properties, curcumin gives twice. It is a potent anti-inflammatory agent, without the potential side effects of anti-inflammatory drugs. These include damage to the lining of the stomach and intestines and a greater risk for kidney and liver problems, heart attack, and stroke. Next, curcumin is a powerful antioxidant. It tracks down and reduces free radicals, insidious molecules that otherwise would cause damage in the body. Both of these properties are important when it comes to preventing or slowing the progression of Alzheimer's disease.

In healthy people, immune cells attack and destroy beta-amyloid plaques—a buildup of proteins between neurons in the brain. But in people with Alzheimer's, this immune response is less efficient and allows plaques to form. Plaque triggers inflammation and free radicals, both of which cause cell damage in the brain. Curcumin slows this harmful process in a number of ways: it forms a powerful bond with the amyloid protein that prevents the protein from clumping; it may break down plaques as well, preliminary research demonstrates; and finally, as I noted before, curcumin reduces the oxidative damage and brain inflammation that are linked to Alzheimer's disease.

CHOLESTEROL BLASTER

Elevated cholesterol is thought to be involved in the development of Alzheimer's, and studies demonstrate that curcumin reduces cholesterol. In one study, healthy volunteers took 500 mg of curcumin supplements every day for one week.

Result: Reduced levels of total cholesterol and also lipid peroxides (markers of free radical damage to fats).

SPICE UP YOUR DIET

In the meantime, I encourage all my patients, especially those over age fifty, to consume one or two teaspoons a day of turmeric. There are many ways to incorporate this spice into your regular diet. You can sprinkle it into egg salad or over vegetables while sautéing, add it to soups or broths, put it on fish or meat, and use it to flavor rice or a creamy vegetable dip. And of course, turmeric adds zing to curries. If you want to make the most healthful curry dishes, it is important to purchase turmeric as a separate spice—lab tests show that many curry powders in this country contain almost no turmeric.

Anyone taking blood-thinning drugs should discuss using turmeric or curcumin supplements with a doctor, because curcumin is a natural blood thinner. Turmeric also can cause gallbladder contractions, so those with a history of gallstones or gallbladder problems should consult a doctor. There is no risk in mixing curcumin with pharmaceutical drugs for Alzheimer's disease.

....

› Mark A. Stengler, NMD, naturopathic doctor and founder of the Stengler Center for Integrative Medicine in Encinitas, California. He is author and coauthor of numerous books, including *The Natural Physician's Healing Therapies* and *Bottom Line's Prescription for Natural Cures*, and is the author of the newsletter *Health Revelations*. MarkStengler.com.

....

Shakespeare's Herb for Better Memory

It turns out that Shakespeare's Ophelia wasn't all that far off when she said that rosemary is for remembrance. According to a study in the *Journal of Neurochemistry*, rosemary contains the compound carnosic acid (CA), which helps protect the brain.

This savory herb also contains phytochemicals that can reduce the formation of cancer-causing compounds known as heterocyclic amines (HCAs). HCAs can form when the proteins in meat are heated to high temperatures.

Preliminary research also indicates that rosemary may enhance insulin sensitivity, improving the action and efficiency of insulin in the body, aiding in a healthy metabolism and slowing the aging process.

Suggested uses: I always add one teaspoon of dried rosemary or a tablespoon or two of fresh to a pound of ground meat before grilling burgers. Rosemary also is good in lamb and potato dishes, soups, and stews.

› Ann Kulze, MD, primary care physician and founder and CEO of Just Wellness, LLC. She is author of *Dr. Ann's 10-Step Diet: A Simple Plan for Permanent Weight Loss and Lifelong Vitality.* DrAnnsWellness.com.

Sharpen Your Memory with Music

Imagine yourself giving a toast, making a speech, or delivering a big presentation at work, only to forget midway through what you wanted to say. If the mere thought makes you cringe, you'll be intrigued by a book that reveals how to use music to improve your recall. The best part is that whatever type of music appeals most to you is what will be most effective, so you don't have to suffer through music you find boring or annoying.

Because music permeates all areas of the brain, it has a tremendous capacity to deposit any memories you attach to it in assorted locations. This embeds them deeper into your brain and makes it possible to retrieve them from multiple memory banks.

You may remember the buzz back in the 1990s when a small study reported that listening to a Mozart piano sonata produced a temporary improvement in spatial reasoning skills. These modest findings were blown out of proportion in the popular press, which disseminated the exaggerated idea that "Mozart makes you smart." Subsequent research has shown that music can indeed have cognitive benefits, but it's not about Mozart. In fact, my method works with any type of music—country, classical, reggae, rock, rap, pop, opera, or whatever—provided you enjoy it. The more you like the music, the more it activates brain networks and functions that amplify and sustain the effects you are working toward, such as increased concentration and alertness.

CHOOSING YOUR MUSIC

Getting back to memorizing that toast, speech, or presentation, here's what you do. First, create three lists of musical selections:

1. **Calming songs.** On this list, include songs that you know from experience make you feel relaxed and balanced because they are associated with pleasurable, peaceful events from your past. For instance, one song might remind you of a blissful solitary stroll in the woods, and another might bring back memories of a glorious sunset sail.

   Tip: Research shows that songs with a slower tempo of 100 beats per minute (BPM) or less tend to bring on relaxation and calm.

   Examples: "New York, New York" sung by Frank Sinatra or "American Pie" by Don McLean.

2. **Fast-paced, "activating" songs.** Activating songs are mentally energizing. They might remind you of a time

when you zoomed through a challenging task, celebrated an accomplishment, or won a race. Generally, songs that work well in this category have a tempo of 130 BPM or faster—for instance, "Beat It" by Michael Jackson or "Jailhouse Rock" sung by Elvis Presley. Such rhythms tend to boost motivation and endurance.

3. **Medium-paced, activating songs.** Here, select songs that recharge your batteries yet have a slightly slower tempo, typically 100 to 130 BPM. Examples include "Stayin' Alive" by the Bee Gees or the Beatles' "Lady Madonna." These types of songs help your brain lock in whatever you're trying to commit to memory.

   Choose half a dozen or more selections for each list.

   Reason: Feelings shift from day to day. For example, you might normally feel relaxed by a song you and your husband slow-danced to at your wedding, but if you two just had an argument, that song might upset you today. Assess your current emotions each time you use your playlists, selecting the songs that feel appropriate for the particular moment.

   Once you've selected your songs, create your three playlists on your cell phone or record the songs onto CDs or cassettes.

PUTTING YOUR PLAYLISTS TO WORK

Now you're ready to use your music to enhance your ability to memorize whatever it is that you want to commit to memory. Follow these steps in order:

+ **Listen to one or more calming songs to prepare your brain to be receptive to learning.** As you listen, recall as vividly as possible the relaxing, positive memories associated with each song. Continue listening until you reach that state of relaxed mental alertness.

+ **Play fast-paced activating songs to shift your brain into remembering mode.** Again, as you listen, visualize in detail the upbeat memories linked with that music. Continue listening until you feel energized and ready to approach your task.

+ **Turn the music off and focus on what you want to remember.** For instance, read your speech aloud from start to finish, moving around or gesturing as you read. The sound of your voice and your physical movements provide additional anchors that help cement the speech in your memory.

+ **When you finish rehearsing, listen to one or more midtempo activating songs.** This serves as a mental cooldown to further fix the material in your mind.

+ **For maximum effect, use this technique daily.** The amount of time you spend depends on the material you're trying to remember, but generally, the music portion of the activity takes about ten to fifteen minutes per session.

Key: Remember to have fun with this—it should not be a chore but instead a source of enjoyment.

› Galina Mindlin, MD, PhD, medical director at Alpha Healing Center in Jersey City. Dr. Mindlin is coauthor of *Your Playlist Can Change Your Life: 10 Proven Ways Your Favorite Music Can Revolutionize Your Health, Memory, Organization, Alertness, and More.* AlphaHealingCenter.com.

For a Better Memory, Just Make a Fist

Do you struggle to remember your mental shopping list or forget people's names right after you're introduced? Research reveals a "handy" trick that can help—and all you need to be able to do is make a fist.

Background: Previous research has shown that when a person clenches his or her right fist, the frontal lobe on the left side of the brain shows increased activity.

Similarly, clenching the left fist activates the right side of the brain.

There is a lot we don't know about how the brain works, but some experts believe that the left frontal lobe is important to encoding (creating) memories, while the right frontal lobe is associated with retrieving (recalling) memories.

So if hand clenching increases activity in different parts of the brain, would clenching the right hand activate the left side of the brain, where memories are encoded, and would clenching the left hand activate the right side of the brain, where memories are recalled?

To test the concept: Fifty-one right-handed people were recruited to participate in the study. (Left-handed people already have superior memories, according to research, so they weren't included in this study.) All the participants were shown a series of thirty-six random words, with each word being displayed for five seconds. Later, they were asked to write down as many of the words as they could.

Prior to reading and recalling the words, however, the participants were divided into five groups. In one group, each member was told to tightly squeeze a small rubber ball (to ensure a fist-clenching action) in his right hand for ninety seconds before seeing the words, then squeeze the ball in his left hand for

ninety seconds before trying to recall the words. A second group did the opposite (left before reading, right before recalling). Two other groups used their right hands both times or used their left hands both times. The fifth group didn't clench their fists at all—they simply cupped the ball gently in both hands.

Results: People who were able to recall the most words correctly were those who had squeezed with their right hands before trying to memorize the words and with their left hands before trying to recall the words. These people remembered almost 15 percent more words, on average, than the second-best performing group, which was the group that did not clench their fists at all. You don't consider a 15 percent improvement in memory such a big deal? Well, think of it in test-scoring terms—it could be the difference between an A and a C. Curiously, the three groups that did the "wrong" kind of clenching did even worse than the nonclenching group.

Give it a whirl: You don't need a ball. If you want to remember things better, simply clench your right hand for a minute and a half before you try to commit something to memory—a shopping list, a to-do list, a train schedule, or parking spot. Then clench your left hand for a minute and a half before you try to recall that list, train schedule, or parking spot number.

Just remember to clench right to learn, left to recall (ironically, the *R* and the *L* mnemonics are opposite). Careful—if you swap those, you could wind up recalling less than you would have if you had done no clenching at all.

....

› Ruth E. Propper, PhD, associate professor, department of psychology, and director, cerebral lateralization laboratory, Montclair State University, New Jersey. Her study was published in *PLOS One*.

....

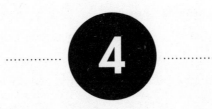

Cancer

Magical Food Combos That Fight Cancer

Researchers know that some foods can help prevent cancer. Now there is growing evidence that certain food combinations may offer more protection against cancer than any one specific food.

The following combinations of foods are especially beneficial. Eat them regularly—either at the same meal or separately throughout the week.

TOMATOES AND BROCCOLI

Results of an animal study presented at the American Institute for Cancer Research International Research Conference showed that rats with tumors that were given a diet of tomatoes and broccoli had significantly smaller tumors than animals fed only one of these foods.

The lycopene in tomatoes is an antioxidant. Antioxidants are crucial for preventing cancer because they help prevent unstable molecules, called free radicals, from damaging cell structures and DNA. Broccoli contains chemical compounds known as glucosinolates, which may be effective in flushing carcinogens from the body.

Also helpful: Combine broccoli or other cruciferous vegetables, such as brussels sprouts and cabbage, with foods that are high in selenium, such as shellfish and Brazil nuts. A study published by the UK's Institute of Food Research found that the combination of broccoli's glucosinolates and selenium has more powerful anticancer effects than either food eaten alone.

BRUSSELS SPROUTS AND BROCCOLI

These potent cancer-fighting vegetables also are rich in vitamin C and folate, as well as phytonutrients that deactivate carcinogens. When eaten in combination, brussels sprouts and broccoli may provide more protection than either one eaten alone.

Brussels sprouts have the phytonutrient crambene, which stimulates phase-2 enzymes, substances that help prevent carcinogens from damaging DNA. Broccoli is high in indole-3-carbinol, a phytonutrient that also stimulates phase-2 enzymes but in a different way.

ORANGES, APPLES, GRAPES, AND BLUEBERRIES

Each of these foods is very high in antioxidants. In a laboratory analysis, researchers measured the amount of antioxidants in each of these fruits individually. Then they combined them and took additional measurements.

Result: The mixture of fruits was more powerful against free radicals than any one fruit alone.

CURCUMIN AND QUERCETIN

Curcumin is a phytonutrient found in the spice turmeric. Quercetin is a phytonutrient that is abundant in yellow onions, especially in the outermost rings. According to a small study in *Clinical Gastroenterology and Hepatology*, people who consumed large amounts of these two phytonutrients had a reduction in the number of colon polyps, growths that may turn into cancer.

The study looked at a small number of people with familial adenomatous polyposis, a hereditary condition that increases the likelihood of developing polyps. The phytochemical combination reduced the number of polyps by 60 percent. It also caused some polyps to shrink.

The researchers used concentrated forms of curcumin and quercetin. You would have to eat two and a half tablespoons of turmeric daily to get a comparable amount. To get the necessary amount of quercetin, you would need to have about two-thirds of a cup of chopped onions daily.

Recommended: Eat a variety of herbs and spices to get the most phytonutrient protection. Even small amounts used frequently will impact your health over time. Among herbs, rosemary and oregano rank among the best phytonutrient sources. Ginger is another powerful spice.

TOMATOES AND FAT

The lycopene in tomatoes is particularly effective against prostate cancer, but only when it's consumed with a small amount of fat. Lycopene, like other members of the carotenoid chemical family, is a fat-soluble substance. The body can't absorb it efficiently in the absence of fat.

It takes only three to five grams of fat (about one teaspoon of oil) to improve the absorption of lycopene from tomatoes. For example, you could have a salad with an oil-based dressing. The type of fat doesn't matter for absorption of lycopene and other carotenoids, but you might as well choose a fat that promotes health. Olive oil and canola oil are good choices.

MORE VARIETY, LESS CANCER

In a study published in the *Journal of Nutrition*, researchers divided 106 women into two groups. All the women were asked to eat eight to ten servings of fruits and vegetables daily for two weeks. However, one of the groups (the high-diversity group) was told to include foods from eighteen different botanical groups, including onions and garlic from the allium family, legumes, cruciferous vegetables, etc. The other group (the low-diversity one) was asked to concentrate all its choices among only five major groups.

Results: Women in both groups showed a decrease in lipid peroxidation— important for reducing the risk of cancer and heart disease. However, only the women in the high-diversity group showed a decrease in DNA oxidation, one of the steps that initiates cancer development.

The ways that chemicals work in the body, known as metabolic pathways, have a rate-limiting effect. This means that beyond a certain point, eating more of a specific food won't provide additional protection. Eating a wide variety of foods brings more metabolic pathways into play, thus bypassing this limiting effect.

....
› Karen Collins, MSRD, registered dietitian and nutrition adviser to the American Institute for Cancer Research (www.aicr.org). A syndicated newspaper columnist and public speaker, she maintains a private nutrition counseling practice in Washington, DC.
....

Complementary Therapies Before, During, and After Cancer Treatment

A diagnosis of cancer presents a difficult battle not only with the disease, but also with the side effects of treatment. To destroy cancer, chemotherapy and radiation basically poison the body, which can bring on a host of miseries. Treatment may be essential, of course, but its side effects can be minimized with natural therapies that strengthen and support the body.

A study in *Breast Cancer Research and Treatment* found that 86 percent of newly diagnosed breast cancer patients incorporated complementary and alternative medicine (CAM) into their treatment. To discuss which CAM therapies are most effective, we contacted Roberta Lee, MD, vice chair of the department of integrative medicine at the Continuum Center for Health and Healing at Beth Israel Medical Center.

Helpful: Look at life after cancer diagnosis as three separate phases—pretreatment, active treatment, and posttreatment—because different CAM approaches work best during different phases.

Important: Before trying any complementary therapies, ask your oncologist which ones are safe and appropriate for you.

BEFORE TREATMENT BEGINS

The focus now is on ensuring that you will be as healthy and strong as possible, physically and emotionally, when treatment begins.

Work with a dietitian who specializes in oncology nutrition. Visit www. OncologyNutrition.org (a practice group of the American Dietetic Association) for a referral. Eat lots of fruits and vegetables, whole grains, and fish; low-fat organic chicken breast if desired; no red meat; and plenty of water.

Consider strengthening supplements. Folic acid and vitamin B-12 help with proper cellular division and tissue recovery. Vitamin D is good for immune regulation, bone health, and mood. Probiotics help optimize immune function and reduce production of cancer-promoting chemicals. Ask your doctor about dosages.

Learn relaxation techniques. An analysis published in *Psycho-Oncology* found that, when learned prior to rather than during cancer treatment, relaxation techniques were significantly more effective at reducing anxiety. Studies show that progressive muscle relaxation and guided imagery can improve cancer treatment–related nausea, pain, depression, and anxiety. Practice a relaxation technique for fifteen to twenty minutes daily.

Exercise appropriately. Gentle movements (simple stretches, leisurely walks) help you stay calm and centered. As for more vigorous workouts, listen to your body—this is not the time to exhaust yourself.

If you work outside the home, plan ahead. Calculating how long a leave you can afford and making arrangements now for your duties to be covered in your absence will give you less to worry about during treatment and ease your transition back to work afterward.

DURING TREATMENT

The primary consideration now is to avoid any CAM therapies that might lessen the effectiveness of your cancer treatment, so your doctor may instruct you to discontinue certain herbs and supplements. However, the following CAM approaches generally are safe during cancer treatment.

Try acupuncture to minimize hair loss. Chemotherapy drugs attack cells that are in the process of reproducing, but the drugs can't distinguish between rapidly dividing cancer cells and normal cells. In the body, hair follicle cells are among those that multiply fastest, which is why many patients experience hair loss. Acupuncture helps stimulate hair growth at a cellular level and reduces the stress that can exacerbate hair loss.

Bonus: Acupuncture can ease chemo-related dry mouth.

Drink herbal teas for digestive woes. Because digestive tract cells also multiply rapidly, chemo patients often develop gastrointestinal troubles. Drink chamomile tea, ginger tea, and/or slippery elm tea as needed to reduce nausea and help smooth over any ulcerations in the intestinal tract. To ease cramping, try fennel tea.

For nerve damage, consider glutamine. Ask your doctor about supplementing with this amino acid to relieve tingling, burning, or numbness from chemo-induced neuropathy.

Soothe skin with massage. Skin exposed to radiation treatment often becomes sensitive, warm, and red, as if sunburned. For relief, try gentle massage with oils, acupressure, reiki (an energy healing technique in which the practitioner's hands are placed on or above certain spots on the patient's body), or reflexology (massage of pressure points on the feet). To find a practitioner who works with cancer patients, check the Society for Oncology Massage (www.s4om.org).

Make each bite count. You probably won't feel like eating much during treatment, so focus on foods that are easy to digest and nutritionally dense, such as protein shakes, soups, and whole-grain breads. Avoid high-fat or acidic foods likely to aggravate nausea.

Do gentle yoga. An analysis published in *Cancer Control* linked yoga to improvements in sleep quality, mood, physical function, and overall quality of life.

Ease emotional distress. Teas made with valerian, chamomile, or hops flowers are calming, as are meditation and massage. Also consider hypnosis, which can help you process and release fear.

Referrals: American Society of Clinical Hypnosis (630-980-4740, www.asch.net, click on "Public" and "Member Referral Service").

AFTER TREATMENT

Once chemo and radiation are over, attention shifts to restoring your health.

Have your doctor assess your nutrient levels. Chemotherapy can deplete nutrients. Blood tests can reveal whether a special diet and/or supplementation is appropriate to support your recovery. Ask your doctor and/or dietitian about magnesium, vitamin D, folic acid, and vitamin B-12, which, in addition to the aforementioned benefits, helps with mood and memory. Also discuss milk thistle, which helps your liver get rid of lingering toxins from chemotherapy.

To encourage hair growth, continue with acupuncture. Folic acid and vitamin B-12 also can help with this, as can zinc and biotin. Ask your physician about dosages.

As strength returns, gradually increase physical activity. Tai chi, Pilates, and yoga are not too taxing.

Benefits for recovery: Exercise relieves stress, fortifies your body against further illness, and improves overall well-being, all of which make it easier to get on with your life.

> › Roberta Lee, MD, vice chair of the department of integrative medicine at the Continuum Center for

Health and Healing at Beth Israel Medical Center in New York City. She also is a member of the board of trustees for the American Botanical Council, the ethnomedical specialist for a multidisciplinary team studying the traditional use of medicinal plants in Micronesia, coeditor of *Integrative Medicine: Principles for Practice*, and author of *The SuperStress Solution*. SuperStressSolution.com.

Supplements That Fight Side Effects of Cancer Treatment

The American Cancer Society estimates that more than one million Americans will be diagnosed with some form of cancer each year. The vast majority will choose to be treated with conventional therapies, such as chemotherapy, radiation, surgery, or a combination. I often advise patients who are undergoing these treatments and want to reduce their risk of side effects and optimize their outcome. It is gratifying to help these people who are in physical and emotional turmoil. An example is Yolanda, a sixty-two-year-old woman who was diagnosed with a form of lymphoma (cancer of the lymphatic system). A program of nutrition and dietary supplements gave her more energy, promoted bowel regularity, and boosted her immunity. Her oncologist was quite surprised with how well she tolerated her chemo treatments and remarked on her quick recovery.

UNDERSTANDING CHEMOTHERAPY AND RADIATION

Chemotherapy involves the use of one or more drugs to destroy cancer cells. The treatments are given intravenously through a vein, orally, or by injection into a muscle. These medications not only attack cancer cells but also harm healthy cells. This causes a variety of side effects, depending on the chemotherapeutic agents being used and the individual's response. Examples of short-term side effects include loss of appetite, memory impairment, constipation, diarrhea, hair loss, nausea, mouth sores, easy bruising, fluid retention, and pain in muscles, bones, nerves, and joints. It also can result in bone marrow suppression, which can lower white and red blood cell counts, causing fatigue and increasing a patient's susceptibility to infection. Long-term side effects can include infertility, chronic fatigue, and continued bone marrow suppression. In addition, chemotherapy can result in secondary cancers. For example, a breast cancer patient might develop acute leukemia.

Radiation therapy also kills cancer cells and shrinks tumors. It is mainly used to attack localized cancers as opposed to cancer that has spread. Radiation treatments can be administered externally by a machine, internally through radioactive material placed in the body near cancer cells, or via radioactive substances that are injected and circulate throughout the body. Side effects can be similar to those caused by chemotherapy, but symptoms such as redness, swelling, and a burning sensation often are specific to the region being treated. Burned or reddened skin also can develop at the treated area.

SUPPLEMENTS THAT HELP

The following supplements are recommended for people undergoing chemotherapy or radiation therapy. You can take all of them at once, with the exception of the mushrooms listed, which are typically taken one at a time, as directed. Always consult with your oncologist before taking any supplement. Supplements work best in conjunction with a healthful diet and lifestyle.

Detoxification Therapies

Toxic by-products are formed by cancer treatments. You can help eliminate these toxins from your body by supporting liver and kidney detoxification.

Milk thistle is an excellent herb that supports liver detoxification and protects against liver and kidney cell damage.

Studies show that it actually helps liver cells regenerate. I recommend a 175- to 250-mg capsule of standardized extract (70 to 85 percent silymarin) taken three times daily. It can also be taken in liquid form. An excellent product is Thisilyn by Nature's Way, available in capsule form at most health-food stores, or you can contact the manufacturer to find a retailer.

Chlorella, spirulina, wheatgrass, and other "super greens" are nature's great detoxifiers. You can take chlorella by itself—it contains chlorophyll and a host of other detoxifying nutrients. A good choice, Sun Chlorella A, is available at health-food stores or from Sun Chlorella USA (800-829-2828, www.sunchlorellausa.com). Follow label instructions. Kyo-Green Energy by Kyolic is a good formula that contains a mixture of greens. It is available in tablet or powder form. To locate a store or mail-order company, contact Wakunaga (800-421-2998, www.kyolic.com).

Boosting Immunity

Because cancer treatments, especially chemotherapy, have a suppressive effect on the immune system—which makes you more vulnerable to infection—immunity boosting is critical. The following natural therapies can be used to support normal immune function without interfering with treatment.

Coriolus versicolor **mushroom extract** is routinely used in Japan and China to support the immune function of people with cancer. It also is helpful in reducing the side effects of chemotherapy and radiation.

A 1994 study published in *The Lancet* examined the effects of coriolus on patients undergoing chemotherapy after surgical removal of stomach cancer. The 262 patients were randomly assigned chemotherapy alone or with coriolus extract. The survival rate of the group using the combination was 73 percent after five years, while the chemotherapy-only group had a survival rate of 60 percent. Researchers concluded that coriolus had "a restorative effect in patients who had been immunosuppressed by both recent surgery and subsequent chemotherapy." The recommended dose is 2,000 to 3,000 mg daily.

The Mushroom Science brand of coriolus duplicates the formula that was used in the study and is available at health-food stores or by contacting Mushroom Science (888-283-6583, www.mushroom-science.com).

Maitake mushroom extract is one of the most-studied mushroom extracts. Since the 1980s, Hiroaki Nanba, MD, a professor of microbiology at Kobe Pharmaceutical University, Kobe, Japan, has been researching maitake extract.

It has been shown to enhance the activity of the body's natural killer cells against cancer cells. In addition, maitake extract has been shown to reduce the side effects of chemotherapy. A survey of 671 patients showed that the use of maitake during chemo reduced adverse effects such as hair loss, pain, and nausea. Maitake Gold 404 is the form recommended by Dr. Nanba. Typical dosage is 1 mg per two pounds of body weight daily. It is available in capsule or liquid form at health-food stores. For a store locator, consult Natural Factors (800-322-8704, www.naturalfactors.com). Or you can buy Cellular Essentials NK-5, which contains Maitake Gold 404, from Swanson Health Products (800-824-4491, www.swansonvitamins.com).

Note: Choose either coriolus or maitake based on the type of cancer being treated. Coriolus is a good general choice, especially for people with cancers of the throat, lungs, and digestive tract. Maitake is better studied for cancers of the breast, prostate, and liver.

Curcumin is the yellow pigment found in turmeric, a prime ingredient in curry. It has been shown to have anticancer properties and to enhance the effectiveness of some chemotherapy drugs, such as cisplatin. It has no known side effects. The recommended supplement dose is 400 mg twice daily. Many brands are available at health-food stores.

Whey protein, derived from cow's milk, supplies all the essential amino acids the body needs for repair, including the amino acid glutamine, which prevents mouth sores and strengthens immunity. Take 20 g of whey protein powder twice daily, in water or a shake.

Digestive Help

Digestive function often is compromised by cancer treatments, particularly chemotherapy and radiation for cancers in the abdominal area. These treatments destroy "friendly" bacteria, which are important for digestion, detoxification, and immune function.

Probiotics contain beneficial bacteria, such as *Lactobacillus acidophilus* and *Lactobacillus bifidus*. Take a daily dose of 10 billion or more active organisms.

Ginger helps relieve indigestion, nausea, bloating, and diarrhea. Sip ginger tea throughout the day, or take two 300 mg capsules twice daily.

Homeopathic nux vomica, derived from the poison nut tree, combats nausea and constipation. Take two pellets of a 30C potency twice daily until symptoms subside, usually within two to three days.

SKIN SOOTHER

Aloe vera gel can be applied topically to areas irritated or burned by radiation therapy. Choose a product that is 95 to 100 percent pure aloe vera. Aloe vera gel is available at health-food stores and pharmacies.

ANTIOXIDANTS MAY HELP

*Antioxidants—such as vitamins A, C, and E, selenium, and coenzyme Q10—*are controversial cancer treatments. Because conventional cancer treatments work in part by producing free radicals and because antioxidants attack free radicals, the fear is that antioxidant supplements may neutralize the effects of chemotherapy or radiation. This is an area that needs to be better studied.

In my opinion, low doses of antioxidants are more helpful than harmful. In their excellent book *How to Prevent and Treat Cancer with Natural Medicine,* naturopathic doctors Michael Murray, Tim Birdsall, Joseph Pizzorno, and Paul Reilly state, "Antioxidant supplementation…offers about as much protection to the cancer cell as a bulletproof jacket would during a nuclear attack. However, normal cells are able to utilize the antioxidant to protect against the toxicity and

damage caused by standard cancer treatments."* I recommend consulting your oncologist on this issue. Certainly, multivitamins and an antioxidant formula (containing CoQ10, mixed vitamin E, green tea extract, and vitamin C) should be used after the completion of treatment for optimal recovery.

> › Mark A. Stengler, NMD, naturopathic doctor and founder of the Stengler Center for Integrative Medicine in Encinitas, California. He is author and coauthor of numerous books, including *The Natural Physician's Healing Therapies* and *Bottom Line's Prescription for Natural Cures,* and is the author of the newsletter *Health Revelations.* MarkStengler.com.

Acupuncture Soothes the Side Effects of Chemotherapy

Nausea and vomiting are two of the most dreaded side effects of chemotherapy. Considering the cure can sometimes feel worse than the cancer it is meant to treat, some patients even elect to discontinue treatment. Although recent advances in antinausea and antivomiting medications have helped many cancer patients, the search for additional and

---

*   Michael Murray, *How to Prevent and Treat Cancer with Natural Medicine* (New York: Riverhead Books, 2002).

more natural methods of relief for these hard-to-tolerate side effects continues. Acupuncture has gotten a lot of attention for this purpose.

STUDY PINPOINTS WHAT WORKS

In a review of eleven studies of acupuncture and its effects on chemotherapy-induced nausea and/or vomiting, the Cochrane Collaboration, an international organization that evaluates medical research, found a mixed bag of results, depending upon which acupuncture method was used and for which side effect.

A REVIEW OF THE FINDINGS

Electroacupuncture (in which a small electrical current is passed through the needle) was effective in reducing vomiting during the first twenty-four hours after chemotherapy.

Traditional manual acupuncture using needles was not shown to be significantly effective for acute (within twenty-four hours of treatment) vomiting or nausea severity.

Based on similar principles but using (highly trained) fingertip pressure on acupuncture points, acupressure was looked at as well. This method showed no benefit for vomiting but did reduce acute nausea, although it was ineffective for delayed nausea (after twenty-four hours of treatment).

It is unclear why electroacupuncture reduced acute vomiting while needles-only acupuncture did not or why one method was successful with nausea while another was successful for vomiting. Of note is that all participants in all the trials reviewed were taking antivomiting drugs, so additional research is needed to determine whether acupuncture alone is effective or whether it should be considered an effective adjunct to medications.

EXPERT OPINION

Surprised by these findings, we asked acupuncturist Matthew D. Bauer, LAc, a former member of the board of directors for the California Acupuncture Association and a practicing acupuncturist with more than twenty years of experience, about these findings. He says it's hard to standardize this sort of study enough to make the findings meaningful. So much depends on the practitioner's skill in placing needles at just the right angle in just the right place. In looking at this many trials, you're obviously dealing with many practitioners at varying levels of skill and experience, which, of course affects outcomes.

Acupuncture can be helpful in many ways for people undergoing treatment for cancer. It's worth a try, since there's little risk and much potential benefit. It's important to work with a seasoned practitioner who has experience with oncology patients. And, of course, all cancer patients should check with their doctors before adding acupuncture or any other treatment to their cancer protocols.

> Matthew D. Bauer, LAc, practicing acupuncturist for more than twenty years. He is a regular contributing columnist to *Acupuncture Today* and formerly served on the executive committee of the California Acupuncture Association. His practice is in La Verne, California.

Acupuncture for Dry Mouth

Radiation for head or neck cancer can damage salivary glands, leading to severe dry mouth, loss of taste, difficulty swallowing, tooth decay, and oral infections. Relief from medication lasts only a few hours and can cause sweating and slow heart rate.

Study: Patients who had completed radiation got twice-weekly acupuncture treatments for four weeks and reported significant improvement in symptoms.

Referrals: American Association of Acupuncture and Oriental Medicine, 866-455-7999, www.aaaomonline.org.

> M. Kay Garcia, DrPH, associate professor and licensed acupuncturist in the department of palliative, rehabilitation, and integrative medicine at MD Anderson Cancer Center in Houston, and leader of a study of nineteen cancer patients. MDAnderson.org.

Six Essential Oils That Help Heal Cancer Patients

Like so many New Age practices and beliefs, aromatherapy has ancient roots. The use of essential oils to affect mood and well-being can be found far back in Egyptian, Greek, and Roman history. While scientific evidence about aromatherapy is scant, its long-standing role in spirituality and healing, along with anecdotal support of its benefits, gives essential oils an important role as a complementary alternative medicine therapy.

BOOSTING IMMUNE FUNCTION

Aromatherapy can be useful for people who are healthy, as well as those with chronic illnesses. Used properly, essential oils can indirectly help bolster immune function in cancer patients, strengthening their ability to fight back against the disease by helping to ease pain, depression, sleeplessness, and stress. The oils can also help relieve anxiety and improve memory, both frequent problems for people in cancer treatment.

ESSENTIALS ABOUT ESSENTIAL OILS

These essential oils have various scents such as floral, minty, citrus, and masculine. Use the ones you like best among the choices indicated for a specific treatment, since more than one oil may address the same problem. The limbic system, which is triggered by the sense of smell, is the emotional seat of the brain. It's the reason why people often respond strongly to certain scents, either positively or negatively. Lavender, for example, might bring back warm memories of a trip to Provence or sour thoughts about a dour relative who wore it as a fragrance.

DILUTION REQUIRED

All oils are highly concentrated distillations of plant parts, including the flowers, leaves, branches, and roots. Because they are so potent (hundreds of times more concentrated than the culinary fresh or dried herb or herbal teas, and therefore easy to overdose on), they should be used only under the supervision of a knowledgeable practitioner, such as a naturopathic physician, registered nurse, massage therapist, clinical herbalist, or aromatherapist. Some of the most popular oils include rosemary, eucalyptus, lavender, and chamomile. Essential oils can be inhaled (safest with a simple diffuser), enjoyed in your bath, or massaged onto your skin (but never directly in their undiluted form, because they can cause a rash or burning sensation).

Oils may come already diluted and will say so on the ingredient label, but you can also dilute a pure oil yourself, with advice from your practitioner. Add three drops of an essential oil to a half tablespoon of scentless organic vegetable oil (such as sunflower or safflower) or to an unscented body lotion. People with sensitive skin should do a skin test before topical use. How much to dilute an oil depends on the type of oil and your skin's sensitivity. Thyme, for example, is quite irritating to some people, so it should be used more sparingly and with caution, whereas lavender is nonirritating to nearly everyone. Citrus oils may cause sensitivity to sunlight, so avoid skin application if you are going to be in the sun. Because they're so pretty and fragrant yet highly toxic if ingested, they should be kept where children cannot reach them.

MENU OF OPTIONS

Here's a list of popular oils that address some common problems, as well as those common among people in treatment for cancer:

+ **Lavender.** Great as a general relaxant, it also treats migraines and relieves stress. It is excellent for insomnia resulting from cancer treatment.

+ **Rosemary.** Use for muscle pain, low blood pressure (do not use if you have high blood pressure), and cold feet and hands. Rosemary stimulates appetite.

+ **Spearmint.** Use to ease nausea and to help digestion. It can help ease gas and other treatment-related digestive problems.

+ **Eucalyptus or peppermint.** Rub on sore muscles. Eucalyptus may also help joints, including arthritic ones. Eucalyptus may increase the absorption of certain cancer drugs that are applied topically, so use caution and try a patch test first, avoiding application to the same area as the cancer drug.

+ **Pink grapefruit or juniper berry.** Use with massage to encourage lymphatic drainage of toxins and waste. Pink grapefruit is a favorite for cancer patients, as it helps energize them and raise their spirits. This and all citrus-type oils should be avoided during chemo and radiation and should not be used until you've spoken with your doctor.

+ **Lemongrass, tea tree, and orange.** Mix together into two cups of Epsom salts. Use five drops of each oil for a total of fifteen drops to make soothing bath salts (use one-half cup per bath).

WHAT TO LOOK FOR

Aromatherapy has become so popular that essential oils are now widely available, including in health-food stores and supermarkets. However, it is far better to purchase them from a shop with a staff knowledgeable in aromatherapy. Oils should come in dark blue or brown glass containers, which prevent light or heat damage. Avoid bottles with rubber droppers—the rubber breaks down and contaminates the oil. Finally, the label should feature both the common and the botanical name of the oil (for example, peppermint/*Mentha piperita*).

HOW TO TRY IT

If you would like to learn more about how to incorporate aromatherapy in your life, read *The Complete Book of Essential Oils & Aromatherapy*, by Valerie Ann Worwood, which is both thorough and easily understood. Again, as in the case with skin sensitivities, people with asthma or allergies need to avoid things that might trigger an attack—for example, chamomile, which is in the ragweed family.

People who want to try inhalation aromatherapy should use only two or three drops of essential oils in a basin of water or diffuser or on a napkin. And always consult with your doctor before using aromatherapy or any complementary therapy.

> Cherie Perez, RN, quality assurance specialist in the department of GU Medical Oncology at MD Anderson Cancer Center in Houston. MDAnderson.org.

Exercise to Fight Cancer

Exercise may help fight the nausea and muscle wasting that sometimes occur with cancer and its treatment. In fact, a meta-analysis of fifty-six studies found that aerobic exercise, including walking and cycling, both during and after treatment, reduced fatigue in cancer patients.

Interestingly, strength training was *not* found to reduce fatigue. But because strength training helps maintain muscle mass, some use of weights or resistance machines should be included for fifteen to twenty minutes twice a week, if possible.

Because cancer patients sometimes have trouble maintaining their body weight, it's especially important for those who are exercising to increase their calorie intake to compensate for what gets burned during their workouts.

Always talk to your doctor before starting a new exercise program. If you have a chronic illness, it may be useful to consult a physical therapist for advice on exercise dos and don'ts for your particular situation.

> John P. Porcari, PhD, program director of the Clinical Exercise Physiology (CEP) program at the University of Wisconsin–La Crosse. A past president of the American Association of Cardiovascular and Pulmonary Rehabilitation, he has authored or coauthored more than 350 abstracts and 150 papers on exercise physiology.

Reduce Swelling after Breast Cancer Surgery with Massage

A technique called lymphatic breast massage, also referred to as manual drainage therapy or manual lymph drainage can reduce swelling after breast cancer surgery, a common complication called lymphedema. It works by promoting the proper function of the lymphatic system, which has the job of breaking down cellular waste, removing impurities from tissues, and maintaining fluid balance. By encouraging the flow of lymph fluid through the lymph vessels, this special massage technique—which uses a press-and-release pumping action—helps prevent lymph fluid from accumulating in tissues near the surgical site. Lymphatic breast massage also can ease breast swelling and tenderness associated with premenstrual syndrome, and, along with antibiotics, it can help treat mastitis (a painful breast tissue infection).

For lymphatic breast massage treatment and instruction, consult a physical therapist. You can ask your doctor for a referral or find a practitioner through the National Lymphedema Network (www. LymphNet.org) or the Lymphology Association of North America (www. clt-lana.org/search/therapists/).

....

> Gwen White, PT, physical therapist and lymphedema specialist with Kaiser Permanente in Portland, Oregon, and coauthor of *Lymphedema: A Breast Cancer Patient's Guide to Prevention and Healing.*

....

Five Supplements That Help Prevent Cancer Recurrence

It's a top question on the minds of many cancer survivors: What will help keep the cancer from coming back? Unfortunately, conventional medicine often doesn't have much of an answer beyond, "Take care of yourself, and try not to worry." Naturopathic medicine, however, does have some specific recommendations for cancer survivors, and dietary supplements play a key role.

The reason: Dietary supplements are able to fit into the "nooks and crannies" of our biochemical pathways, creating specific changes that influence our bodies on a cellular level.

The five supplements listed below comprise a foundational supplement plan for just about every cancer survivor—and for just about every person who wants to reduce the odds of ever getting cancer in the first place. Each of the five supplements helps reduce cancer risk through five key pathways:

+ Boosting immune system function.
+ Reducing inflammation.
+ Improving insulin sensitivity.
+ Supporting digestion and detoxification.
+ Reducing stress-induced hormone imbalances.

Although dietary supplements are available over-the-counter, before you start taking them, it is essential to check with a naturopathic doctor (ideally one with additional board certification in naturopathic oncology) or an integrative medical doctor with specific expertise in integrative cancer care. These providers have training in nutritional biochemistry as it relates to cancer. They can confirm that the following supplements are appropriate for you and determine the dosages and the specific brands that will best suit your needs.

For my own postcancer patients, I typically prescribe all five of the following supplements, to be taken daily starting as soon as conventional treatment is completed. Some patients may be advised to start taking some of these supplements during their conventional treatment, but that should be done only under the guidance of an integrative health-care physician.

OMEGA-3 FATTY ACIDS

These essential fatty acids—found in supplements of fish oil, flaxseed oil, and algae-based oil—positively influence all five of the key pathways mentioned above. However, they are especially important for reducing chronic inflammation, which is one of the precursors of cancer. Think of inflammation as a burning ember in your body that can change your tissues in ways that favor the growth of abnormal cells. Omega-3s quench that fire.

Though omega-3s are helpful for survivors of all types of cancer, studies show particular benefits for patients who have battled colon, prostate, breast, or lung cancer. A typical daily dosage is 1,000 to 3,000 mg of omega-3 oil.

Caveat: Omega-3s can increase bleeding, so it's vital to get your doctor's OK before taking omega-3s if you are on blood-thinning medication or are anticipating any surgery.

PROBIOTICS

Beneficial bacteria in the intestinal tract help metabolize nutrients, bind waste products for removal in stool, and regulate immunity. When beneficial bacteria are depleted, the digestive tract is overrun with harmful bacteria, and a condition called dysbiosis develops. This negatively impacts all five of the body's key pathways, contributing to an increased risk for cancer recurrence. Studies have shown that supplementing with beneficial intestinal bacteria called probiotics can reduce the risk for infection after surgery and improve the immune system's response.

You can get some probiotics from eating yogurt and fermented foods such as fresh sauerkraut, miso, tempeh, and kefir. However, to fully support my patients' beneficial digestive bacteria, I typically prescribe a supplement that combines several types of probiotics at a dosage of at least one billion colony-forming units (CFU) daily.

Caution: Probiotics are not appropriate for people whose white blood cell count is below normal. Some evidence suggests that probiotics can increase the risk for blood infection in those individuals.

POLYPHENOLS

Healthful, colorful fruits and vegetables get their rainbow hues from the naturally occurring plant compounds called polyphenols (also referred to as flavonoids). Three polyphenols are particularly important in the fight against cancer:

+ **Green tea catechins,** which may lower the risk for cancers of the digestive tract, breast, bladder, lung, blood, and prostate.
+ **Curcumin,** the bright yellow flavonoid found in turmeric root, which appears to inhibit cancer formation in a variety of ways, helping protect against the majority of cancer types.
+ **Resveratrol,** which gives color to red grapes and some berries and has shown promise against breast, colorectal, and liver cancers by activating tumor suppressor genes and increasing the rate of apoptosis (normal programmed cell death).

Your doctor may prescribe a combination supplement that contains all three of these polyphenols, or you may take each one separately. Many high-quality brands also include other polyphenols. But watch out for what I call "window-dressing" supplements that list twenty to thirty different polyphenols, because the amount of each one will be so small that you might as well just eat a salad.

ANTIOXIDANTS

Look at metal that's been exposed to rain and sunlight—it starts to rust because it's being oxidized. That's essentially what happens to our bodies from exposure to free radicals, or oxidative toxins. Antioxidants guard against this by binding to oxidative toxins so they can be eliminated, and they also stimulate cell repair and normal apoptosis. Cancer treatment can deplete your antioxidant capacity, because cancer drugs themselves exert their cancer-killing effects via oxidation. A plant-based diet provides antioxidants, but cancer survivors should get additional support by taking the following:

+ **Glutathione,** the body's "master antioxidant," which is critical for the elimination of environmental toxins. A typical dosage is 250 to 500 mg daily.
+ **Coenzyme Q10 (CoQ10),** which is associated with decreased risk for breast and thyroid cancer, as well as melanoma. A typical daily dosage is 30 to 100 mg.

VITAMIN D

Numerous studies have shown the cancer-preventing potential of this vitamin, which promotes proper cell maturation and regulates inflammation, among other activities. Without adequate levels of vitamin D, it's hard for our bodies to maintain good blood sugar control or reduce inflammation.

Although it's often called the sunshine vitamin, many people in the northern hemisphere cannot get enough vitamin D just from being outdoors, especially during cooler seasons. Ask your doctor to measure your blood level of vitamin D—that information will help determine the right dosage for you.

Caution: If you take the heart medication digoxin, be especially sure to talk with your doctor before taking vitamin D, because the combination could lead to abnormal heart rhythms.

Important: Dietary supplements are called "supplements" for a reason—they are meant to supplement the diet, not to replace healthy eating. Over time, they provide targeted molecular support that gently but radically alters the terrain in your body, creating an environment that impedes cancer recurrence, so you can get back to the business of living your life.

> Lise N. Alschuler, ND, board-certified naturopathic oncologist, Naturopathic Specialists (www.listenandcare.com), Scottsdale, Arizona. A breast cancer survivor, she is coauthor of *The Definitive Guide to Thriving After Cancer: A Five-Step Integrative Plan to Reduce the Risk of Recurrence and Build Lifelong Health* and cocreator of www.

FiveToThrivePlan.com, a website about integrative cancer care. Dr. Alschuler also is a past president of the American Association of Naturopathic Physicians, a founding board member of the Oncology Association of Naturopathic Physicians, and former medical director of the Bastyr University Natural Health Clinic. DrLise.net.

Green Tea Combats Skin Cancer

Polyphenols, *a type of antioxidant* found in green tea, protect skin from the sun's damaging ultraviolet radiation and help prevent the formation of skin tumors.

Best: Drink five to six cups of green tea a day—the fresher, the better. Fresh green tea leaves have a light yellow or green color. A brownish hue indicates that the tea has undergone oxidation, which destroys antioxidants. Tea bags and loose leaves are better than instant and bottled teas.

> Santosh Katiyar, PhD, professor of dermatology, University of Alabama, Birmingham, and leader of a study of green tea and skin tumor development in mice, published in the *Journal of Nutritional Biochemistry.*

Three Foods That Fight Prostate Cancer

Many foods that we perceive as nutritional lightweights actually are just as healthy as—and, for many people, more enjoyable than—the so-called superfoods, such as broccoli and spinach.

Bonus: These foods can reduce risk for prostate and other cancers.

WATERMELON

Watermelon contains more water than most fruits. The high liquid content, along with the sugars and fiber, make watermelon the perfect snack before workouts. But it's more than a snack food.

Fact: Watermelon contains 40 percent more lycopene than fresh (uncooked) tomatoes. Lycopene is a potent antioxidant that strengthens the immune system and may lower the risk for breast and prostate cancers.

Helpful: When you take a watermelon home, keep it on the counter even after cutting it open. Room-temperature watermelon continues to produce antioxidants for about two weeks. It will contain up to 40 percent more lycopene and up to 139 percent more beta-carotene than cold watermelon.

SAUERKRAUT

Fresh, minimally processed vegetables are presumed to be the healthiest. Not always.

Fact: One study found that women who ate at least four weekly servings of fermented cabbage, better known as sauerkraut, were 72 percent less likely to develop breast cancer than those who ate less.

Eating fermented cabbage changes gut metabolism and may help to protect the intestinal tract. Isothiocyanates, which are naturally present in all the cruciferous vegetables, appear to inhibit the proliferation of cancer cells and accelerate the death of these cells.

Korean kimchi, a spicy form of fermented cabbage, appears to have similar effects.

ONIONS

Most people use onions mainly as a seasoning ingredient in soups and stews and on burgers and salads. For good health, use a lot of them.

Fact: Onions are high in vitamin C, fiber, vitamin B-6, and folate. They also are rich in quercetin, a flavonoid with powerful anticancer effects, and allyl sulfides, the same protective compounds that are present in garlic.

Studies have found that people who eat between fourteen and twenty-two servings of onions a week can reduce their risk for oral cancer by 84 percent. They have a 56 percent reduced risk for colon cancer, a 25 percent reduced risk for breast cancer, and a 71 percent reduced risk for prostate cancer.

Red onions have the most quercetin. However, pink shallots contain the richest mix of chemical compounds and more antioxidants than other onions.

....

› John La Puma, MD, board-certified specialist in internal medicine and trained chef with a private nutritional medical practice in Santa Barbara, California. He is the author of *ChefMD's Big Book of Culinary Medicine* and *Refuel: A 24-Day Eating Plan to Shed Fat, Boost Testosterone, and Pump Up Strength and Stamina.* DrJohnLaPuma.com.

....

Allspice May Combat Prostate Cancer

Allspice is best known as the flavor powerhouse in pumpkin pie, but researchers have discovered that it also may have the power to shrink prostate cancers.

ALL-POWERFUL ALLSPICE

To understand why allspice might protect the prostate, you must start with the fact that most forms of prostate cancer thrive on androgens (male hormones, such as testosterone). That's why doctors treat prostate cancer with powerful drugs that either stop the production of androgens or block them from being used by the body. But the medications' side effects—severe hot flashes, decreased libido, and increased risk for osteoporosis, diabetes, and coronary artery disease—can be so difficult to tolerate that many men don't remain on the drugs long enough to reap the full benefits.

The study shows that allspice can block androgen receptor molecules that are vital to the growth and spread of prostate cancer, at least in mice. Though preliminary, the research is so encouraging that all men should take note.

Part of the study took place in test tubes. The researchers prepared an allspice extract from the crushed berries and distilled water, then mixed the extract with human prostate cancer cells. Using several different methods, they determined that the allspice extract slowed the growth of prostate cancer cells by half in just forty-eight hours, blocked the progression of the cancer cell cycle, and induced cancer cell death.

Next, the researchers tested allspice in animals. First, mice were injected with human prostate cancer cells to make tumors grow. Then, one group of mice was given allspice extract to drink every day, and a second group was injected with the extract three times per week. Other mice, serving as controls, were not given any of the extract.

Six weeks later: Compared with prostate tumors in the control mice, tumors in the mice that were injected with the allspice extract were 58 percent smaller. Drinking the extract seemed even more beneficial, with tumors in that group of mice being 62 percent smaller than those in the control group. There were no apparent adverse effects from the allspice.

After some trial-and-error testing, the researchers determined that the compound in allspice responsible for the slower tumor growth was ericifolin. Rather than affecting androgens themselves (as antiandrogen drugs do), ericifolin prevents the androgen receptor from being synthesized in the cancer cells. Because it gets to the root cause of the trouble, the researchers said, this mechanism potentially makes ericifolin particularly useful in fighting a deadlier, advanced form of the disease (called hormone refractory prostate cancer) in which the receptor works autonomously, without the androgens.

Bonus: Ericifolin also has been shown to have antioxidant, antibacterial, and pain-relieving effects.

Obviously, since this study was performed in test tubes and mice, it is way too early to suggest that allspice can prevent or cure prostate cancer in men, but the researchers did call it "potentially a unique dietary chemopreventive agent" in the fight against the number-two cause of cancer deaths among men.

Allspice generally is considered safe when consumed in amounts typically used to season foods, but not enough is known about its safety in medicinal amounts, and there is some concern that it may slow down blood clotting or interfere with medications that reduce blood clotting. Clearly, future studies are needed to test allspice's safety and efficacy in reducing prostate tumor size and/or preventing prostate cancer and to determine the most appropriate medicinal dosage. In the meantime, it's worth talking to your doctor about the possibility of adding more allspice to your diet.

Adding more allspice to your diet: To receive a dose of allspice equivalent to that which the mice received, a man would have to consume about two teaspoons of powdered allspice per day. You're probably not going to eat enough pumpkin pie daily to get that much allspice (though you might enjoy trying), but there are lots of other ways to get allspice into your diet. For instance, allspice is frequently used in Asian, Middle Eastern, and Caribbean cuisine, especially Jamaican jerk seasoning and spiced teas. You can use allspice by sprinkling it on green beans, carrots, sweet potatoes, or scrambled eggs; using it to season braised or barbecued meats after cooking; or adding it to ground coffee before brewing. Experiment to see what tastes good to you.

....

> Bal Lokeshwar, PhD, professor of medicine at Augusta University and research career scientist, CN VA Medical Center, Augusta, Georgia. His study was published in *Carcinogenesis*.

....

5

Cardiovascular Health: Preventing Heart Disease and Stroke

Dr. Kahn's Seven-Step Heart-Healthy Regimen

When it comes to keeping your heart healthy, most cardiologists make general recommendations—get regular exercise, eat a balanced diet, and don't smoke. But wouldn't it be nice to know *exactly* what a doctor who specializes in heart disease does to keep his/her own heart healthy?

Here are the personal secrets from cardiologist Joel K. Kahn, MD, that he does to ensure that his heart stays strong. They can help you too—whether you want to prevent heart disease or already have it.

Secret #1: **Drink room-temperature water.** You may not expect an MD who was trained in mainstream Western medicine to practice principles of the ancient Indian wellness philosophy of Ayurveda. But many of these lifestyle habits do carry important health benefits.

For example, according to Ayurvedic medicine, room-temperature water spiked with lemon or lime is good for digestive and cardiovascular health. Because the esophagus is located close to the heart, swigging ice water can cause changes in the heart's normal rhythm in some people.

What I do: If I don't have time to prepare a glass of lemon water, I always drink a big glass of room-temperature water before I get out of bed.

Here's why: We all get dehydrated during the night. Drinking water pumps up the liquid volume of blood, which reduces the risk for blood clots.

I also drink a lot of liquids throughout the day. How much do you need? Divide your weight in half. That's the number of ounces you should drink. A person who weighs, say, 150 pounds, should drink at least seventy-five ounces (about nine cups) of fluids, including water, every day.

Secret #2: **Make time for prayer and reflection.** There's a strong link between stress and cardiovascular disease. One landmark study found that heart patients who experienced high levels of stress—along with depression, which is often fueled by stress—were nearly 50 percent more likely to have a heart attack or die than those with more emotional balance.

What I do: I like meditation and prayer. My routine includes counting my blessings before I get out of bed in the morning and saying a few prayers. I also appreciate the simple miracles of sunrises, hugs, and special friends and family.

Other stress reducers: Listening to music and taking long walks.

Secret #3: **Do fast workouts.** Exercise is crucial to keeping your heart strong, but it's sometimes hard to fit this into a busy schedule. I exercise before breakfast (see below) and eat within thirty minutes after finishing my workout.

What I do: My usual morning workout (six days a week) includes twenty minutes of cardio—on a treadmill, recumbent bike, or rowing machine—followed by about ten minutes of weight lifting.

When I don't have time for a half-hour session, I may do just twelve minutes of high-intensity interval training (HIIT).

This typically includes a two-minute warm-up of fast walking on the treadmill, followed by eight minutes of intervals—running all-out for thirty seconds, followed by thirty seconds of walking. I follow this with a two-minute cooldown of slow walking.

HIIT increases cardiorespiratory fitness, builds muscle, and reduces inflammation and insulin resistance (which promotes diabetes).

Important: HIIT is strenuous, so check with your doctor before trying it.

Secret #4: **Have a healthy breakfast.** Millions of Americans skip this important meal. That's a problem, because skipping meals has been linked to obesity, high blood pressure, insulin resistance, and elevated cholesterol.

Specifically, men who skipped breakfast were found to be 27 percent more likely to develop coronary heart disease than those who ate a healthy breakfast, according to a study in the journal *Circulation*.

What I do: To save time, I get my breakfast ready the night before. I fill a glass container with oatmeal and almond milk and let it soak in the refrigerator overnight. In the morning, all the liquid is absorbed, and it's soft and ready to eat. I stir it well and top with a few tablespoons of chopped dried figs, unsweetened coconut flakes, or sliced berries.

For variety: I have a "super smoothie" with antioxidant-rich ingredients, such as kale, spinach, frozen blueberries, flax, etc., and organic soy or almond milk.

Secret #5: **Use heart-healthy supplements.** Dietary supplements aren't the best way to *treat* cardiovascular disease (although they can help in some cases). Supplements are better for *preventing* heart problems.

Note: Check with your doctor before taking any of those listed here—they can interact with some medications.

+ **Magnesium glycinate,** which is easily absorbed. People who get enough magnesium (millions of Americans are deficient) are less likely to have a heart attack or stroke than those who don't get adequate amounts of the mineral.
+ **Vitamin D.** The evidence isn't yet definitive but suggests that vitamin D may improve heart health.
+ **Coenzyme Q10 (CoQ10).** It is a vitamin-like substance that lowers blood pressure and can improve symptoms of heart failure.

Secret #6: **Eat a plant-based diet.** It's been linked to a reduced risk for diabetes and certain types of cancer as well as heart disease.

What I do: I've been a vegetarian for nearly forty years. I eat foods with a variety of colors, such as berries and peppers. For me, a huge salad can be a meal! I also enjoy a handful of raw nuts every day.

Secret #7: **Get enough sleep.** People who sleep at least seven hours a night are 43 percent less likely to have a fatal heart attack than those who get by on six hours or less.

What I do: I usually get up at 6:00 a.m., so I make sure that I'm in bed by 11:00 p.m. I also *plan* a good night's sleep. For example, I stop drinking caffeinated beverages at least ten hours before bedtime (this means that I have nothing with caffeine after 1:00 p.m.) and usually stop eating three hours before bed—active digestion makes it harder to fall asleep and increases nighttime awakenings.

Another trick: I have a sleep-promoting bulb in the reading lamp on my nightstand. Typical lightbulbs emit high levels of short-wavelength blue light, which suppresses the brain's production of the sleep-inducing hormone melatonin. You can buy bulbs (such as the Good Night LED or the GE Align PM) that emit small amounts of blue light.

> Joel K. Kahn, MD, clinical professor of medicine at Wayne State University School of Medicine in Detroit and founder of the Kahn Center for Cardiac Longevity in Bloomfield Hills, Michigan. He is

also an associate professor at Oakland University William Beaumont School of Medicine in Rochester, Michigan, a founding member of the International Society of Integrative, Metabolic and Functional Cardiovascular Medicine, and the author of *The Whole Heart Solution*. DrJoelKahn.com.

Six Secrets to Holistic Heart Care

These *fun, easy changes really* do help.

You don't smoke, your cholesterol levels look good, and your blood pressure is under control.

This means that you're off the hook when it comes to having a heart attack or developing heart disease, right? Maybe not.

Surprising statistic: About 20 percent of people with heart disease do *not* have any of the classic risk factors, such as those described above.

The missing link: While most conventional medical doctors prescribe medications and other treatments to help patients control the big risk factors for heart disease, holistic cardiologists also suggest small lifestyle changes that over time make a significant difference in heart disease

risk.* Here are some secrets for preventing heart disease.

Secret #1: **Stand up!** You may not think of standing as a form of exercise. However, it's more effective than most people realize.

Think about what you're doing when you're *not* standing. Unless you're asleep, you're probably sitting. While sitting, your body's metabolism slows, your insulin becomes less effective, and you're likely to experience a gradual drop in HDL "good" cholesterol.

A study that tracked the long-term health of more than 123,000 Americans found that those who sat for six hours or more a day had an overall death rate that was higher—18 percent higher for men and 37 percent for women—than those who sat for less than three hours.

What's so great about standing? When you're on your feet, you move more. You pace, fidget, move your arms, and walk from room to room. This type of activity improves metabolism and can easily burn hundreds of extra calories a day. Standing also increases your insulin sensitivity to help prevent diabetes. So stand up and move around when talking on the phone, checking email, and watching television.

* To find a holistic cardiologist, go to the website of the American Board of Integrative Holistic Medicine and search the database of certified integrative physicians.

Secret #2: **Count your breaths.** Slow, deep breathing is an effective way to help prevent high blood pressure—one of the leading causes of heart disease. For people who already have high blood pressure, doing this technique a few times a day has been shown to lower blood pressure by five to ten points within five minutes. And the pressure may stay lower for up to twenty-four hours.

During a breathing exercise, you want to slow your breathing down from the usual twelve to sixteen breaths a minute that most people take to about three breaths. I use the "4-7-8 sequence" whenever I feel stressed.

What to do: Inhale through your nose for four seconds, hold the breath in for seven seconds, then exhale through the mouth for eight seconds.

Also helpful: A HeartMath software package, which you can load on your computer or smartphone, includes breathing exercises to help lower your heart rate and levels of stress hormones.

Secret #3: **Practice "loving kindness."** This is an easy form of meditation that reduces stress, thus allowing you to keep your heart rate and blood pressure at healthy levels.

Research has shown that people who meditate regularly are 48 percent less likely to have a heart attack or stroke than those who don't meditate. "Loving kindness" meditation is particularly effective at promoting relaxation. It lowers levels of the stress hormones adrenaline and cortisol while raising levels of the healing hormone oxytocin.

What to do: Sit quietly, with your eyes closed. For a few minutes, focus on just your breathing. Then imagine one person in your life whom you find exceptionally easy to love. Imagine this person in front of you. Fill your heart with a warm, loving feeling, think about how you both want to be happy and avoid suffering, and imagine that a feeling of peace travels from your heart to that person's heart in the form of white light. Dwell on the image for a few minutes. This meditation will also help you practice small acts of kindness in your daily life—for example, giving a hand to someone who needs help crossing the street.

Secret #4: **Don't neglect sex.** Men who have sex at least two times a week have a 50 percent lower risk for a heart attack than those who abstain. Similar research hasn't been done on women, but it's likely that they get a comparable benefit.

Why does sex help keep your heart healthy? It probably has more to do with intimacy than the physical activity itself. Couples who continue to have sex tend to be the ones with more intimacy in their marriages. Happy people who bond with others have fewer heart attacks—and recover more quickly if they've had one—than those without close relationships.

Secret #5: **Be happy!** People who are happy and who feel a sense of purpose and connection with others tend to have lower blood pressure and live longer than those who are isolated. Research shows that two keys to happiness are to help others be happy—for example, by being a volunteer—and to reach out to friends and neighbors. Actually, any *shared* activity, such as going to church or doing group hobbies, can increase survival among heart patients by about 50 percent.

Secret #6: **Try Waon (pronounced Wa-own) therapy.** With this Japanese form of "warmth therapy," you sit in an infrared (dry) sauna for fifteen minutes, then retreat to a resting area for half an hour, where you wrap yourself in towels and drink plenty of water. Studies show that vascular function improves after such therapy due to the extra release of nitric oxide, the master molecule in blood vessels that helps them relax.

Some health clubs offer Waon treatments, but the dry saunas at many gyms should offer similar benefits. I do *not* recommend steam rooms—moist heat places extra demands on the heart and can be dangerous for some people.

> Joel K. Kahn, MD, clinical professor of medicine at Wayne State University School of Medicine in Detroit and founder of the Kahn Center for Cardiac Longevity in Bloomfield Hills, Michigan. He is also an associate professor at Oakland University William Beaumont School of Medicine in Rochester, Michigan, a founding member of the International Society of Integrative, Metabolic and Functional Cardiovascular Medicine, and the author of *The Whole Heart Solution*. DrJoelKahn.com.

Oregano Fights Heart Disease and Stroke

Two major components of oregano—thymol and carvacrol—have been proven to have healing powers, protecting against heart disease and stroke.

In a study published in the *Journal of International Medical Research*, people with high LDL "bad" cholesterol were divided into two groups. One group ingested oregano extract with every meal, and one group didn't. Three months later, the oregano group had greater decreases in LDL, lower levels of C-reactive protein (a biomarker of artery-damaging inflammation), and greater increases in arterial blood flow.

In other studies, researchers found that oregano is more powerful than any other spice in stopping the oxidation of LDL—the breakdown of cholesterol by unstable molecules called free radicals that drives the formation of arterial plaque. Oregano also stops the activation of cytokines, components of the immune system that attack oxidized cholesterol, sparking the inflammation that worsens heart disease.

How to use: You can buy oregano fresh or dried. I recommend using the dried form because it concentrates the therapeutic compounds. It often is used in salad dressings, marinades, chili, and in Italian and Greek dishes. For optimum benefits, try to use at least one teaspoon of dried oregano daily.

> Bill Gottlieb, CHC, a certified health coach and health journalist. He is the author and coauthor of numerous books, including *Bottom Line's Speed Healing.* BillGottliebHealth.com.

Six Tasty Foods That Protect Your Heart

J ust about everyone knows that a Mediterranean-style diet can help prevent heart disease and stroke. Even if you've already had a heart attack, this style of eating—emphasizing such foods as fish and vegetables—can reduce the risk for a second heart attack by up to 70 percent.

Problem: About 80 percent of patients with cardiovascular disease quit following dietary advice within one year after their initial diagnosis. That's often because they want more choices but aren't sure which foods have been proven to work.

Solution: Whether you already have heart disease or want to prevent it, you can liven up your diet by trying foods that usually don't get much attention for their heart-protective benefits.

Popcorn. It's more than just a snack. It's a whole grain that's high in cholesterol-lowering fiber. Surprisingly, popcorn contains more fiber, per ounce, than whole-wheat bread or brown rice.

Scientific evidence: Data from the 1999–2002 National Health and Nutrition Examination Survey found that people who eat popcorn daily get 22 percent more fiber than those who don't eat it.

Important: Eat "natural" popcorn, preferably air-popped or microwaved in a brown paper bag, without added oil. The commercially prepared popcorn packets generally contain too much salt, butter, and other additives. Three cups of popped popcorn, which contain almost 6 g of fiber and ninety calories, is considered a serving of whole grains. Studies have shown that at least three servings of whole grains a day (other choices include oatmeal and brown rice) may help reduce the risk for heart disease, high cholesterol, and obesity.

Chia seeds. You're probably familiar with Chia pets—those terra-cotta figures that sprout thick layers of grassy "fur." The same seeds, native to Mexico and Guatemala, are increasingly available in health-food stores. I consider them a superfood because they have a nutrient profile that rivals heart-healthy flaxseed.

In fact, chia seeds contain *more* omega-3 fatty acids than flaxseed. Omega-3s increase the body's production of anti-inflammatory eicosanoids, hormonelike substances that help prevent adhesion molecules from causing plaque buildup and increasing atherosclerosis.

Scientific evidence: A study published in the *Journal of the American College of Cardiology*, which looked at nearly forty thousand participants, found that an omega-3-rich diet can prevent and even reverse existing cardiovascular disease.

Other benefits: One ounce of chia seeds has 10 g of fiber, 5 g of alpha-linolenic acid, and 18 percent of the recommended dietary allowance for calcium for adults ages nineteen to fifty.

Chia seeds look and taste something like poppy seeds. You can add them to baked goods, such as muffins, or sprinkle them on salads and oatmeal or other cereals.

Figs. They're extraordinarily rich in antioxidants with an oxygen radical absorbance capacity (ORAC) score of 3,383. Scientists use this ORAC scale to determine the antioxidant capacity of various foods. An orange, by comparison, scores only about 1,819. Fresh figs are among the best sources of beta-carotene and other heart-healthy carotenoids.

Scientific evidence: In a study published in the *Journal of the American College of Nutrition*, two groups of participants were "challenged" with sugary soft drinks, which are known to increase arterial oxidation. Oxidation in the arteries triggers atherosclerosis, a main risk factor for heart disease and stroke. Those who were given only soda had a drop in healthful antioxidant activity in the blood; those who were given figs as well as soda had an *increase* in blood antioxidant levels.

Bonus: Ten dried figs contain 140 mg of calcium. Other compounds in figs, such as quercetin, reduce inflammation and dilate the arteries. Perhaps for these reasons, people who eat figs regularly have much less heart disease than those who don't eat them, according to studies. Most dried figs contain added sulfites, so it's best to buy organic, sulfite-free dried figs.

Soy protein. Tofu, soy milk, and other soy foods are complete proteins—that is, they supply all the essential amino acids that your body needs but without the cholesterol and large amount of saturated fat found in meat.

Scientific evidence: People who replace dairy or meat protein with soy will have an average drop in LDL "bad" cholesterol of 2 to 7 percent, according to research from the American Heart Association. Every 1 percent drop in LDL lowers heart disease risk about 2 percent.

A one-half cup serving of tofu provides 10 g of protein. An eight-ounce glass of soy milk gives about 7 g. Edamame (steamed or boiled green soybeans) has about 9 g per half cup. Avoid processed soy products, such as hydrogenated soybean oil (a trans fat), soy isoflavone powders, and soy products with excess added sodium.

Lentils. I call these "longevity legumes," because studies have shown that they can literally extend your life.

Best choices: Brown or black lentils.

Scientific evidence: In one study, published in the *Asia Pacific Journal of Clinical Nutrition*, the eating habits of five groups of older adults were compared. For every 20 g (a little less than three-fourths of an ounce) increase in the daily intake of lentils and/or other legumes, there was an 8 percent reduction in the risk of dying within seven years.

Lentils contain large amounts of fiber, plant protein, and antioxidants along with folate, iron, and magnesium, all of which are important for cardiovascular health.

Similarly, a Harvard study found that people who ate one serving of cooked beans (one-third cup) a day were 38 percent less likely to have a heart attack than those who ate beans less than once a month.

Caution: Beans have been shown to cause gout flare-ups in some people.

Important: Lentils cook much faster than other beans. They don't need presoaking. When simmered in water, they're ready in twenty to thirty minutes. You need about one-half cup of cooked lentils, beans, or peas each day for heart health.

Pinot noir and cabernet sauvignon. All types of alcohol seem to have some heart-protective properties, but red wine offers the most.

Scientific evidence: People who drink alcohol regularly *in moderation* (one five-ounce glass of wine daily for women, and no more than two for men) have a 30 to 50 percent lower risk of dying from a heart attack than those who don't drink, according to research published in *Archives of Internal Medicine*.

Best choices: Pinot noir, cabernet sauvignon, and tannat wines (made from tannat red grapes). These wines have the highest concentrations of flavonoids, antioxidants that reduce arterial inflammation and inhibit the oxidation of LDL cholesterol. Oxidation is the process that makes cholesterol more likely to accumulate within artery walls.

Bonus: Red wines also contain resveratrol, a type of polyphenol that is thought to increase the synthesis of proteins that slow aging. Red wine has ten times more polyphenols than white varieties.

In a four-year study of nearly 7,700 men and women nondrinkers, those who began to drink a moderate amount of red wine cut their risk for heart attack by 38 percent compared with nondrinkers.

If you are a nondrinker or currently drink less than the amounts described above, talk to your doctor before changing your alcohol intake. If you cannot drink alcohol, pomegranate or purple grape juice is a good alternative.

> Janet Bond Brill, PhD, RDN, FAND, nutrition, health, and fitness expert specializing in cardiovascular disease prevention. Brill is a columnist for *Bottom Line Health Insider* and is the author of *Blood Pressure DOWN, Cholesterol DOWN,* and *Prevent a Second Heart Attack.* DrJanet.com.

Green Tea Lowers Risk of Heart Attack and Stroke

Green tea has remarkable powers to combat disease. We all should include green tea in our daily health regimen.

The leaves of the evergreen shrub *Camellia sinensis* are used to make green, black, and oolong tea, but green tea contains the most epigallocatechin gallate (EGCG). EGCG (a type of plant compound called a polyphenol, flavonoid, or catechin) is a powerful anti-inflammatory and antioxidant. Research shows that chronic low-grade inflammation (produced by an immune system in overdrive) and oxidation (a kind of internal rust that damages cells) are the two processes that trigger and advance most chronic diseases. Evidence shows that green tea can prevent and treat many of these diseases, especially heart disease and stroke.

Researchers studied fourteen thousand people ages sixty-five to eighty-four for six years. They found that men who drank seven or more cups of green tea a day had a 30 percent lower risk of dying from heart disease or stroke, and women had an 18 percent lower risk, compared with those who drank less than one cup of green tea a day.

How it works: Green tea can do the following:

+ Lower blood levels of LDL "bad" cholesterol and reduce the oxidation of LDL, which generates the small, dense particles that can clog arteries and cause a heart attack or stroke.

+ Reduce the activity of platelets, blood components that clump and form artery-plugging clots.

+ Prevent ventricular arrhythmia, a spasm of the heart muscle that can trigger or worsen a heart attack.

+ Reduce high blood pressure, a risk factor for stroke.

+ Improve the flexibility of the endothelium (the lining of the arteries), boosting blood flow to the heart and brain.

Green tea also helps protect against other cardiovascular risks, including diabetes, weight, and gum disease.

TYPE 2 DIABETES

Type 2 diabetes is a major risk factor for cardiovascular disease and can lead to many other disastrous health problems, including kidney failure, blindness, and lower-limb amputation.

In a study of sixty people with diabetes, those who took a daily supplement of green tea extract for two months significantly reduced hemoglobin A1C, a biomarker of blood sugar levels.

How it works: People with diabetes who drank green tea for twelve weeks boosted their levels of insulin (the hormone that helps move sugar out of the blood and into muscle cells) and decreased their levels of A1C.

OVERWEIGHT

More than 65 percent of Americans are overweight. Those extra pounds are a risk factor in dozens of health problems, including cardiovascular disease, cancer, osteoarthritis, and type 2 diabetes. Researchers from the Netherlands reviewed forty-nine studies on green tea and weight loss and analyzed the results of the eleven most scientifically rigorous. They found that those who drank green tea significantly decreased body weight and significantly maintained body weight after a period of weight loss.

Why it works: EGCG blocks the action of an enzyme that breaks down noradrenaline (NA). This hormone and neurotransmitter stimulates the sympathetic nervous system, which controls heart rate, muscle tension, and the release of energy from fat. By preserving NA, EGCG triggers your metabolism to stay more active and burn more calories.

GUM DISEASE

Research links the chronic bacterial infection of gum (periodontal) disease to many health problems, including heart disease and diabetes. Japanese researchers studied nearly one thousand men ages forty-nine to fifty-nine and found that those who regularly drank green tea had fewer cases of or less severe periodontal disease. For every additional daily cup of tea the men drank, there was a significant decrease in the depth of periodontal pockets (the grooves around the teeth that deepen as gum disease advances), a decrease in the loss of attachment of the gum to the tooth, and a decrease in bleeding.

How it works: The polyphenols in green tea may decrease the inflammatory response to oral bacteria.

THE RIGHT AMOUNT

To guarantee a sufficient intake of EGCG, I recommend one or more of the following strategies. You can safely do all three.

Drink green tea. Five to ten eight-ounce cups a day of regular or decaf.

Best: For maximum intake of EGCG, use whole-leaf loose tea rather than a teabag, using one teaspoon per cup. Steep the tea for at least five minutes.

Take a supplement of green tea extract.

Minimum: 400 mg a day of a supplement standardized to 90 percent EGCG.

Add a drop of green tea liquid extract to green tea or another beverage.

Look for a product that is standardized to a high level (at least 50 percent) of EGCG, and follow the dosage recommendation on the label.

SAFE USE

Talk to your doctor if you use:

- **An antiplatelet drug** (blood thinner), such as warfarin, because green tea also thins the blood.
- **A bronchodilator** for asthma or chronic obstructive pulmonary disease, because green tea can increase its potency.
- **An antacid,** because green tea can decrease the effect.

> Patrick M. Fratellone, MD, executive medical director of Fratellone Medical Associates in New York City, professor at the University of Bridgeport College of Naturopathic Medicine, and former chief of medicine and director of cardiology at Atkins Center for Complementary Medicine. He is coauthor of a comprehensive review article on the health benefits of green tea in *Explore.* FratelloneMedical.com.

Why Cheese Is Surprisingly Good for Your Heart

You dutifully eat your fat-free yogurts, unbuttered veggies, and other virtuously low-fat (and low-flavor) fare.

After all, you want to protect your cardiovascular system from harmful saturated fats.

But what if a nice chunk of cheese—yes, that deliciously decadent dairy delight that comes in so many mouthwatering varieties—was also good for your heart?

Well, it's true, according to research from the UK, which revealed some previously unknown properties of cheese.

And the findings may help explain a mystery that has confounded scientists for decades.

The conundrum is called the French paradox. People in France have remarkably low rates of cardiovascular disease despite the fact that their diets typically are quite high in saturated fat. By some estimates, saturated fats contribute up to *40 percent* of their total calories! Based on that, you'd expect Frenchmen to be dropping like flies from heart disease. But they aren't. Instead, they have the third-lowest rate of cardiovascular mortality in the world.

Some people attribute this to French folks' fondness for red wine, which contains the antioxidant resveratrol. But inhabitants of other countries also drink lots of red wine, yet their heart health can't compare to that of the French.

So researchers wondered what other dietary factors might help explain the French paradox. Since cheese consumption in France is among the highest in the world, they took a close look at cheese—not only a laboratory analysis of the biochemical properties of cheese, but also a clinical trial that directly examined how cheese consumption affects people. What they discovered was extremely promising—and startling.

NEWLY REVEALED HEALTH BENEFITS

Cheese's heart-protective properties may derive from its beneficial effects on the following.

Inflammation. A complex enzymatic transformation that occurs as cheese ripens leads to the formation of substances known to reduce inflammatory markers such as C-reactive protein. This is extremely important, because high levels of inflammation are closely associated with cardiac and other vascular diseases.

Blood pressure. Cheese contains compounds capable of inhibiting the angiotensin-converting enzyme (ACE) that controls blood pressure. The effects could be similar to ACE inhibitor medications used to control hypertension.

Cholesterol and bacteria. Cheeses with mold (such as Roquefort) may be particularly advantageous to cardiovascular health. When these cheeses are ripened through fermentation with fungi such as *Penicillium roqueforti*, they form substances that combat bacteria. What do these bacteria have to do with heart disease? In more than half of adults, bacteria acting as parasites in the liver and blood vessels are responsible for increases in cholesterol synthesis.

Nutrient status. Cheese also provides numerous nutrients that the body needs for overall good health—including heart health—such as protein, calcium, and vitamins A, D, B-6, and B-9.

THE BEST OF THE BUNCH

The researchers' analysis was quite extensive, encompassing nine blue-veined cheeses from six different countries, eight white fungi-fermented cheeses from three countries, seven bacteria-fermented cheeses from five countries, and two processed "cheeses" from two countries. Most were made from cow's milk, but some were made from ewe's milk or goat's milk. The various cheeses were evaluated for anti-inflammatory activity using a proprietary patented lab test.

Based on the researchers' discoveries, some cheeses rate as more heart-healthy than others. Here are the ones that top the list. All are available at supermarkets, cheese shops, and/or online.

- **Blue-veined cheeses,** such as Roquefort, Danish Blue, Gorgonzola, and mature Stilton.
- **White fungi-fermented cheeses,** such as Camembert (from cow's or goat's milk) and mature Brie.
- **Bacteria-fermented cheeses,** such as mature cheddar, mature Emmental (which is similar to Swiss and made with two types of bacteria to produce the characteristic holes), and Ossau-Iraty (a ewe's milk cheese with a toasted-wheat aroma and nutty, grassy-sweet flavor). While all cheeses are bacteria-fermented, the study suggested that these three are among the most beneficial for your heart.

You'll notice that the processed "cheese" (such as American cheese) so common in the United States does not appear on the list above, because it was not found to have heart-healthy properties.

How much cheese should you eat? Aim for a total of 15 to 25 grams (about one-half to one ounce) per day, choosing from the selections above. Don't go overboard—cheese has around one hundred calories per ounce.

To keep the calorie count under control, forget about pairing cheese with bread or crackers. Instead, place slivers of cheese on slices of apple or pear, tuck cheese into celery sticks, or sprinkle cheese over a chopped-veggie salad. If you like your cheese melted, go ahead—melting it will not diminish its beneficial properties.

....

› Ivan Petyaev, MD, PhD, CEO and founder of Lycotec Ltd., Cambridge, UK. His study was published in *Medical Hypotheses.*

....

Nondrug Approaches to Prevent Killer Blood Clots

Millions of Americans take anticlotting medications, or blood thinners, including aspirin and warfarin, to prevent clots and reduce the risk for such conditions as heart attack and stroke.

These drugs are extremely effective. Daily aspirin, for example, can reduce the risk for a first heart attack by 44 percent, according to data from the Physicians' Health Study.

The downside: Even at low doses, every anticlotting agent can cause bleeding—often from the stomach, gums, or intestines—as a side effect. Sometimes, gastrointestinal bleeding can occur even without causing noticeable symptoms.

In addition, warfarin, one of the leading blood thinners, doubles the risk

for intracerebral hemorrhage (bleeding in the brain).

NATURAL BLOOD THINNERS

Certain herbs and other supplements can be used for their anticlotting properties and may have a reduced risk for side effects, such as bleeding.

This approach is not intended to replace medications. Patients with a high risk for clotting need to take such drugs. Under a doctor's supervision, these supplements can be combined with blood-thinning medications to boost the drugs' effectiveness and potentially allow you to take a lower dose, thus reducing the risk for bleeding.

Those with only a slight risk for clots (due to family history, for example) may want to consider using natural anticoagulants alone, under a doctor's supervision, to promote better circulation.

Bonus: Natural blood thinners usually have anti-inflammatory properties. This is important because most chronic diseases, including heart disease, rheumatoid arthritis, and stroke, are caused in part by inflammation.

The supplements below can be taken alone or in combination, depending on the degree of protection that's required.

Some of these supplements may interact with prescription medications, so consult a doctor who is knowledgeable about supplement use.*

Fish oil. Studies of large populations show that people who eat a lot of cold-water fish, such as salmon and mackerel, tend to have lower heart attack death rates than people who don't eat fish.

The omega-3 fatty acids in cold-water fish are strong anticlotting agents. Fish oil is thought to inhibit platelet aggregation (clumping), part of the clotting process. One report, published in the *Annals of Pharmacotherapy*, found that taking fish oil along with warfarin caused an increase in anticlotting activity.

Typical dose: Depending on other risk factors, such as elevated cholesterol and high blood pressure, one tablet twice daily of Vectomega Whole Food Omega-3 DHA/EPA Complex, which provides 292 mg of omega-3s (DHA and EPA balanced) in a phospholipid peptide complex, in which the fish oil is bound to peptides to increase absorbability. Or one teaspoon twice daily of Nordic Naturals Ultimate Omega Liquid, which provides 1,626 mg of EPA and 1,126 mg of DHA.

Ginger and curcumin. Ginger reduces levels of fibrinogen, a precursor to fibrin, a protein that is a major component of blood clots. Curcumin has only modest effects on coagulation but is a stronger anti-inflammatory agent. That's why I advise patients to take these herbs together. Studies have shown that both ginger and curcumin can reduce inflammation in the body. An Australian study found that substances in ginger inhibited the activity of arachidonic acid, part of the chemical sequence involved in clotting. In the study, ginger compounds were more effective than aspirin at blocking platelet activity.

Typical dose: Twice daily, 50 to 100 mg of ginger and one or two 375-mg capsules of curcumin.

Nattokinase. Extracted from soybeans, nattokinase is an enzyme that helps prevent clot formation. It also makes platelets less likely to clump together. Unlike warfarin, which only prevents clots, nattokinase appears to break down clots that already have formed.

Typical dose: Depending on other risk factors, one to two capsules or tablets (2,000 fibrin units per 100 mg) twice daily.

Important: I recommend taking nattokinase between meals. The anticlotting properties are strongest when it is taken without food.

....

* To find a doctor who has experience treating patients with supplements, consult the American Association of Naturopathic Physicians, 866-538-2267, Naturopathic.org.

Vinpocetine. This supplement is extracted from periwinkle. It's extremely important to take vinpocetine under a doctor's supervision. Vinpocetine is the most potent natural substance for preventing clots, and, like prescription anticlotting agents, it can cause internal bleeding in some patients. For this reason, I recommend it mainly for high-risk patients who are unable to take warfarin because of side effects and/or complications.

Typical dose: 2 mg total, in divided doses twice daily. Higher doses (5 mg total in divided doses) might be needed, but don't increase from the starting dose without talking with your doctor. Should be taken without food.

Ginkgo. The extract from the dried leaves of the ginkgo biloba tree has traditionally been used to treat intermittent claudication, leg pain caused by insufficient blood flow, as well as cognitive impairments (such as memory problems) due to poor blood circulation in the brain.

Ginkgo is effective at reducing clots and also acts as a vasodilator that helps improve blood flow to the brain, heart, and other parts of the body. I don't recommend it as often as other anticoagulants, because it has little effect on inflammation. If you use ginkgo, ask your doctor about combining it with curcumin or other anti-inflammatory herbs/supplements.

Typical dose: About 40 mg, three times daily.

Garlic. Studies have shown that patients who take garlic supplements have a lower risk for clots. Use only those products that list a high allicin content—the main active ingredient in garlic. This can be found frequently in fresh garlic supplements.

Typical dose: The optimal dose for garlic hasn't been definitively established. However, some studies indicate that you need at least 180 mg of allicin twice daily.

Important: In general, natural therapies should be started at low doses that are slowly increased, under a doctor's supervision, over time. I recommend that the supplements described in this article be used at least twice daily to ensure that adequate levels of the therapeutic compounds are maintained in the body.

› Decker Weiss, NMD, naturopathic medical doctor who specializes in integrative cardiology. He is founder and owner of Weiss Natural Medicine, in Scottsdale, Arizona, and author of *The Weiss Method: A Natural Program for Reversing Heart Disease and Preventing Heart Attacks.* DrDeckerWeiss.com.

Sunlight Helps Prevent Heart Attacks

A*h, sunlight.*
There's nothing like being outdoors on a summer morning.

What you may not know is that sunshine doesn't just boost your mood and your vitamin D level. It also may help you ward off a heart attack or minimize the damage that one can cause, according to a first-of-its-kind study.

Here, the study's lead author, Tobias Eckle, MD, PhD, an associate professor of anesthesiology, cardiology, and cell and developmental biology at the University of Colorado School of Medicine in Denver, tells how we can all harness the power of light to brighten our heart health.

FASCINATING RHYTHM
Our circadian rhythm—the physical, mental, and behavioral changes prompted by light and darkness that occur over each twenty-four-hour period—helps determine the level of a certain protein that can minimize the cell damage and cell death caused by a heart attack. This protein might even stop a heart attack in its tracks. Dr. Eckle and his colleagues were eager to see whether exposure to certain kinds of light at a certain time might be effective at boosting levels of this protein.

In the study, researchers divided mice into two groups. One group was exposed to light boxes emitting light that was the same level of brightness as daylight ("bright light"), and others were exposed to regular room lighting ("regular light"). Both groups were exposed to the light first thing in the morning at 6:00 a.m.

Then the mice were given anesthesia, and heart attacks were triggered in them. Researchers found that mice that had been exposed to three hours of bright light had three times the amount of the protective protein as the mice that had been exposed to regular light, and incredibly, the bright light mice's hearts had experienced only one-fifth as much damage!

HOW SUNNY ARE THE FINDINGS?
There are, of course, unanswered questions—for example, how the findings might apply to humans and how lasting the benefit of the protein might be.

That said, the results are promising. What's especially interesting is that it's the light exposure on the *eyes*—not the *skin*—that affects the protein levels. So humans wearing sunscreen or long sleeves wouldn't blunt the effect.

SAFE WAYS TO LET IN THE LIGHT
Several forces have conspired over recent decades to keep people out of the

sun during the day, such as indoor work and fear of skin cancer. But many people would be likely to benefit from getting more sunlight exposure as early in the morning as possible.

Here are some safe ways to shed more light on your daily routine.

Take a daily walk outdoors, and keep wearing sunscreen. Even ten to twenty minutes a day is better than nothing. Since, as I mentioned earlier, it's the way that light affects your eyes (not your skin) that matters, apply sunscreen—that won't dampen the benefits. The added exercise will boost your heart health too.

Get sunlight while indoors. Sit near large, bright windows.

Use a light therapy box. If you can't follow either of the first two tips or if you're at high risk for skin cancer and want to avoid UV rays at all costs, this may be the best option for you. Available online for about fifty dollars and up, light therapy boxes mimic the brightness of sunlight while filtering out most damaging UV rays.

> Tobias Eckle, MD, PhD, associate professor of anesthesiology, cardiology, and cell and developmental biology, University of Colorado School of Medicine, Denver. His study was published in *Nature Medicine*.

Natural Ways to Effectively Reduce Heart Attack Risk without a Statin

More seniors than ever are being advised to take statins to lower their cholesterol. But plenty of people don't like to take any type of prescription medication if they can avoid it.

Most integrative physicians, who prescribe natural therapies (and drugs when needed), agree that the majority of people who take statins—and most of those who will be recommended to do so—could get many of the same benefits, such as lower cholesterol and inflammation levels, with fewer risks by relying on targeted food choices and supplements. Exercise—ideally, about thirty minutes at least five days a week—should also be part of a healthy-heart regimen.

THE BEST CHOLESTEROL-LOWERING SUPPLEMENTS

Fish oil (a typical daily dose of 1,000 mg total of EPA and DHA) fights inflammation, lowers LDL "bad" cholesterol, and is part of most good heart-protective regimens.* In addition, I recommend using the first supplement below and adding the other three supplements if total cholesterol levels don't drop below 200 mg/dL.

Red yeast rice. You have probably heard of this rice, which is fermented to produce monacolins, chemical compounds with statin-like effects. It can lower LDL cholesterol by roughly 30 percent.

Red yeast rice can be a good alternative for people who can't tolerate statins due to side effects such as muscle aches and increased risk for diabetes. Red yeast rice also has other natural protective substances, such as isoflavones, fatty acids, and sterols, not found in statins.

Typical dosage: 1.2 to 2.4 g daily. I advise starting with 1.2 g daily. The dose can be increased as needed, based on your physician's advice.

What I tell my patients: Unfortunately, red yeast rice has gotten a bad rap because of the way some products were labeled. The supplements that I recommend are manufactured with high standards of quality control and contain therapeutic levels of active ingredients.

When taking red yeast rice, some people have heartburn, gastrointestinal (GI) upset, or mild headache. These effects usually are eliminated by taking the supplement with food.

Niacin. Few doctors recommend niacin routinely, even though it's one of the most effective cholesterol remedies. Although one publicized study questioned the effectiveness of niacin, most research finds it beneficial. It may lower LDL by about 10 percent and increase HDL "good" cholesterol by 15 to 35 percent. It can lower levels of triglycerides and lipoprotein A, a sticky cholesterol particle that causes atherosclerosis.

Typical dosage: 1 to 3 g of time-released niacin daily, divided into two doses and taken with food.

What I tell my patients: Start with 250 mg daily, and increase the dose by 250 mg every two weeks until you are taking the amount recommended by your doctor. People who take high doses of niacin too quickly often have uncomfortable facial flushing and sometimes stomach upset or other GI disturbances. "Flush-free" niacin is available, but it doesn't lower cholesterol as effectively as the regular version.

Pantethine. You may not be familiar with this supplement, a form of pantothenic acid (vitamin B-5). Studies show

---

* A recent study linking fish oil to increased risk for prostate cancer is not supported by other medical research, so most men can take fish oil supplements under a doctor's supervision.

that it raises HDL cholesterol, and it prevents LDL from oxidizing, the process that causes it to cling to arteries.

Typical dosage: 900 mg, divided into two or three doses daily.

What I tell my patients: Take pantethine with meals to reduce the risk for indigestion and to aid absorption.

Sterols and stanols. These cholesterol-lowering plant compounds are found in small amounts in many fruits, vegetables, and grains. But sterol and stanol supplements are much more powerful. In supplement form, the plant compounds reduce LDL by about 14 percent and cause no side effects.

Typical dosage: Take 3 g of a sterol/stanol supplement daily. Pure Encapsulations makes a good product (PureEncapsulations.com).

Most integrative physicians are very knowledgeable about natural remedies. To find one in your area, consult the American College for Advancement in Medicine.

YUMMY CHOLESTEROL FIGHTERS

For years, oat bran and oatmeal were touted as the best foods for high cholesterol. Rich in soluble fiber, these foods help prevent cholesterol from getting into the bloodstream. A daily serving of oats, for example, can lower LDL by 20 percent. Other good foods rich in soluble fiber include barley, beans, pears, and prunes. But research has now gone beyond these old standby food choices. Here are some other fiber-rich foods that have been found to give cholesterol the heave-ho.

All nuts. Walnuts and almonds are great cholesterol fighters, but so are pistachios, peanuts, pecans, hazelnuts, and other nuts, according to research. Eat a handful (1.5 ounces) of nuts daily.

Popcorn actually contains more fiber per ounce than whole-wheat bread. Just go easy on the salt and butter, and stay away from store-bought microwave popcorn (it can contain harmful chemicals).

Smart idea: Put one-quarter cup of organic plain popcorn in a lunch-size brown paper bag, and pop in the microwave. It's delicious—and there's no cleanup.

....

› Allan Magaziner, DO, osteopathic physician and founder and director of the Magaziner Center for Wellness in Cherry Hill, New Jersey. One of the country's top specialists in nutritional and preventive medicine, Dr. Magaziner is coauthor of *The All-Natural Cardio Cure: A Drug-Free Cholesterol and Cardiac Inflammation Reduction Program.* DrMagaziner.com.

....

Five Foods That Fight High Blood Pressure

Is your blood pressure on the high side? Your doctor might write a prescription when it creeps above 140/90, but you may be able to forgo medication. Lifestyle changes still are considered the best starting treatment for mild hypertension. These include not smoking, regular exercise, and a healthy diet. In addition to eating less salt, you want to consume potent pressure-lowering foods, including the following.

RAISINS

Raisins are basically dehydrated grapes, but they provide a much more concentrated dose of nutrients and fiber. They are high in potassium, with 220 mg in a small box (1.5 ounces). Potassium helps counteract the blood pressure–raising effects of salt. The more potassium we consume, the more sodium our bodies excrete. Researchers also speculate that the fiber and antioxidants in raisins change the biochemistry of blood vessels, making them more pliable—important for healthy blood pressure. Opt for dark raisins over light-colored ones, because dark raisins have more catechins, a powerful type of antioxidant that can increase blood flow.

Researchers at Louisville Metabolic and Atherosclerosis Research Center compared people who snacked on raisins with those who ate other packaged snacks. Those in the raisin group had drops in systolic pressure (the top number) ranging from 4.8 points (after four weeks) to 10.2 points (after twelve weeks). Blood pressure barely budged in the no-raisin group. Some people worry about the sugar in raisins, but it is natural sugar (not added sugar) and will not adversely affect your health (though people with diabetes need to be cautious with portion sizes).

My advice: Aim to consume a few ounces of raisins every day. Prunes are an alternative.

BEETS

Beets are also high in potassium, with about 519 mg per cup. They're delicious, easy to cook, and very effective for lowering blood pressure.

A study at the London Medical School found that people who drank about eight ounces of beet juice averaged a ten-point drop in blood pressure during the next twenty-four hours. The blood pressure–lowering effect was most pronounced at three to six hours past drinking but remained lower for the entire twenty-four hours. Eating whole beets might be even better because you will get extra fiber.

Along with fiber and potassium,

beets also are high in nitrate. The nitrate is converted first to nitrite in the blood, then to nitric oxide. Nitric oxide is a gas that relaxes blood vessel walls and lowers blood pressure.

My advice: Eat beets several times a week. Look for beets that are dark red. They contain more protective phytochemicals than gold or white beets. Cooked spinach and kale are alternatives.

DAIRY

In research involving nearly forty-five thousand people, researchers found that those who consumed low-fat "fluid" dairy foods, such as yogurt and low-fat milk, were 16 percent less likely to develop high blood pressure. Higher-fat forms of dairy, such as cheese and ice cream, had no blood pressure benefits. The study was published in the *Journal of Human Hypertension.*

In another study, published in the *New England Journal of Medicine,* researchers found that people who included low-fat or fat-free dairy in a diet high in fruits and vegetables had *double* the blood pressure–lowering benefits of those who just ate the fruits and veggies.

Low-fat dairy is high in calcium, another blood pressure–lowering mineral that should be included in your diet. When you don't have enough calcium in your diet, a "calcium leak" occurs in your

kidneys. This means that the kidneys excrete more calcium in the urine, disturbing the balance of mineral metabolism involved in blood pressure regulation.

My advice: Aim for at least one serving of low-fat or nonfat milk or yogurt every day. If you don't care for cow's milk or can't drink it, switch to fortified soy milk. It has just as much calcium and protein and also contains phytoestrogens, compounds that are good for the heart.

FLAXSEED

Flaxseed contains alpha-linolenic acid (ALA), an omega-3 fatty acid that helps prevent heart and vascular disease. Flaxseed also contains magnesium. A shortage of magnesium in our diet throws off the balance of sodium, potassium, and calcium, which causes the blood vessels to constrict.

Flaxseed also is high in flavonoids, the same antioxidants that have boosted the popularity of dark chocolate, kale, and red wine. Flavonoids are bioactive chemicals that reduce inflammation throughout the body, including in the arteries. Arterial inflammation is thought to be the trigger that leads to high blood pressure, blood clots, and heart attacks.

In a large-scale observational study linking dietary magnesium intake with better heart health and longevity, nearly fifty-nine thousand healthy Japanese people were followed for fifteen years. The scientists found that the people with the highest dietary intake of magnesium had a 50 percent reduced risk for death from heart disease (heart attack and stroke). According to the researchers, magnesium's heart-healthy benefit is linked to its ability to improve blood pressure, suppress irregular heartbeats, and inhibit inflammation.

My advice: Add one or two tablespoons of ground flaxseed to breakfast cereals. You also can sprinkle flaxseed on yogurt or whip it into a breakfast smoothie. Or try chia seeds.

WALNUTS

Yale researchers found that people who ate two ounces of walnuts a day had improved blood flow and drops in blood pressure (a 3.5-point drop in systolic blood pressure and a 2.8-point drop in diastolic blood pressure). The mechanisms through which walnuts elicit a blood pressure–lowering response are believed to involve their high content of monounsaturated fatty acids, alpha-linolenic acid, magnesium, and fiber and their low levels of sodium and saturated fatty acids.

Bonus: Despite the reputation of nuts as a "fat snack," the people who ate them didn't gain weight.

The magnesium in walnuts is particularly important. It limits the amount of calcium that enters muscle cells inside artery walls. Ingesting the right amount of calcium (not too much and not too little) on a daily basis is essential for optimal blood pressure regulation. Magnesium regulates calcium's movement across the membranes of the smooth muscle cells, deep within the artery walls.

If your body doesn't have enough magnesium, too much calcium will enter the smooth muscle cells, which causes the arterial muscles to tighten, putting a squeeze on the arteries and raising blood pressure. Magnesium works like the popular calcium channel blockers, drugs that block entry of calcium into arterial walls, lowering blood pressure.

My advice: Eat two ounces of walnuts every day. Or choose other nuts such as almonds and pecans.

....

› Janet Bond Brill, PhD, RDN, FAND, nutrition, health, and fitness expert specializing in cardiovascular disease prevention. Brill is a columnist for *Bottom Line Health Insider* and is the author of *Blood Pressure DOWN, Cholesterol DOWN,* and *Prevent a Second Heart Attack.* DrJanet.com.

....

More Magnesium, Please!

Consuming an additional 100 mg of magnesium a day may reduce your risk for stroke by 9 percent. And magnesium isn't an expensive drug with side effects—it's a natural mineral that's already in many of the foods we eat. Most of us, especially those of us at high risk for stroke, high blood pressure, or diabetes, would benefit from eating more magnesium-rich foods, such as:

+ **Pumpkin seeds** (191 mg per ¼ cup)
+ **Almonds** (160 mg per 2 ounces)
+ **Spinach** (156 mg per cup)
+ **Cashews** (148 mg per 2 ounces)
+ **White beans** (134 mg per cup)
+ **Artichokes** (97 mg per one large artichoke)
+ **Brown rice** (84 mg per cup)
+ **Shrimp** (39 mg per 4 ounces)

You can also supercharge your cooking with magnesium if you use oat bran (221 mg per cup) and buckwheat flour (301 mg per cup).

Should anyone be concerned about overdosing on magnesium? It's hard to eat too much magnesium. If you do, your kidneys excrete the extra through urine, so only those with kidney failure need to make sure they don't consume too much.

> Roger Bonomo, MD, neurologist in private practice, stroke specialist, and former director, Stroke Center, Lenox Hill Hospital, New York City.

Dietary Fiber Cuts Stroke Risk

In one analysis, for every 7 g of fiber daily, the risk for a first-time stroke decreased by 7 percent. One serving of whole-wheat pasta or two servings of fruits and vegetables contain about 7 g of fiber. Other top fiber sources include brown rice, spelt, quinoa, and other whole-grain foods, almonds and other nuts, and lentils and other dried beans.

Recommended daily fiber intake: People age fifty or younger, 38 g (men) and 25 g (women); over age fifty, 30 g (men) and 21 g (women).

> Victoria J. Burley, PhD, associate professor in nutritional epidemiology at University of Leeds, England, and coauthor of an analysis of eight studies, published in *Stroke*.

Animal Protein for Stroke Prevention

You already know what not to eat to protect yourself from stroke, so you stay away from foods that are high in salt and artery-clogging fats. And you probably know that you should be eating lots of fruits, vegetables, and whole grains for their fiber and healthful antioxidants. But there's another nutrient that you need for stroke protection. Protein—yes, protein. And here's the surprise—although nuts, beans, and grains are all protein sources known for helping heart health, the results of a recent study suggest that a certain kind of animal protein may be the best for stroke protection.

You're probably thinking that makes no sense. Many studies have shown that protein-rich diets, particularly diets in which the protein mostly comes from animals, are not beneficial for stroke prevention. At the same time, other studies have shown that protein-rich diets can reduce stroke risk.

Researchers from China who tried to make sense of conflicting studies about protein and stroke risk found that people whose diets included a moderate to moderately high amount of protein—particularly animal protein (up to 2.19 ounces per day, compared with the average U.S. recommended amount of 1.6 to 2 ounces of protein from any source)—were less likely to have a stroke than people who included only a little bit of protein in their diets. In looking at a group of studies

that, in total, included 254,489 people, the researchers discovered that people who ate the most protein from any source had a 20 percent lower risk of stroke compared with those who consumed the least protein. Also, interestingly, the more protein eaten from any source, the lower the risk of stroke. That is, for every 0.7 ounces more of protein (moderately) consumed, stroke risk dropped by 26 percent.

In studies that specifically looked at either animal protein or vegetable protein, the researchers discovered that eating more, rather than less, animal protein reduced risk by 29 percent, and eating more, rather than less, vegetable protein reduced risk by 12 percent. The range between high and low consumption in the studies on vegetable protein wasn't that wide though, which may be why a larger difference in stroke risk reduction wasn't seen in them.

THE BEST SOURCE OF PROTEIN

Here's the most valuable takeaway from the meta-study—the greatest benefit for stroke protection, by far, seemed to come from getting animal protein from fish.

When the Chinese researchers looked more closely at the individual scientific studies, they noticed something striking about cultural and regional differences that put the puzzle about protein and stroke risk all together for them. Studies from Japan—a country in which fish consumption is particularly high—showed that people who ate the most protein had half the stroke risk of people who ate the least. And a research paper from Sweden—another country big on fish-eating—showed that stroke risk was reduced by 26 percent in higher consumers of protein. Compare these risk numbers to the one pooled from four studies from the United States, whose residents, on average, get the least amount of their protein from fish. Stroke risk reduction from higher protein consumption was only 9 percent.

How does protein reduce stroke risk? One theory is that it does so by lowering blood pressure, a well-known risk factor for stroke. Red meat, poultry, fish, and dairy all contain L-arginine, an amino acid that our bodies convert to nitric oxide. Nitric oxide causes blood vessels to open wider, which improves blood flow and reduces blood pressure. But this good effect might be countered by the types of fat (and cholesterol) in red meat and dairy. This is why fish, which contains other heart-healthy nutrients such as omega-3 fatty acids, looks like the better choice.

This study makes a strong case that fish should be our main source of protein. The Mediterranean diet—a diet high in whole grains, vegetables, olive oil, fish, and

fruit and low in red meat—is beneficial for stroke reduction. So if you're already fortifying your diet with vegetables and protein and especially substituting fish for red meat, you're doing it right. If not, consider making this heart-healthy change now.

› Xinfeng Liu, MD, PhD, professor and chairman, department of neurology, Jinling Hospital, Nanjing University School of Medicine, China. His study was published in *Neurology*.

A Grapefruit a Day Helps Keep Stroke Away

Mmm, *citrus. There's nothing like* a refreshing orange, a tangy tangerine, or a sweet pink grapefruit. It really does taste like sunshine.

But these juicy fruits aren't just delicious. They may actually help you ward off a stroke.

And you may be surprised to hear that it's not because of the vitamin C.

HONING IN ON FLAVONOIDS

A zillion studies have shown the health benefits of eating fruit, including studies that have shown that people who eat five or more servings of fruits and vegetables have a 25 percent lower risk for stroke (both ischemic and hemorrhagic) compared with those who eat three or fewer servings. Researchers have suspected that flavonoids, antioxidant compounds found in many fruits and vegetables, are one key to their power since they reduce inflammation and improve blood vessel function.

But there are six different types of flavonoids found in foods, and each has a subtly different chemical structure. Given the variety, researchers from England, Italy, and the United States wanted to learn which specific flavonoids and which fruits or vegetables in particular are most beneficial for preventing stroke.

THE FLAVONOID THAT CAME OUT ON TOP

The research used information from seventy thousand women who were followed for fourteen years as part of the Nurses' Health Study. Every two years, the participants completed questionnaires that covered their medical histories and lifestyles. And every four years, the women completed food questionnaires, which asked how much of certain foods and drinks they consumed and how often they consumed them.

The women's diets were analyzed for the six different types of flavonoids, and their medical histories were reviewed for the number and type of strokes that the women had.

Findings: High consumption—more than about 63 mg per day of a certain subclass of flavonoids called flavanones (the amount found in about one to two servings of citrus per day)—was associated with a 19 percent reduced risk for ischemic stroke (the type caused by a clot, not by a bleed), compared with low flavanone consumption (under 13.7 mg per day). And this was after adjusting for other stroke risk factors, such as smoking, age, body mass index, and others. The other five flavonoids studied reduced stroke risk too, but not by as much (only by 4 to 13 percent).

One reason that the flavanones may have been associated with decreased risk for ischemic stroke is that flavanones may inhibit platelet function and clotting factors. The study didn't look at whether citrus affected risk for hemorrhagic stroke, but it's unlikely that eating citrus would lead to an increased risk for hemorrhagic stroke. It takes a relatively small amount of clotting to cause an ischemic stroke, but on the other hand, it takes a relatively large amount of excessive bleeding to cause a hemorrhagic stroke.

Although this study, which was published in *Stroke*, looked only at women, there is no reason to think that these findings wouldn't apply to men too.

PICK YOUR CITRUS

You can get all the flavanones you need (about 63 mg) from eating one or two servings of citrus each day. Whole fruits are always better than juices or smoothies, because the bulk of the flavanones are found in the inner membranes of the fruit and the pith or white part of the fruit. The pith is generally removed when the fruit is juiced or cleaned for smoothies.

The USDA provides information about the amount of flavanones in every 100 grams of edible fruit, so to save you the trouble of weighing your fruits, here are estimates of the flavanone content for some common citruses:

+ **Grapefruit** (one-half of a four-inch diameter) 47 mg
+ **Orange** (2 ⅝ inch diameter) 42 mg
+ **Tangerine** (2 ½ inch diameter) 18 mg

Sticking to whole fruit is better than taking supplements. And don't overdo it on citrus, or else your stomach or teeth might suffer from the acid. Just a serving or two a day is all you need!

› Kathryn M. Rexrode, MD, MPH, physician, division of preventive medicine, Brigham and Women's Hospital, and assistant professor of medicine, Harvard Medical School, both in Boston.

Tomato Sauce Reduces Stroke Risk

People with the highest blood levels of the antioxidant lycopene had 55 percent lower risk for stroke than people with the lowest levels. Lycopene is found in tomatoes, red peppers, carrots, papaya, and watermelon. It is even more concentrated in cooked tomato products, such as tomato sauce.

› Rafael Alexander Ortiz, MD, chief, Neuro-Endovascular Surgery and Interventional Neuroradiology, Lenox Hill Hospital, New York City.

Stroke Fighter: Red Peppers

Eating red peppers and other vitamin C–rich fruits and veggies may reduce your risk for intracerebral hemorrhagic stroke (a blood vessel rupture in the brain). And what's so great about red peppers? At 190 mg per cup, they contain three times more vitamin C than an orange. Other good sources of vitamin C include broccoli and strawberries. Researchers believe that this vitamin may reduce stroke risk by regulating blood pressure and strengthening collagen, which promotes healthy blood vessels.

› Stéphane Vannier, MD, neurologist, Pontchaillou
University Hospital, Rennes, France, from research
presented at the annual meeting of the American
Academy of Neurology.

Olive Oil Can
Keep Strokes Away

Peaple who consistently added olive oil to their food in cooking and salad dressings were 41 percent less likely to suffer from an ischemic stroke than people who did not use olive oil. An ischemic stroke, in which blood flow to a part of the brain is blocked, is the most common kind of stroke.

› Cécilia Samieri, PhD, researcher, department of
epidemiology, Université Bordeaux Segalen, France,
and leader of two studies on olive oil consumption
and stroke risk, published in *Neurology*.

6

Colds, Flu, and Pneumonia

Boost Your Immunity to Fight Colds, Flu, and Pneumonia

Colds are potentially more danger-ous than most people realize. That's because they often weaken an already compromised immune system, making the sufferer more vulnerable to the flu and pneumonia.

A nutritional deficiency is the most common cause of depressed immunity, but even people who make a point to eat a well-balanced diet often fall short when it comes to getting enough key nutrients. For this reason, many Americans turn to dietary supplements for extra protection.

But which ones really work?

Michael T. Murray, ND, is a leading naturopathic physician who has spent more than thirty years compiling a database of more than sixty thousand scientific articles on the effectiveness of natural medicines, including supple-ments. Here are some of the most effective supplements for preventing and treat-ing colds and related upper-respiratory ailments. Start with the first supplement and add others (all are available at health-food stores), based on specific symptoms.*

Mixed antioxidants. When it comes to fortifying your body to fight off colds, it's wise to start with a high-potency multisupplement. I recommend one that combines zinc, selenium, beta-carotene (or other carotenes), and vitamins C and E.

---

* Consult your doctor before trying these supplements, especially if you have a chronic medical condition and/or take medication. Some of these remedies may interact with medication. Most supplements need to be taken for at least six weeks to reach their full effect.

This antioxidant mix helps prevent oxidative damage to the thymus gland—a robust thymus is needed to produce T lymphocytes, a type of white blood cell that recognizes and attacks viruses and other infectious agents.

Typical daily dose: 20 to 30 mg zinc, 200 micrograms (mcg) selenium, 25,000 international units (IU) beta-carotene, 500 mg vitamin C, and 200 IU vitamin E. You'll find roughly these amounts in any high-potency multisupplement. Many people take a multisupplement year-round.

Astragalus. Few Americans know about this herb, although it's a standard treatment in traditional Chinese medicine (TCM). It is getting more attention these days because scientists have learned that it contains polysaccharide fraction F3 and other substances that stimulate different parts of the immune system.

Test-tube and animal studies have found that astragalus has potent antiviral effects—important for preventing colds and the flu. In one study, 115 patients who took the herb for eight weeks showed significant improvement in their counts of infection-fighting white blood cells.

Typical daily dose: 100 to 150 mg of powdered extract combined with any liquid, three times daily, whenever you have a cold or the flu or throughout the winter months if your immunity is low (for example, due to extra stress).

Caution: If you have rheumatoid arthritis or some other autoimmune disease, use astragalus only under a doctor's supervision—the increase in immune activity could worsen your autoimmune symptoms.

South African geranium. Also known as *umckaloabo*, this herbal remedy is commonly used for bronchitis, an upper-respiratory infection that often follows colds, particularly in winter.

In a study of 205 patients with bronchitis, those taking it had reduced bronchitis-related symptoms, such as a cough and shortness of breath. Other studies have shown similar effects.

Although doctors who specialize in herbal medicine typically recommend this supplement for patients who have been diagnosed with bronchitis or sinusitis, I advise taking it if you have a cold, because it reduces symptoms and helps prevent a secondary bronchial infection.

Typical daily dose: 20 mg, three times daily, until the symptoms subside.

Beta-glucan. This class of compounds is found in baker's yeast, medicinal mushrooms (such as maitake), and a variety of grains. Supplemental forms have been shown to stimulate the activity of immune cells. They also stimulate immune signaling proteins, which help the body fight viral infections.

In a study of fifty-four firefighters (who are susceptible to colds because of frequent exposure to smoke and other fumes), those who took a beta-glucan supplement had 23 percent fewer upper-respiratory infections compared with those who took a placebo.

Typical daily dose: 250 to 500 mg daily. This dose is effective for treatment of viral infections as well as prevention (for example, when you feel a cold coming on). I recommend Wellmune WGP (it contains a substance derived from yeast that has been shown to strengthen immune cells) or Maitake Gold beta-glucan supplements—the research is more solid with these than with other products.

Echinacea. This herb has been the subject of more than nine hundred studies. A few years ago, researchers reported that it was not effective for colds—probably because these scientists were using products that had insufficient amounts of active compounds. In my experience, echinacea is very effective both for prevention and treatment.

Example: One study, involving 120 patients who had just started to experience cold symptoms, found that only 40 percent of those taking echinacea went on to develop a full-fledged cold compared with 60 percent of those not taking the herb. When patients in the echinacea group did get sick, their symptoms started to improve after four days versus eight days in those taking placebos.

Typical daily dose: One-half to one teaspoon of liquid extract, which can be added to a glass of water or taken straight, three times daily, when you have a cold or feel one coming on. Buy a product that is made from the fresh aerial portion of the plant. This information will be printed on the label. You will receive a higher concentration of active compounds. People who have allergies to plants in the daisy family (which includes ragweed) should not take echinacea.

ADD A DOSE OF STRESS RELIEF

It's important to remember that virtually everyone is more likely to get sick during times of stress.

Reasons: Stress increases blood levels of adrenal hormones, which suppress the immune system. In addition, stress triggers the release of cytokines and other substances that decrease the activity of white blood cells and inhibit the formation of new ones.

What to do: In addition to getting regular exercise and sleeping at least seven hours a night, make a habit of doing activities that improve your mood. Deep breathing, meditation, or simply having a good time with friends will all help you stay healthier.

DITCH THE SUGAR!

If you want to stay healthy, cut way back on sugar. This is important, because the simple sugars in sweets and sweet beverages (including fruit juices) diminish the ability of lymphocytes to fight off viruses. When you consume sugar, the immune system weakens within just thirty minutes, and it remains in a depressed state for more than five hours.

It's not clear why sugar has such serious effects on immunity. It's possible that elevated blood sugar prevents vitamin C from attaching to and entering white blood cells, which makes the immune system less effective.

My advice: Have no more (and preferably less) than 15 to 20 g of sugar in any three-hour period. Sugar content information is, of course, found on food labels. A four-ounce glass of fruit juice, for example, will have about 12 g of sugar.

> › Michael T. Murray, ND, one of the country's best-known naturopathic physicians. He serves on the Board of Regents of Bastyr University in Seattle and has written more than thirty books, including *The Encyclopedia of Natural Medicine* with coauthor Joseph Pizzorno, ND. DoctorMurray.com.

Fight Colds the Way Performers Do

When you catch a cold, the sneezing, runny nose, sore throat, and coughing will most likely make you feel miserable for a week or so, yet you probably manage to go about your business.

But what if you were an opera singer or a Broadway actor and started sniffling a few days before opening night? Or a politician or a preacher? For these so-called voice professionals (individuals whose jobs require the use of their voices), a cold wreaks havoc on their ability to work. They can take cortisone (an anti-inflammatory steroid) to quickly relieve laryngitis, but congestion and other symptoms don't give up so easily.

As it turns out, there are a number of effective, unique therapies that voice pros use to prevent and treat colds and related illnesses.

COLDS

The average American catches two to four colds a year. Avoiding the common cold involves well-known precautions such as getting enough rest, drinking plenty of fluids, eating a nutritious diet, and frequent hand washing. But these don't always work. Here are some therapies performers use:

+ **Slippery elm tea.** Derived from the inner bark of the slippery elm tree, this traditional remedy eases coughs and sore throat pain. The bark contains mucilage, a substance that becomes slick and gel-like when mixed with water. It's a highly effective remedy for coating and soothing the throat.

    To make this tea: Pour two cups of boiling water over about two tablespoons of powdered bark. Steep for five minutes and drink. Do this several times a day.

    Or try slippery elm lozenges.

+ **Lots of black pepper.** It's an expectorant that quickly thins mucus to reduce congestion. Add generous amounts to your meals whenever possible until you've gotten over your stuffy nose.

+ **Fruit smoothies.** These tasty drinks will replenish lost fluids, and the antioxidants may even help you recover from a cold more quickly.

    What to do: Once or twice a day, blend fruits—such as pineapple, blueberries, and/or bananas—with a cup or two of fruit juice and some ice. Do not add anything else. The key is to get a potent shot of antioxidants and a lot of liquid. (If you have diabetes, be sure to check with your doctor before using this remedy, since fruit contains high amounts of natural sugar.)

+ **Zinc.** Used within twenty-four hours after symptoms start, zinc lozenges can shorten the duration of a cold by at least a day. Use the lozenges until the cold is gone, but don't take more than four lozenges a day.

+ **Vitamin C.** Throughout cold season, take 500 mg of vitamin C twice a day to prevent colds or 1,000 mg twice a day to recover from a cold more quickly. (If you get diarrhea from this dose, reduce the amount you take accordingly.)

LARYNGITIS

Most colds clear up in a week or so, but they're sometimes followed by laryngitis, inflammation of the larynx (voice box) that can last for several weeks.

In addition to resting your voice as much as possible, try this:

+ **Steam with eucalyptus oil.** Few remedies are better than steam and eucalyptus, a powerful decongestant, for quick relief of laryngitis.

    What to do: After boiling a couple of cups of water in a saucepan, turn off the heat and add a few drops of eucalyptus oil (available at health-food stores). Lean over the pan with a towel draped over your head to trap the steam. Being careful not to burn yourself, breathe the steam for a few minutes, two to three times a day.

SORE THROAT

A sore throat is usually due to a viral infection. If the pain is not severe and the soreness starts to go away within a few days, you probably won't need medical treatment. If the pain doesn't go away or it seems to be getting worse, see your doctor to check for strep throat.

For a simple sore throat, try this:

+ **Gargle.** Use a salt and baking soda solution. The salt draws fluids from the tissues and reduces swelling and pain. Baking soda makes the gargle more soothing.

  What to do: Add about one-half teaspoon each of salt and baking soda to one cup of warm water, and gargle for thirty to sixty seconds.

  Important: Do *not* gargle with commercial antiseptic mouthwash. Even though it temporarily reduces bacteria in the mouth, it may damage mucous membranes in the throat and increase the risk for infection.

A SURPRISING CAUSE OF HOARSENESS

If you're hoarse but it's not due to a cold or overuse of your voice (as is often the case with singers, politicians, preachers, and sports fans), there may be another cause—and it's often overlooked.

Laryngopharyngeal reflux (LPR) is a condition in which stomach acid backs up into the larynx or throat (pharynx). It's similar to what happens with heartburn but without the typical burn in the chest. Here's what to do:

+ **Follow heartburn-prevention strategies.** The same steps that you follow to prevent heartburn—eating smaller meals, avoiding greasy, fatty foods, not eating within a few hours of going to bed, and raising the head of the bed a few inches—will also help prevent LPR.

+ **Neutralize stomach acid.** Alginate is a compound that neutralizes acid and helps prevent it from surging out of the stomach. It is an active ingredient in heartburn products such as Gaviscon.

+ **Try DGL.** Taken in pill or powder form before meals when you're feeling hoarse, deglycyrrhizinated licorice (DGL) helps prevent stomach acid from damaging the larynx. Drugs such as Prilosec have a similar effect, but they increase osteoporosis risk. DGL is a safer remedy.

> Len Horovitz, MD, internist, pulmonary specialist, and director of Carnegie Medical PC, a private practice in New York City. *New York Magazine* has included him among "The Best Doctors in New York" for both pulmonary and internal medicine. He is a contributor to the medical anthology *The Singer's Guide to Complete Health.*

How to Stop a Cold in Its Tracks

Uh oh. It's around noon, and you detect a slight sore throat and your nose is getting stuffy—signs of an impending cold. But instead of giving in, you can equip your body with the tools it needs to knock back a cold virus before it fully develops. I find an hour-by-hour approach to be most effective—it gives the body time to gradually make use of the healing therapies described below—but you can also use as many of them as possible any time throughout the day. To help eliminate the virus, start by drinking eight ounces of water and repeat every hour until you go to bed. Also try the following:

Hour 1: **Gargle.** This kills germs that would otherwise collect and multiply in the back of the throat. I use Alka-Thyme, an old-fashioned, saline-based formula with menthol and eucalyptus. It is available at health-food stores

and Heritage Products. Listerine (the original version) or a mouthwash that contains essential oils including eucalyptus and menthol (such as Tom's of Maine) will also work.

Hour 2: **Try a neti pot.** To further reduce germs and congestion, use a neti pot.

What to do: Add Alka-Thyme or Listerine (one-quarter teaspoon per pot) to four to six ounces of saline solution. Neti pots are sold in pharmacies and natural-medicine stores. Use a few times throughout the day.

Hour 3: **Use herbs.** Try the cold-fighting herbs echinacea, Oregon grape root, licorice, and ginger in liquid extract form, alone or combined.

Typical dose: 60 drops in total in one ounce of water, every three hours while awake and again in the middle of the night if you wake up. Use for no more than three days.

Hour 4: **Add a homeopathic remedy.** My two go-to cold remedies are gelsemium 30C (when you feel dull and tired, with heavy eyes and nasal or sinus congestion) and aconite 30C (when symptoms include chills, achy pain, dry eyes, and anxiousness). Choose the remedy that matches most of your symptoms and take two pellets, under the tongue, fifteen minutes before or after eating or drinking. Repeat four hours later.

Hour 5: **Consume soup and citrus.** During the first twelve hours of a cold, limit food to warm, salty, broth-based soups such as chicken with rice. Also have oranges or grapefruits and tea sweetened liberally with honey. This regimen provides electrolytes and vitamin C and helps keep the body hydrated. Avoid mucus-producing foods such as dairy and soy.

Hour 6: **Warm your body.** A hot bath can help kill a virus, and breathing in the steam of a bath or sauna reduces congestion. Ginger tea has antiviral properties and augments the warming process.

Hour 7: **Sleep.** Get in bed early, and sleep for nine full hours, if possible, to boost your immune system. These steps should also speed the healing of an existing cold.

....

› Jamison Starbuck, ND, naturopathic physician in family practice and a guest lecturer at the University of Montana, both in Missoula. She is past president of the American Association of Naturopathic Physicians. Starbuck is a columnist for the *Bottom Line Health Insider* and hosts *Dr. Starbuck's Health Tips for Kids* on Montana Public Radio. DrJamisonStarbuck.com.

....

Amazing Folk Remedies for Colds, Coughs, Flu, and More

Not every winter illness requires a trip to the doctor's office. The following time-tested folk remedies offer effective, inexpensive treatments for minor health complaints.

Important: Consult your doctor if your condition persists or grows worse.

COLDS

The average adult contracts between two and four colds each year, mostly between September and May. Medical science has no cure for these highly contagious viral infections, but the following folk remedies can help ward off colds, ease symptoms, and possibly shorten a cold's duration.

Garlic. Garlic contains allicin, which has been shown to reduce the severity of a cold. Eat four cloves of freshly crushed raw garlic three times a day until you have recovered.

Cinnamon, sage, and bay. Cinnamon contains compounds believed to reduce congestion. Sage can help sooth sore throats. Some Native American cultures have used bay leaves to clear breathing passages. Steep one-half teaspoon each of cinnamon and sage with a bay leaf in six ounces of hot water. Strain and add one tablespoon of lemon juice. Lemon helps reduce mucus buildup. If you like your tea sweet, add honey.

Chicken soup. The Mayo Clinic has said in its health newsletter that chicken soup can be an excellent treatment for head colds and other viral respiratory infections for which antibiotics are not helpful.

FLU

Influenza is a potentially serious viral infection. People often mistake colds for the flu. Colds take hold gradually and are not usually accompanied by severe aches or a fever. The onset of the flu is sudden, and symptoms include fever, severe muscle aches, and fatigue.

Garlic and cognac. A shot of cognac is a popular flu remedy in Germany, where it's thought to ease symptoms and help the body cleanse itself. Garlic helps clear mucus, among other potential benefits.

To prepare: Peel and dice a half-pound of garlic. Add one quart of 90-proof cognac, and seal the mixture in an airtight bottle. Store in a cool, dark place for two weeks. Strain out the garlic, and reseal the liquid in the bottle. Prepare a new batch each year.

To treat the flu: Add twenty drops to eight ounces of water. Drink three glasses a day, one before each meal.

For prevention: Use ten to fifteen drops, instead of twenty, per glass during flu season.

Important: This treatment is not advisable for people who have drinking problems or for children.

Sauerkraut. Sauerkraut's concentration of lactic acid bacteria may weaken infections. Have two tablespoons of sauerkraut juice or about one-half cup of sauerkraut each day during flu season to reduce the chances of infection.

SORE THROATS

Experiment with these remedies until you find what works best for you.

Apple cider vinegar. Vinegar is a powerful anti-inflammatory, and its acidity might help kill the bacteria that cause some sore throats. Add two teaspoons of apple cider vinegar to six ounces of warm water. Gargle with a mouthful, spit it out, then drink a mouthful. Continue this until the mixture is gone. Rinse your mouth with water to prevent the vinegar from eroding your teeth. Repeat the vinegar gargle every hour for as long as your sore throat persists.

Sage. Sage is an anti-inflammatory. Add one teaspoon of dried sage to one six-ounce cup of boiling water. Steep for three to five minutes, strain, then gargle and swallow.

Lemon and honey. Honey coats

the throat, while lemon can temporarily reduce the mucus buildup that often accompanies a sore throat. Squeeze one lemon, add a teaspoon of honey, and drink. Repeat every two hours.

Tongue stretching. Stick out your tongue for thirty seconds, relax it for a few seconds, then repeat four times. This is believed to increase blood flow to the throat, speeding the healing process.

COUGHS

Try these folk remedies to figure out which works best for you:

Lemon, honey, and olive oil. Honey and olive oil coat and soothe, while lemon reduces mucus. Heat one cup of honey, one-half cup of olive oil, and the juice of one lemon over a medium flame for five minutes. Turn off the heat, and stir for two minutes to blend the ingredients. Consume one teaspoon of the mixture every two hours.

Vinegar and cayenne pepper. Cayenne pepper contains capsaicin, a proven painkiller, while vinegar serves as an anti-inflammatory. Add a half cup of apple cider vinegar and one teaspoon of cayenne pepper to one-half cup of water. Add honey if desired. Take one tablespoon when your cough acts up and another tablespoon before bed.

Horseradish and honey. Horseradish can help loosen mucus, while honey coats the throat. Grate one teaspoon of fresh, peeled horseradish into two teaspoons of honey. Consume one teaspoon every two to three hours.

Ginger. Ginger is an anti-inflammatory that contains gingerols, which provide pain-reducing and sedative benefits. Chew a piece of fresh, peeled gingerroot when you feel the cough acting up, usually in the evening before bed. Chew until the ginger loses its kick.

Licorice-root tea. Licorice relieves the pain of irritated mucous membranes. Drink licorice-root tea as long as your cough persists.

Note: Don't try licorice root if you have high blood pressure or kidney problems.

> Joan Wilen and Lydia Wilen, health investigators and folk-remedy experts based in New York City who have spent decades collecting "cures from the cupboard." They are authors of *Bottom Line's Treasury of Home Remedies & Natural Cures, Bottom Line's Household Magic,* and *Bottom Line's Secret Food Cures.*

Drug-Free Solution to a Lingering Cough

A very common cause of a lingering cough is an upper respiratory infection that has come and gone. You and your doctor may run a gamut—and run up a huge medical bill—in search of an exotic, life-threatening cause of a die-hard cough that's really happening because cough-triggering nerves have become overly irritated and hypersensitive from that cold you had.

Nature's cure for an aggravating cough is honey, of course, but it still might not be a match for a cough that has lingered for weeks. It turns out that having some coffee with your honey (instead of the other way around) does the trick.

HOMEMADE COUGH RELIEF

A team of Iranian researchers ran across this seeming marvel when they compared a honey-coffee remedy with a steroid solution and an expectorant cough suppressant. They performed the comparison in ninety-seven adults whose cough had lingered for more than three weeks after a respiratory infection came and went. Smokers and any other potential study participants whose coughs could be diagnosed as something other than a persistent postinfectious cough were not allowed to participate in the study.

Participants were divided into three groups. One group received a "jam" made of honey and coffee (the honey-to-coffee ratio was about five parts honey to one part instant coffee). Another group received a jam containing the steroid prednisolone, which is sometimes prescribed to people with persistent cough, and the third group received a jam containing guaifenesin— the active ingredient in expectorants such as Mucinex and Robitussin. All three remedies were made by a pharmacist to look and taste the same by adding food coloring, coffee essence, artificial honey flavor, and liquid glucose to the products containing the steroid and expectorant.

The participants drank one table-spoon of their jam dissolved in about seven ounces of warm water three times per day (every eight hours) for a week. All the participants knew what remedies were being compared, but none knew which one he or she was taking. And they all agreed not to use any other anti-inflammatory drugs or cough suppressants or otherwise consume any honey or coffee during the study.

Results: The honey and coffee combo strongly beat out the steroid, with the combo reducing cough frequency by 93 percent compared with 20 percent for the steroid. And it obliterated the expectorant cough suppressant, which had virtually no effect on the frequency of persistent cough.

WORTH A TRY?

If a lingering cough that set in after a cold is driving you crazy, having some coffee with your honey (by mixing instant coffee granules with honey) might be worth a try. But this is definitely a remedy you shouldn't take several times a day before speaking to your doctor, since the short- and long-term adverse effects, such as effects on blood sugar levels, aren't known.

> Study titled "Honey Plus Coffee Versus Systemic Steroid in the Treatment of Persistent Post-infectious Cough: A Randomized Controlled Trial," published in *Primary Care Respiratory Journal.*

Don't Catch Pneumonia from Your Dentures

Could you be giving yourself pneumonia because of some innocent thing that you do each and every night? A study from Japan says that's exactly what may be happening to denture wearers around the globe. Here's what everyone who wears dentures needs to know.

WHAT NOT TO WEAR TO BED

The Japanese study included 524 men and women who ranged in age from 85 to 102. At the beginning of the study, each participant had a dental exam and a

face-to-face interview to answer questions about his or her general and oral health. The participants who wore dentures were also asked questions such as how and how often they cleaned their dentures. And they were asked if they wore their dentures to bed.

Over the course of the next three years, twenty of the participants died of pneumonia. Another twenty-eight were hospitalized with pneumonia but eventually recovered. When the researchers analyzed the data, they found that factors associated with increased risk of pneumonia included difficulty swallowing, cognitive impairment, whether the person had ever had a stroke or a serious or chronic respiratory disease, and *whether he or she wore dentures to bed.*

Sleeping with dentures was the *only* risk factor directly related to behavior. In fact, people who wore dentures to bed had *double* the risk of pneumonia of those who removed their dentures at night.

People who slept wearing dentures also tended to clean their dentures less frequently. As you can guess, bacteria can easily congregate on dentures. When it does, a bacterial film forms, similar to the layer of soap scum that accumulates in a bathtub that doesn't get cleaned. Eventually, the bacteria find their way from a person's mouth to the throat.

From there, the organisms can be inhaled (aspirated) into the lungs, and this is what the researchers think is happening among people who sleep wearing dentures. Bacteria inhaled in this way can result in aspiration pneumonia, pneumonia caused by breathing in particles of any type that enter the throat. Older people are much more vulnerable to aspiration pneumonia because their immune systems aren't as strong as those of younger people.

GOOD DENTURE HYGIENE AND SLEEP

But is the problem wearing dentures to sleep or wearing *dirty* dentures to sleep? Some American dentists think that overnight denture-wearing helps prevent sleep apnea because it helps keep the airways open. Rather than dentures though, the American Academy of Dental Sleep Medicine recommends that people with sleep apnea be fitted for an oral appliance specifically made to be worn at night and designed to prevent sleep apnea. You can find dentists certified in dental sleep medicine in your area through the academy.

If you wear dentures (full or partial) or know someone who does and are concerned about health risks of sleeping with dentures—or health risks of sleeping without them—talk to your dentist. Most

importantly, especially if you choose not to remove them while sleeping, make sure to keep them clean, as suggested in the Japanese study, by washing them daily in peroxide-based cleaner, such as Polident.

> Study titled "Denture Wearing During Sleep Doubles the Risk of Pneumonia in the Very Elderly," published in *Journal of Dental Research.*

Heal Pneumonia Faster with Osteopathic Manipulation

Pneumonia is a serious problem in the elderly. When hospitalized for it, they are there longer and also are at greater risk of dying from the illness compared with younger people. In a study of 306 pneumonia patients, researchers found that when osteopathic manipulative treatment (OMT) was added to the antibiotic therapy pneumonia is always treated with, it resulted in one full day reduction in the length of hospital stay.

THE STUDY

The patients were divided into three groups. Those receiving only conventional medical treatment (antibiotics) were hospitalized an average of 3.9 days, while patients who received conventional treatment plus OMT spent only 2.9 days (on average) in the hospital. A third group that received a placebo treatment of light touch and antibiotics was discharged in an average of 3.5 days. A provocative and intriguing finding was that patients aged seventy-five and older who received either OMT or light touch had no deaths, compared with a 9 percent death rate for those receiving antibiotics alone.

In the study, the OMT and light touch groups received two fifteen-minute treatment sessions daily, six hours apart. The OMT session consisted of standardized osteopathic treatment techniques designed to improve chest wall mobility and circulation, plus five minutes of nonstandardized treatment. The light touch treatments mimicked the OMT treatments but with only minimal movement of tissue, lymph flow, etc.

MOBILIZING THE IMMOBILE

Research has already established that when hospitalized patients are able to get out of bed and walk around, they recover faster. However, many elderly patients with pneumonia are too sick to get out of bed. Osteopathic manipulation can accomplish many of the same physiological benefits of early mobilization. It's a way to mobilize the immobile.

Osteopathic physicians treat various ailments by manipulating soft tissue and joints. For this study, the researchers used techniques designed to influence the respiratory system—for example, rib raising, which helps patients take deeper breaths and therefore relieves congestion. The techniques used in the study are gentle ones that older people can tolerate, similar to massage, but more focused and based on each patient's physical examination.

To find an osteopathic physician in your area, log onto www.osteopathic.org.

› Donald R. Noll, DO, internist and geriatrician in Stratford, New Jersey, and member of the faculty of Rowan University School of Osteopathic Medicine's New Jersey Institute for Successful Aging.

7

Digestion

Natural Ways to Improve Digestive Health

Gastrointestinal (GI) health is fundamental to overall wellness. The GI tract, also known as the gut, allows us to draw nourishment from our food and eliminate toxins. A variety of medications claim to promote intestinal health, but I prefer my own eight-step natural approach, which is both inexpensive and easy to follow. Add one new step each day. If you're like most people, your GI tract will be healthier within two weeks.

1. **Avoid foods that cause indigestion.** Indigestion is your body's way of telling you that a certain food is not readily digestible. Instead of trying to make a food digestible by taking drugs, choose foods that you can easily digest, such as fish, brown rice, and steamed vegetables.

2. **Shortly after awakening in the morning, drink an eight-ounce glass of room-temperature water.** This "wakes up" the GI tract, preparing you for both digestion and elimination. Repeat this step five to ten minutes before each meal. Avoid iced beverages, including water, with meals and fifteen minutes before and afterward. Some research suggests that cold beverages decrease the secretion of digestive enzymes.

3. **Squeeze fresh lemon or sprinkle vinegar on your food.** For most people, one-half teaspoon of lemon or vinegar per meal fights indigestion by increasing stomach acidity and improving the digestion of fats.

4. **Take a fifteen-minute walk after meals.** Doing so will improve your

digestion and elimination. If you can't do this after every meal, do so following the largest meal of the day.

5. **Practice simple home hydrotherapy.** This practice increases blood flow to your intestines, which helps them function properly.

    What to do: Finish your daily shower or bath with a thirty-second spray of cool or cold water to your entire abdomen. Towel dry with brisk strokes immediately after the cool water spray.

    Caution: If you have a history of stroke, check with your doctor before trying hydrotherapy.

6. **Drink chamomile or peppermint tea after dinner.** These herbs soothe the lining of the stomach and intestines. Add one tea bag or two teaspoons of loose herb to eight ounces of water.

7. **Use foot reflexology to relieve intestinal pain.** Massaging reflexology points on the feet is thought to help increase blood flow to and improve the function of corresponding organs or body parts.

    What to do: Whenever you have GI discomfort, firmly massage (for five to seven minutes) with your thumb and forefinger the outside portion of the middle one-third of the soles of the feet. According to reflexologists, this area corresponds to the colon. Your strokes should move toward the heel.

8. **Never eat when you are stressed.** Our bodies are not designed to simultaneously manage both stress and digestion. Studies show that just a few moments of relaxation, such as deep breathing or prayer, before a meal will improve the digestive process.

› Jamison Starbuck, ND, naturopathic physician in family practice and a guest lecturer at the University of Montana, both in Missoula. She is past president of the American Association of Naturopathic Physicians. Starbuck is a columnist for the *Bottom Line Health Insider* and hosts *Dr. Starbuck's Health Tips for Kids* on Montana Public Radio. DrJamisonStarbuck.com.

The Right Way to Chew (It's Not as Simple as You Think)

Mastication, or chewing, begins the digestive process and prepares food for swallowing. Front teeth cut and tear the food, and back teeth crush and grind it, increasing its surface area so that digestion of carbohydrates can begin. Here are some things to avoid when chewing.

Too little. Often the result of eating too fast, this can cause choking or pain upon swallowing. Additionally, heartburn or stomach pain can occur because saliva's digestive enzymes don't have time to work. And because gobbling food inhibits the release of hormones that tell you when you're full, you may overeat.

Solution: Start with smaller bites, and use your molars more—you should barely feel food going down when you swallow.

To slow down: Put your fork down between bites, and take a deep breath after each swallow.

Too long. Once a bite is ready to be swallowed, teeth should separate and not touch. Chewing past the point when the normal swallowing reflex occurs can overload jaw muscles, resulting in muscle pain and/or dysfunction. This is one reason why gum chewing—in which teeth touch during chewing—can lead to disorders of the temporomandibular joint (TMJ) or jaw joint.

On just one side of your mouth. If you have a full set of teeth and a normal diet, having a favorite side on which to chew—as many people do—is not a problem. But if you wear full dentures, food must be distributed during the chewing process from one side of the mouth to the other to maintain the dentures' stability.

Important: If you avoid chewing on one side because it is painful, see your dentist.

› Karyn Kahn, DDS, staff member of the Head and Neck Institute in the dentistry department and consultant for craniofacial pain and jaw dysfunction at Cleveland Clinic and associate professor at Case Western Reserve University School of Dentistry, both in Cleveland.

The Power of Enzymes for Better Digestion

Healthy digestion is at the core of wellness—the nutrients in your food fuel your body and help build strong defenses against illness. But what is the key to healthy digestion? Believe it or not, despite all those TV ads you see about heartburn pills that fight stomach acid, it's stomach acid that you really need for healthy digestion.

What makes having acid in your stomach a good thing? Many of your body's digestive enzymes won't work properly unless they're in an acidic environment, and if your enzymes aren't working well, your digestion isn't working well either.

ENZYME BASICS

Enzymes are natural chemicals manufactured by the body and present in many foods to make some kind of chemical reaction happen faster. Digestive enzymes work by breaking down the chemical bonds in your food and releasing the nutrients so you can absorb them. Without the enzymes, proper digestion doesn't happen. There are three major types:

+ **Proteolytic enzymes digest proteins.** The major proteolytic enzyme is pepsin, which breaks down the complex bonds in protein like a rock crusher.
+ **Lipolytic enzymes digest fats.** Lipase is a major enzyme in this category.
+ **Amylolytic enzymes digest carbohydrates.** Amylase, a major enzyme in this category, is primarily found in saliva, where it starts digesting as soon as you start chewing.

In your stomach, pepsin is the primary digestive enzyme. The others play a much bigger role later, when the food moves on to your small intestine. You make pepsin in your stomach lining, but it starts out in a preliminary form called pepsinogen.

The acid connection: Only when pepsinogen encounters sufficient stomach acid does it get converted to pepsin so it can do its job. Not enough acid in your stomach can prevent you from digesting protein, or anything else, well.

NOT ENOUGH STOMACH ACID

Another naturally occurring and vital substance in the stomach is hydrochloric acid. By the time most people hit age forty, they no longer make as much hydrochloric acid as they used to. By then, most people aren't making enough to trigger proper pepsin production, and digestion and nutrient absorption begin to suffer. Low stomach acid can lead to trouble with gas and heartburn from incomplete breakdown of protein and other nutrients in the stomach.

The B connection: Animal protein is most people's major dietary source of B vitamins. When you don't digest it well, the B vitamins aren't released to be absorbed, so you can start to run low on these vitamins. Serious consequences include anemia, poor healing, low resistance to illness, and memory problems that can even resemble dementia.

Stomach acid production continues to drop gradually with stress and as you get older, to the point where many elderly people produce far less than they need for good nutrition.

What can you do to restore a good level of stomach acidity? My recommendations fall into two areas—better eating habits and acid-producing supplements.

EATING AND ENZYMES

How and what you eat has a lot to do with how well you digest it. Some simple changes in the way you eat can have a big positive effect.

Chew more. Digestion begins in your mouth. Chewing coats your food with saliva, which contains carbohydrate-digesting amylase. Chewing also breaks your food down into smaller pieces that can be digested more thoroughly.

What to do: Chew your food thoroughly. Consciously spend a little time on each mouthful.

Bonus: You'll enjoy your food more and feel more satisfied by it, and you'll probably eat less. If you need to lose weight, this is a painless way to do it while improving your digestion at the same time.

Drink less. Cut back on the liquids you drink while consuming a meal. When you chase your bites with sips, you dilute the acid in your stomach and the enzymes themselves, which keeps them from working as well.

What to do: Limit the amount you drink during a meal. Skip sodas and drinks with caffeine. Sodas cause gassiness, and caffeine slows down your digestion of carbohydrates. Stick to plain water, well after you finish eating (wait at least a half hour).

Combine your foods carefully. Different foods need to spend different amounts of time in your stomach to be fully digested. Simple carbohydrates, such as bread, pasta, rice, potatoes, and sugary foods, are digested quickly. Complex carbohydrates, such as whole grains, beans, and nuts, as well as proteins and fats, take longer. When you combine simple carbs with these complex foods, your stomach can empty too slowly, promoting fermentation (and growth of yeast) from improper carbohydrate digestion.

What to do: Eat small amounts of simple carbs along with more complex foods. For example, have only a small portion of French fries along with a steak and salad. Skip prepared desserts completely. For a sweet treat, have fresh fruit—but fruit is sugary, so wait at least an hour after finishing your meal or eat it a half hour before.

ENZYME SUPPLEMENTS

Even with dietary changes, if you're older than age forty, you're probably not making enough stomach acid for good digestion and are likely to experience such symptoms as increased irregularity and intestinal gas. I often prescribe the following effective, safe supplements to help restore healthy stomach acid levels.

Betaine HCL. This generic supplement (available at health-food stores) works well to turn on the acid switch in your stomach. A 500-mg dose just before each meal is often prescribed.

DuoZyme. This combination supplement (available only through a health-care practitioner) contains betaine HCL, pepsin, and other enzymes that help increase stomach acid, combined with additional enzymes that help later in the digestive process.

Gastri-Gest. Another combination supplement but made with plant-derived enzymes, Gastri-Gest helps increase stomach acid and also helps in the later phase of digestion.

Digestive enzymes can be helpful to nearly anyone older than age forty, particularly those who experience acid stomach, mild nausea, gas, irregularity, and other digestive upsets. Often, betaine HCL is prescribed for a few weeks. If symptoms still persist, DuoZyme or Gastri-Gest may follow. Both can help, but some people respond better to one or the other.

Vegetarians and vegans will prefer Gastri-Gest, which doesn't contain animal products.

You'll probably need to take the supplements for a few weeks before you notice improvement. Digestive enzymes are generally very safe. But to avoid possible interactions, don't take them if you're taking an antibiotic or medication for an ulcer or other digestive problem, such as Crohn's disease. As with all medication, inform your doctor or other prescriber and follow his/her directions.

....

› Andrew L. Rubman, ND, medical director of Southbury Clinic for Traditional Medicines in Southbury, Connecticut. He is a founding member of the American Association of Naturopathic Physicians. His blog, *Nature Doc's Patient Diary*, is published on BottomLineInc.com. SouthburyClinic.com.

....

Natural Cures for Heartburn and Ulcers

Doctor, I have heartburn, but I don't want to take a prescription drug. What can I do?" Many people have asked me for such advice, especially since the media have publicized risks associated with popular heartburn and ulcer medications called proton pump inhibitors (PPIs). These drugs, including omeprazole, lansoprazole, and esomeprazole, offer short-term relief by reducing stomach acid, but they do not cure the underlying problem. Even worse, long-term use (more than a year) of PPIs increases risks for hip fracture (because of decreased mineral absorption) and the bacterial intestinal infection *Clostridium difficile* (because stomach acid is needed to fight bacteria). For my patients, I use a different approach that focuses on improving digestion and healing the lining of the stomach and the esophagus.

If you suffer from heartburn and/or have an ulcer, avoid any foods that may irritate your condition, such as fried foods, citrus, tomato-based foods, and spicy meals. Don't overeat. Large meals increase the demand for stomach acid. Chew thoroughly, and eat nothing within two hours of going to bed. Avoid smoking and pain relievers, such as aspirin or ibuprofen, that can cause gastrointestinal irritation.

Herbal tea also can be surprisingly effective for heartburn and ulcers. Chamomile and licorice root are two herbs with a long medicinal history for treating the digestive tract lining.* Drink three cups of either tea daily on an empty stomach. Use two teaspoons of dried plant or one teabag per eight ounces of water.

For heartburn (without ulcer), I suggest that you add stomach acid, which is necessary for good digestion, rather than reduce it with an acid blocker. At the end of your meal, sip on a four-ounce glass of water to which you have added one teaspoon of either apple cider vinegar or fresh lemon juice.

Caution: Do not drink vinegar or lemon water if you have an ulcer or gastritis (inflammation of the lining of the stomach). Discontinue this practice if it causes pain or worsens symptoms.

If you have an ulcer (with or without heartburn), I recommend adding other botanical medicines. The antiseptic herbs echinacea, cranesbill root, and Oregon grape root (50 mg each) help reduce bacteria associated with ulcers. The herbs cabbage leaf, marshmallow root, and slippery elm bark (200 mg each) help restore the gut's protective lining. Take these herbs three times daily on an empty stomach until the ulcer symptoms have eased, usually for two to eight weeks.

If you take a PPI but want to stop using it, gradually wean yourself off the drug while you add this protocol. Consult your doctor about your plan and schedule a follow-up visit in a month. You can review your condition and discuss what I hope will be good news about your progress.

HEARTBURN REDUCED

I advise patients to start with natural approaches, including sleeping on their left side (sleeping on the right side makes heartburn worse), avoiding trigger foods, such as onions and chocolate, and

---

* If you have high blood pressure, avoid licorice tea.

maintaining a healthy weight (excess weight makes stomach acid more likely to enter the esophagus and cause heartburn). Melatonin, a supplement that is often used for insomnia, also is effective for heartburn. A study published in the *Journal of Pharmacology* found that melatonin reduces the amount of acid produced in the stomach without blocking it altogether. This is important, because you need stomach acid for good digestion— you just don't want too much of it.

Dose: 3 to 6 mg, taken daily at bedtime.

> › Mark A. Stengler, NMD, naturopathic doctor and founder of the Stengler Center for Integrative Medicine in Encinitas, California. He is author and coauthor of numerous books, including *The Natural Physician's Healing Therapies* and *Bottom Line's Prescription for Natural Cures*, and is the author of the newsletter *Health Revelations*. MarkStengler.com.

Pectin for Heartburn Relief

For relief proven in clinical studies, try pectin, a substance found in the outer skin and rind of fruits and vegetables. Apples and bananas are among the best sources of pectin. If you suffer from heartburn, try eating an apple (do not choose green or other tart varieties) or a banana to see if it relieves your symptoms.

Pectin supplements, which are available at most health-food stores, are another option. Take at the onset of heartburn until it subsides. For dosage, follow label instructions. Pectin supplements are generally safe but may interfere with the absorption of some medications, so check with your doctor before trying them.

Caution: Chronic heartburn (more than twice a week) may indicate gastroesophageal reflux disease (GERD), a condition that should be treated by a gastroenterologist.

> › Ara DerMarderosian, PhD, professor emeritus of pharmacognosy (the study of natural products used in medicine) and Roth chair of natural products at the University of the Sciences in Philadelphia. He also is the scientific director of the university's Complementary and Alternative Medicines Institute.

Marshmallow Root for Heartburn

When acid from the stomach backs up into the esophagus, the result is often heartburn (a burning pain behind the breastbone).

Best herbal treatment: Marshmallow root. It coats and soothes the esophageal lining.

How to use: Make an infusion by

adding one heaping teaspoon of powdered marshmallow root to a cup of cold water and letting it sit at room temperature for twelve hours. Drink the entire mixture when heartburn occurs. If you get heartburn more than three times a week, drink one infusion in the morning and another at bedtime until the heartburn eases. If you make more than one cup in advance, you can refrigerate the unused portion for twenty-four hours.

Important: Do not use hot water. It will provide only about one-fourth of the soothing mucilage (lubricating substance) of a cold-water infusion.

› David Hoffmann, clinical medical herbalist based in Sonoma County, California, fellow of Britain's National Institute of Medical Herbalists, advisory board member of the American Botanical Council, and founding member and past president of the American Herbalists Guild. He teaches at the California School of Herbal Studies in Forestville, is a visiting faculty member at Bastyr University in Kenmore, Washington, and is the author of seventeen books, including *Herbal Prescriptions After 50.*

Sleep on Your Left Side

Sleeping on your right side worsens heartburn. People who sleep on their right side suffer reflux for longer periods than people who sleep on their left side. Left-side sleeping may keep the junction between the stomach and esophagus above the level of gastric acid, reducing heartburn symptoms.

Also helpful: If you have heartburn, sleep on an incline so that gravity helps keep stomach contents in place.

› Donald O. Castell, MD, professor, division of gastroenterology at Medical University of South Carolina, Charleston, and leader of two studies of acid reflux, published in the *Journal of Clinical Gastroenterology* and the *American Journal of Gastroenterology.*

Homeopathy for Indigestion

A *good remedy to keep in* your medicine cabinet is nux vomica. It effectively treats indigestion as well as constipation, especially when these uncomfortable problems are caused by overindulgence. When you experience symptoms, dissolve three 30C pellets of nux vomica under your tongue. If you do not feel better within forty-five minutes, repeat the dosage once or twice more. Do not exceed three doses in a day. Homeopathic remedies are sold at health-food stores and online.

› Edward Shalts, MD, DHt (diplomate in homeothera-peutics), private practitioner in New York City and author of two books, including *Easy Homeopathy: The 7 Essential Remedies You Need for Common Illness and First Aid*. HomeopathyNewYork.com.

Constipation: Why More Fiber Isn't Always the Answer

Constipation is one of those ailments that most people think they know how to treat. The majority believe that simply eating more fiber is the answer. But this often doesn't work.

What few people realize: Chronic constipation can have some very surprising causes, and dietary changes alone help only about one-third of those with the condition. What's more, if overused, some of the same laxatives that relieve constipation initially can exacerbate it in the long run, so most people need additional help to really get rid of their constipation.

WHAT'S NORMAL?

Most people have one to three bowel movements daily, while others have as few as three a week. This variability is normal.

What's more important are changes in bowel habits, particularly if you're having fewer bowel movements than usual and also are experiencing other symptoms that could indicate a more serious problem, such as blood in stool (colon cancer), unexplained weight loss (diabetes or colon cancer), or weight gain (low thyroid function).

The first step: Even though not all people with constipation will improve by eating a fiber-rich diet, it's still wise to start by eating more fruits, vegetables, legumes, and whole grains that are high in fiber. In general, people who consume 20 to 35 g of dietary fiber daily—and who exercise regularly—are less likely to suffer from constipation than those who mainly eat a meat-and-potatoes diet.

Examples of fiber sources: One cup of oatmeal or a bran muffin provides 4 to 5 g of fiber.

Helpful: Be sure to eat the vegetables and fruits that are most likely to draw water into the stool to facilitate soft, bulky bowel movements.

Best vegetables to ease constipation: Those in the brassica family, such as broccoli, asparagus, brussels sprouts, cauliflower, and cabbage.

Best fruits to ease constipation: Peaches, pears, cherries, and apples (or apple juice).

If your constipation doesn't improve within a few weeks, then try the following.

Check your medications. Many prescription and over-the-counter medications slow intestinal movements and cause constipation. Narcotic painkillers, such as oxycodone and the combination of acetaminophen and oxycodone, are among the worst offenders. Tricyclic antidepressants, such as amitriptyline, also can cause it. So can medications that treat high blood pressure (calcium channel blockers) and Parkinson's disease.

Helpful: Constipation also can be triggered by the antihistamines used in allergy medications, such as cetirizine (Zyrtec) and diphenhydramine (Benadryl), if used daily. Lowering the dose of an antihistamine drug or taking it less often may reduce constipation.

Get your magnesium and potassium levels tested. Most people get sufficient amounts of both minerals in their diets. But if you take a daily diuretic or laxative or have an intolerance to gluten (a protein found in wheat, barley, and rye), you may be deficient. Low magnesium or potassium decreases the strength of intestinal contractions—this may contribute to diarrhea or constipation.

Important: If constipation doesn't improve within a month of boosting your fiber intake, see your doctor. The problem could be due to a deficiency of either or both minerals. If a blood test shows that you have low magnesium and/or potassium, supplements can restore normal

levels within a week or two (ask your doctor for the appropriate dosage).

Be cautious with calcium. High-dose calcium often causes constipation, particularly in people who take antihistamines or other drugs that slow intestinal transit time (how long it takes food to pass through the bowel).

My advice: Get most of your calcium from calcium-rich foods. If your constipation is related to high-dose calcium supplements, talk to your doctor about limiting the supplement dose to 500 to 1,000 mg daily, and be sure to eat plenty of high-fiber foods and drink lots of fluids.

Drink at least two quarts of fluids daily—more if you exercise or engage in activities that cause you to perspire heavily.

Drinking this much fluid increases lubrication and makes stools larger, which helps them pass more easily (and frequently). Water is best—it has no calories and usually is the most readily available fluid.

Avoid laxatives. Some of the most popular products actually can increase constipation. So-called stimulant laxatives, such as Dulcolax and castor oil, cause the intestinal muscles to stretch and weaken with continued use. People who use these products frequently may become dependent—they can't have a bowel movement without them.

Important: It's fine to use these products occasionally—when, for example, you haven't had a bowel movement for several days and are feeling uncomfortable. But if you use them more than once or twice a week, it's too much. Talk to your doctor about healthier methods such as those described in this article.

Relax and reregulate. If you get enough fiber and drink enough fluids but still are constipated, see your doctor. You may have a type of constipation known as dyssynergic defecation (different parts of the anorectal area—pertaining to the anus and rectum—contract and relax at the wrong time).

This type of constipation can be diagnosed by giving patients oral radiopaque markers that allow the doctor to view intestinal movements on an abdominal X-ray. Normally, people initiate a bowel movement by instinctively contracting the upper part of the rectum while relaxing the lower part. People with dyssynergic defecation constipation often do the opposite. Stools aren't propelled through the colon, or they get hung up due to inappropriate muscle movements.

People with this type of constipation usually are referred to a gastroenterologist, who often uses biofeedback, along with exercises such as Kegels (a type of pelvic-muscle exercise), to help them learn to relax

and contract different parts of the anorectal area. They're also taught not to strain during bowel movements—this decreases the force of intestinal contractions and impairs one's ability to have a bowel movement.

> Norton J. Greenberger, MD, clinical professor of medicine at Harvard Medical School and senior physician at Brigham and Women's Hospital, both in Boston. He is a former president of the American Gastroenterological Association and coauthor, with Roanne Weisman, of *4 Weeks to Healthy Digestion: A Harvard Doctor's Proven Plan for Reducing Symptoms of Diarrhea, Constipation, Heartburn, and More.*

Homemade Tea Relieves Gas

G*as happens to everyone! But* if you despise stomach discomfort and you enjoy the company of others, gas is a good thing to get rid of. Here's an easy remedy from your kitchen.

Crumble up one-half teaspoon of dried bay leaves, and add to a six-ounce cup of just-boiled water. Let it steep for five minutes, then strain out the leaves, and drink the liquid slowly. You should feel relief before you finish your tea.

> Joan Wilen and Lydia Wilen, health investigators and folk-remedy experts based in New York City

who have spent decades collecting "cures from the cupboard." They are authors of *Bottom Line's Treasury of Home Remedies & Natural Cures*, *Bottom Line's Household Magic*, and *Bottom Line's Secret Food Cures*.

....

How to Never Have Another Hemorrhoid

Hemorrhoids are swollen veins, similar to varicose veins, in or around the anus or lower rectum. Often, they itch, bleed, and cause significant pain, especially when a blood clot forms and creates a hard lump. Anything that puts pressure on or strains the rectum can trigger hemorrhoids. Here are some tips for avoiding them.

Adopt an anticonstipation diet so that you won't have to strain to push out stool. Most importantly, get plenty of fiber, which softens and bulks up stool. Good sources include whole-grain breads and cereals, vegetables and fruits, and ground flaxseeds. Increase your fiber intake gradually so that you don't have problems with gas. Avoid or limit consumption of foods that contribute to constipation, such as those that are high in fat (cheeses, meats) or low in fiber (white rice, pasta, white bread).

Also: Drink at least six to eight glasses of water each day.

Check the side effects of your medications and supplements. Many commonly used drugs (such as statins and hypertension medications) and dietary supplements (including calcium and iron) can contribute to constipation. To find out if any of your drugs do this, check the labels and literature that come with the medications, then talk to your doctor about trying different drugs or natural alternatives. If constipation persists, take an over-the-counter stool softener, such as Colace, or a psyllium fiber supplement, such as Metamucil, following the instructions on the package, or lubricate stools by taking one to two tablespoons of flaxseed oil daily with meals.

Spend the right amount of time on the toilet. If you're in too big a hurry, you're likely to strain, so allow time for nature to take its course, if necessary. But if you sit there too long, that spread-open position puts extra pressure on the rectal area, so break the habit of reading or doing a crossword puzzle while on the toilet.

Go when the urge strikes. Many women resist the urge to go to the bathroom in a public restroom or at a friend's house, but suppressing a bowel movement can contribute to hemorrhoids by making the stool hard and dry and placing pressure on the anal opening. Remind yourself that a moment's self-consciousness is a small price to pay to prevent a real pain in the you-know-what.

....

> Richard C. Sheinbaum, MD, assistant clinical professor of medicine at Columbia University College of Physicians and Surgeons, New York City, and gastroenterologist in private practice in Stamford, Connecticut.

....

Heal Your Digestive Tract to Heal Your Inflammation

P*ain anywhere in the body* is almost always accompanied, and made worse, by inflammation. The inflammatory response, which includes the release of pain-causing chemicals, can persist in the body for decades, even when you don't have redness or other visible signs.

Common cause: A damaged mucosa in the innermost lining of the intestines. The damage can be caused by food sensitivities, a poor diet with too much sugar or processed foods, or a bacterial imbalance, among many other factors. A weakened mucosal lining can allow toxic molecules to enter the body, where they then trigger persistent inflammation.

If you suffer from chronic pain—particularly pain that's accompanied by intermittent bouts of constipation and/or diarrhea—your first step should be to heal the damaged intestinal tissue. Here are the best ways to do this.

Eat a variety of fermented foods. They are rich in probiotics, which will help the mucosa heal. Most people know that live-culture yogurt is a good source of probiotics, but yogurt alone doesn't supply enough. You can and should get more probiotics by eating one or more daily servings of fermented foods such as sauerkraut or kimchi (Asian pickled cabbage).

Because highly processed fermented foods—such as canned sauerkraut—will not give you the live probiotics you need, select a product that requires refrigeration even in the grocery store. You also can take a probiotic supplement, which is especially important for people who take antibiotics or who don't eat many fermented foods.

Cut way back on sugar. A high- or even moderate-sugar diet, which includes the simple sugars in refined carbohydrates such as bread and other baked goods as well as white rice, many breakfast cereals, and most juices, increases levels of cytokines, immune cells that cause inflammation.

Limit red meat. Red meat, especially the organic, grass-fed kind, does have valuable nutrients and can be part of a healthy diet. But eaten in excess (more than three ounces daily), red meat increases inflammation. If you eat more than the amount mentioned earlier, cut back. At least half of each meal should be foods grown in the ground—such as vegetables, nuts, and seeds. One-quarter should be whole grains, and the rest should be protein, which doesn't always mean animal protein. Other good protein sources include lentils, beans, and tempeh.

EAT OTHER FOODS THAT TURN OFF THE FIRE

Avoiding inflammatory foods is only half the equation. The other half, if you want to reduce pain, is to eat foods that can reduce the inflammation in your body.

If you are expecting an exotic recommendation here, sorry. What you really need to eat to reduce inflammation in your body is lots and lots of vegetables— raw, steamed, sautéed, baked, or roasted. Vegetables contain cellulose, a type of fiber that binds to fats and some inflammatory substances and carries them out of the body in the stools. The antioxidants in vegetables, such as the lycopene in tomatoes and the indole-3-carbinol in crucifers such as broccoli, cabbage, and brussels sprouts, further reduce inflammation.

This part of your pain-reduction strategy is pretty simple, really. There is not a vegetable on the planet that will worsen your pain, and most of them, if not all, will help reduce your pain. For easy, general dietary guidelines, just follow the well-known, traditional Mediterranean-style diet, which includes lots of vegetables, fish (fish oil is anti-inflammatory), small amounts of red meat, and olive oil.

Helpful: It's good to avoid sweets, but make an exception for an ounce or two of dark chocolate daily. Chocolate that contains at least 70 percent cocoa is very high in antioxidants. It reduces inflammation, improves brain circulation, and lowers blood pressure, according to research. And because it's a sweet treat, it will make it easier for you to say no to the nasty stuff like cake, cookies, and ice cream.

DON'T FORGET SPICES

Turmeric and ginger are great spices for pain relief and can replace salty and sugary flavor enhancers. Ginger tea is a delicious pain fighter. Also, garlic and onions are high in sulfur, which helps in healing.

COFFEE: YES...BUT

Even though some people can stop a migraine by drinking a cup of coffee when their symptoms first start, too much coffee (the amount varies from person to person) can have a negative effect on other types of pain. It increases the body's output of adrenaline, the stress hormone, as well as inflammation. It also masks fatigue, so you're more likely to push yourself too hard.

Do not drink more than one or two cups of coffee daily. Give it up for about a week once every three months to keep from getting addicted. Reducing coffee gradually over several days also helps prevent a caffeine-withdrawal headache.

....

› Heather Tick, MD, Gunn-Loke Endowed professor for integrative pain medicine, University of Washington, Seattle, where she is a clinical associate professor in the department of family medicine and the department of anesthesiology and pain medicine. She is author of *Holistic Pain Relief: Dr. Tick's Breakthrough Strategies to Manage and Eliminate Pain.*

....

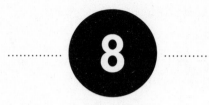

Eyes

Say Goodbye to Reading Glasses

When it comes to signs of aging, different people have different pet peeves. Some of us really don't like those gray hairs. Others sigh over a lost silhouette. Still others hate needing reading glasses to see what's on the menu.

Since exercise improves the strength, flexibility, and function of our bodies, it makes sense that eye exercises could improve our ability to see close up. Yet this is a controversial topic. Though various studies have found no clear benefit from eye exercises, many holistic practitioners and their patients say that vision can indeed be improved.

The challenge with aging eyes: Many people first become farsighted—meaning that nearby objects look blurry even though more distant objects are clear—starting in their forties. This is due to presbyopia, a condition in which the aging lens of the eye becomes too stiff to focus clearly up close.

Detractors of eye exercise say that it won't restore lens elasticity. But that's not the point. Eye exercises can improve the strength, flexibility, and adaptability of muscles that control eye movement and encourage a mental focus that helps the brain and eyes work better together. This can slow the progression of farsightedness and possibly improve vision.

So can eye exercises help us say good riddance to reading glasses? The answer is yes for some people—and it certainly can't hurt to try.

The following four exercises will help you improve close-up vision. While you do the exercises, remember to keep breathing and keep blinking. And smile! Smiling reduces tension, which helps your muscles work optimally and your brain focus on what's around you.

Try to do the exercises while not wearing any reading glasses—or if your close-up vision is not good enough for that, wear weaker reading glasses than you normally do. If you usually wear glasses or contacts for distance vision, it is OK to wear those while doing the exercises.

How long to practice: Do each exercise for three to four minutes, for a total practice time of about fifteen minutes per session, at least three times weekly. If you get headaches while exercising your eyes, reduce the time spent on each exercise, and see your eye doctor if the problem persists.

Letter reading: for better scanning accuracy and conscious eye control when reading or using a computer.

Preparation: Type up a chart with four rows of random letters, just large enough that you can read them while holding the page at a typical reading distance (type size will vary depending on an individual's vision). Leave space between each row. In row one, type all capitals, one space in between each letter; row two, all lowercase, one space in between each letter; row three, all lowercase, no spaces; row four, word-like groups of random letters arranged as if in a sentence.

Exercise: Hold the chart with both hands. Looking at row one, read each letter

aloud left to right, then right to left. Then read every second letter, then every third letter. If your mind wanders, start over.

Over time: When you master row one, try the same techniques with row two, then row three, then row four. If you find that you have memorized parts of the chart, make a new one using different letters.

Near and far: for improved focus and focusing speed when switching your gaze from close objects to distant objects (such as when checking gauges on a car as you drive).

Preparation: Type a chart with six to eight rows of random capital letters, each letter about one-half inch tall (or as tall as necessary for you to read them from ten feet away). Tack the chart to a wall and stand back ten feet.

Exercise: Hold a pencil horizontally, with its embossed letters facing you, about six inches from your nose (or as close as possible without it looking blurry). Read any letter on the pencil, then read any letter on the chart. Keep doing this, switching back and forth as fast as you can without letting the letters blur.

Over time: Do this with one eye covered, then the other.

Pencil pushups: to promote eye teamwork. All you need is a pencil.

Exercise: Hold a pencil horizontally at eye level twelve inches from your face (or as far as necessary to see the pencil clearly). With both eyes, look at one particular letter on the pencil. Keep looking while bringing the pencil closer to your face. If the letter blurs or doubles, it means that one eye is no longer accurately on target. Move the pencil back until the letter is clear once more, then try again to slowly bring the pencil closer while keeping the letter in focus.

The "hot dog": for improved flexibility of the muscles within the eye that allow the lens to change shape. No props are needed.

Exercise: With your hands at chest height about eight inches in front of you, point your index fingers and touch the tips together, so that your index fingers are horizontal. Gaze at any target in the distance and, without changing your focus, raise your fingers into your line of sight. Notice that a "mini hot dog" has appeared between the tips of your fingers. Still gazing at the distant object, pull your fingertips apart slightly, and observe that the hot dog is now floating in the air.

Keep the hot dog there for two breaths, then look directly at your fingers for two breaths, noticing that the hot dog disappears. Look again at the distant object, and find the hot dog once again. Continue switching your gaze back and forth every two breaths.

As your close-up vision improves, you may find that you need less-powerful reading glasses—or none at all—for your day-to-day activities.

› Marc Grossman, OD, LAc, holistic developmental/behavioral optometrist, licensed acupuncturist and medical director, Natural Eye Care, New Paltz, New York. He is coauthor of *Greater Vision: A Comprehensive Program for Physical, Emotional, and Spiritual Clarity* and *Natural Eye Care: An Encyclopedia.* NaturalEyeCare.com.

How to See Better in the Dark

Night vision has two elements. First, the pupils must dilate to let in as much light as possible. Normally, this happens within seconds of entering a darkened environment—but as we age, the muscles that control pupil dilation weaken, slowing down and/or limiting dilation. Second, chemical changes must occur in the light-sensitive photoreceptors (called rods and cones) of the retina at the back of the eyeball. Some of these changes take several minutes, and some take longer, so normally, full night vision is not achieved for about twenty minutes. Even brief exposure to bright light (such as oncoming headlights) reverses these chemical changes, so the processes must start over. With age, these chemical changes occur more slowly, and some of our photoreceptors may be lost.

While we cannot restore the eyes' full youthful function, we can take steps to preserve and even improve our ability to see in low light.

First, see your eye doctor to investigate possible underlying medical problems. Various eye disorders can cause or contribute to reduced night vision, including cataracts (clouding of the eye's lens), retinitis pigmentosa (a disease that damages the retina's rods and cones), and macular degeneration (in which objects in the center of the field of vision cannot be seen). Night vision also can be compromised by liver cirrhosis or the digestive disorder celiac disease, which can lead to deficiencies of eye-protecting nutrients, or diabetes, which can damage eye nerves and blood vessels. Diagnosing any underlying disorder is vital, because the sooner it is treated, the better the outcome is likely to be.

Adopt an eye-healthy diet. Eat foods rich in the vision-supporting nutrients below, and ask your doctor whether supplementation is right for you.

+ **Lutein,** a yellow pigment and antioxidant found in corn, dark leafy greens, egg yolks, kiwi fruit, oranges, and yellow squash.

  Typical supplement dosage: 6 mg daily.
+ **Vitamin A,** found in carrots, Chinese cabbage, dark leafy greens, pumpkin, sweet potatoes, and winter squash.

  Typical supplement dosage: 10,000 IU daily.
+ **Zeaxanthin,** a yellow pigment and antioxidant found in corn, egg yolks, kiwi fruit, orange peppers, and oranges.

  Typical supplement dosage: 300 micrograms daily.
+ **Zinc,** found in beans, beef, crab, duck, lamb, oat bran, oysters, ricotta cheese, turkey, and yogurt.

  Typical supplement dosage: 20 mg daily.

Update prescription lenses. Many people just keep wearing the same old glasses even though vision tends to change over time, so new glasses with the correct prescription often can improve night vision.

Keep eyeglasses and contacts clean. Smudges bend rays of light and distort what you see.

Wear sunglasses outdoors on sunny days, especially between noon and three p.m. This is particularly important for people with light-colored eyes, which are more vulnerable to the sun's damaging ultraviolet rays. Excessive sun exposure is a leading cause of eye disorders (such as cataracts) that can impair eyesight, including night vision. Amber or gray lenses are best for sunglasses, because they absorb light frequencies most evenly.

Do not use yellow-tinted lenses at night. These often are marketed as "night driving" glasses, implying that they sharpen contrast and reduce glare in low light. However, *any* tint only further impairs night vision.

Safest: If you wear prescription glasses, stick to untinted, clear lenses—but do ask your optometrist about adding an antireflective or antiglare coating.

Exercise your night vision. This won't speed up the eyes' process of adjusting to the dark but may encourage a mental focus that helps the brain and eyes work better together, thus improving your ability to perceive objects in a darkened environment.

What to do: For twenty minutes four times per week, go into a familiar room at night and turn off the lights. As your eyes are adjusting, look directly toward a specific object that you know is there. Focus on it, trying to make out its shape and details and to distinguish it from surrounding shadows. With practice, your visual perception should improve.

For an additional challenge, do the exercise outdoors at night, while looking at unfamiliar objects in a dark room, or while using peripheral vision rather than looking directly at an object.

When driving at night, avoid looking directly at oncoming headlights. Shifting your gaze slightly to the right of center minimizes the eye changes that would temporarily impair your night vision yet still allows you to see traffic.

Also: Use the night setting on rearview mirrors to reduce reflected glare.

Clean car windows and lights. When was the last time you used glass cleaner on the inside of your windshield or on rear and side windows or on headlights and taillights? For the clearest possible view and minimal distortion from smudges, keep all windows and lights squeaky clean.

....

› Marc Grossman, OD, LAc, holistic developmental/behavioral optometrist, licensed acupuncturist and medical director, Natural Eye Care, New Paltz, New York. He is coauthor of *Greater Vision: A Comprehensive Program for Physical, Emotional, and Spiritual Clarity* and *Natural Eye Care: An Encyclopedia.* NaturalEyeCare.com.

....

Nutrients That Reverse Cataracts

A*re cataracts no big deal?* Cataract surgery has become so quick and effective that many people now ignore opportunities to protect themselves from getting cataracts in the first place. They assume that their eyes can be made good as new one day with some simple surgery, so why worry about it now?

Please don't think that way. While cataract surgery has been well perfected, there is always potential for problems—including retinal detachment. There are very simple ways to ward off the cloudiness of cataracts.

Cataracts begin forming in the eyes shortly after you pass the age of fifty and currently affect some 22.3 million Americans. One of the keys to cataract prevention is a combination of diet and supplements that boost the body's level of glutathione, a powerful antioxidant that is distinguished by its ability to interfere with the development of cataracts.

Several studies show that glutathione can prevent the further formation of cataracts, and in my own experience, I've seen glutathione reverse the development of cataracts that have already formed. That's pretty extraordinary.

A CLOSER LOOK

To appreciate how glutathione works, it's important to understand how cataracts develop. The lenses in your eyes are made up of proteins arranged in a very orderly way so that light passes easily through them. But as we age—especially if we lapse into poor diets, smoke, drink too much alcohol, or develop diabetes or other chronic diseases—oxygen interacts with these proteins, creating highly reactive free radicals that cause the proteins to clump together. As they do, it becomes more difficult for light to pass through the lenses, and the result is cataracts and vision that's increasingly blurry.

Here's where antioxidants come into play. These substances can protect cells against the effects of free radicals. Vitamins A, C, and E are antioxidants that we all know about. Those that are somewhat less well known include beta-carotene, lutein, lycopene, and selenium. All these help to slow the development of cataracts, but when it comes to the eye lens, the most powerful antioxidant is glutathione.

If glutathione—which is made up of three amino acids (cysteine, glycine, glutamic acid)—were easy for the body to absorb, preventing cataracts would be a simple matter of taking regular supplements. Unfortunately, we have the opposite scenario—glutathione is far more difficult to absorb than the more familiar antioxidants.

The solution is twofold. First, eat foods that boost your body's ability to create glutathione, primarily in your liver. The list includes asparagus, eggs, broccoli, avocados, garlic, onions, cantaloupe, watermelon, spinach, and strawberries. However, it's doubtful that diet alone can raise glutathione to sufficient levels for preventing the formation of cataracts. You should also eliminate or at least reduce the amount of refined sugar in your diet (including milk sugar, which is found in dairy products) and take supplements, not of glutathione itself but of substances known to encourage production of the body's level of glutathione—N-acetylcysteine (NAC), alpha-lipoic acid, and vitamin C. Alpha-lipoic acid is particularly effective. You can buy it and NAC at some drugstores, many health-food outlets, and online.

NAC and alpha-lipoic acid are generally OK for everyone as long as the safe dosage is not exceeded—up to 300 mg for alpha-lipoic acid and up to 600 mg for NAC. However, it's best to talk to your doctor before taking either supplement, because they may lower thyroid hormone levels, adversely affect people with certain kidney conditions, as well as strengthen the effects of certain medications, including ACE inhibitors for high blood pressure and immunosuppressive drugs.

Ultraviolet light encourages the proteins in the lens to clump together. So in addition to increasing levels of glutathione by eating the foods above and taking supplements, be sure to wear quality sunglasses that block UV light and a wide-brimmed hat whenever you're out on a sunny day.

....

> Marc Grossman, OD, LAc, holistic developmental/behavioral optometrist, licensed acupuncturist and medical director, Natural Eye Care, New Paltz, New York. He is coauthor of *Greater Vision: A Comprehensive Program for Physical, Emotional, and Spiritual Clarity* and *Natural Eye Care: An Encyclopedia*. NaturalEyeCare.com.

....

Simple Steps to Avoid Age-Related Macular Degeneration Vision Loss

While *an advanced age and* a family history of the disease cannot be changed, there are many things you can do to prevent age-related macular degeneration (AMD) or slow its progression. Here are a few tips:

+ **Practice healthy lifestyle habits.**

Maintain normal blood pressure, watch your weight, exercise, and don't smoke.

+ **Eat a well-balanced diet** that includes lots of fruits and vegetables rich in nutrients known to protect against AMD—vitamins C (found in citrus fruits) and E (found in whole grains and wheat germ), lutein (found in dark, leafy green vegetables), zeaxanthin (found in yellow and orange fruits and vegetables), and zinc (found in dairy products, meat, whole grains). If your eating habits aren't what they ought to be, take an antioxidant supplement that contains the recommended dietary intake levels of these nutrients.

+ **Eat foods that contain omega-3 fatty acids** (salmon and sardines), which are also associated with a reduced risk of AMD.

+ **Limit intake of readily digested carbohydrates,** especially those that are high on the glycemic index, since these may increase the risk of developing AMD. Examples of foods to avoid include those containing high fructose corn sweeteners, as well as white breads, candy, and soda, which contain sugar.

+ **Protect your eyes from exposure to direct sunlight** by wearing sunglasses

and a wide-brimmed hat when you are outside, even on overcast days.

› Allen Taylor, PhD, professor, Friedman School of Nutrition Science and Policy, and senior scientist and director, Laboratory for Nutrition and Vision Research, Tufts University, Boston. Nutrition.Tufts.edu.

Supplements That Help Safeguard Sight for People with Retinitis Pigmentosa

Imagine how scary it would be, as a teen or young adult, to be told that you were slowly going blind. Now imagine how relieved you would be to learn that two common nutrients could help you hang onto your sight well into old age. Well, that is exactly what Harvard researchers discovered.

With retinitis pigmentosa (RP), the light-sensitive retina (which converts images to electrical signals and sends them via the optic nerve to the brain) slowly loses the ability to do its job. RP sufferers typically report night blindness in adolescence, loss of side vision in young adulthood, tunnel vision with advancing age, and in some cases, blindness by age sixty.

The study drew on data from earlier clinical trials in which RP patients took a supplement of vitamin A palmitate (*not* beta-carotene) at 15,000 IU daily for four to six years. They also filled out yearly questionnaires about their dietary habits. That initial research revealed that vitamin A supplementation helped to slow the rate of decline of retinal function across the whole retina, as shown by a test called an electroretinogram. For the newer study, the researchers further analyzed the data on 357 RP patients who were taking vitamin A to see whether their intake of omega-3 fatty acids had any effect on their disease.

Findings: Compared with RP patients who consumed less than 200 mg of omega-3s daily, those whose diets included 200 mg or more per day of omega-3s experienced a *40 percent slower* rate of decline in their distance central vision. The study authors also noted that, in their earlier research, the vitamin A/omega-3 combination helped preserve some side vision too.

Based on this evidence, the researchers made an encouraging projection. A typical RP patient who starts by age thirty-five to supplement with 15,000 IU per day of vitamin A palmitate and eats an omega-3-rich diet—for instance, one or two three-ounce servings per week of cold-water oily fish (such as salmon, mackerel, herring, tuna, or sardines)—could, on average, gain *eighteen additional years* of relatively preserved central vision. That would be enough to keep him/her seeing fairly well for most if not all of his life.

RP patients: Even if you're already older than thirty-five, it's worthwhile to talk to your ophthalmologist to see whether this nutritional treatment is safe and appropriate for you. Do not self-treat—researchers noted that this dose of vitamin A is not appropriate for children under age fifteen, people with liver disease, or women who are or plan to become pregnant.

> › The late Eliot L. Berson, MD, who was William F. Chatlos Professor of Ophthalmology, Harvard Medical School, and director, Berman-Gund Laboratory for the Study of Retinal Degenerations, Massachusetts Eye and Ear Infirmary, both in Boston, and lead author of a study on omega-3 fatty acids and vision loss published in *Archives of Ophthalmology*.

Natural Remedies for Dryness, Styes, "Computer Eye," and More

Best overall remedy: Eat fish high in omega-3 fatty acids, such as salmon, anchovies, mackerel, and herring. People who eat fish regularly produce less arachidonic acid, a substance that can lead to chronic inflammation and eye damage. Aim for two to three fish meals a week. If you are not a fish lover, take a fish oil supplement.

Here are some common eye problems and the best home treatments.

"COMPUTER EYE"

The average American spends up to seven hours each day looking at digital images on computers, TVs, etc.

Result: Eyes that are irritated and dry.

Studies show that we blink at only about one-third of the normal rate when using a computer or watching TV. This causes eye dryness and an increase in muscle tension. Prolonged sitting also reduces respiration and oxygen saturation in eye tissues.

Natural care: Practice the "three Bs." Blink more often, take deep breaths every minute or two to relax your eyes and your body, and take a break every twenty minutes. Look away from the TV or computer screen, and focus on various objects at varying distances for about twenty seconds—preferably while standing—to get your eyes moving more fluidly.

DRY-EYE SYNDROME

Dry-eye syndrome usually is due to a decline in the quality and quantity of tear film, the oily liquid that coats the eyes when you blink.

Natural care: Practice the "three Bs" described earlier.

Also helpful: An oral supplement called BioTears, which improves the quality of the tear film. It contains a blend of omega-3 and omega-6 fatty acids and other natural ingredients, such as vitamin E and curcumin. The use of preservative-free eyedrops, such as Tears Naturale Forte, also can help.

Important: Don't smoke. Cigarette smoke is a leading cause of dry-eye syndrome.

BLOODSHOT EYES

Redness typically occurs when blood vessels in the clear covering of the sclera, the white part of the eyes, dilate.

Main cause: Irritation from allergies, dust, and/or excessive sunlight.

Natural care: Take 250 mg of vitamin C, four times daily. It strengthens blood vessels and helps with the formation and maintenance of collagen in the cornea, the transparent dome that covers the iris and pupil.

I also advise patients to take a B-complex supplement. B-vitamin deficiencies have been linked to bloodshot eyes.

Important: Do not use over-the-counter eye whiteners, such as Visine. These products reduce redness by temporarily shrinking blood vessels. The next day, most patients experience a rebound phenomenon, in which the blood vessels dilate even more.

FLOATERS

These are the squiggles, dots, strands, and other shapes that drift in and out of your field of vision. They're the remnants of old, broken-down blood vessels that float in the vitreous, the transparent gel of the eye. Floaters also can occur when protein fibers in the gel clump together.

Floaters tend to get worse with age—not because they increase in number, but because the vitreous becomes more fluid and less gel-like. This allows the floaters to move more freely.

Natural care: An antioxidant-rich diet that includes fruits, vegetables (especially leafy greens), and whole grains. The antioxidants in these foods make the vitreous less watery.

Important: See an eye doctor if you notice a sudden increase in floaters or if floaters are accompanied by flashes of light. These additional symptoms could indicate inflammation of the retina or a retinal detachment.

BLEPHARITIS

This is an inflammation of the small glands and/or eyelash follicles on the surface of the eyelids. In addition to eyelid swelling, some patients may develop small sores. Also, some eyelashes may fall out.

Blepharitis that is accompanied by sores usually is caused by a bacterial infection. Other cases are caused by seborrheic dermatitis, a form of dandruff that also may affect the eyelids and eyebrows, along with the ears and the area around the nose and lips. Environmental irritants, such as allergens and smog, also can cause it.

Natural care: For blepharitis, apply a warm, moist washcloth to the eye. Keep it in place until it cools. Continue using compresses three or four times a day until the inflammation is gone. Heat and moisture increase circulation and the flow of nutrients to the eye. They also flush away inflammatory chemicals.

Also helpful: Use green or black tea to moisten the washcloth. The polyphenols in teas shrink swollen tissues and reduce inflammation.

If the condition doesn't improve in two to three days, see your doctor. Bacterial blepharitis can be treated with an over-the-counter antibiotic ointment such as Neosporin.

STYES

Caused by a bacterial infection in one of the tiny glands on the edges of the eyelids, a stye is a small pimple that can be painful as well as unsightly. Styes almost always clear up on their own within a week. Those that last longer (or that hurt a lot) may need to be drained by a doctor who also may prescribe antibiotics.

Natural care: Steam. Boil some water, and pour it into a cup. Close the affected eye, and bring it close to the cup to let the steam rise toward the stye. Be careful not to burn yourself. Repeat three or four times a day. Or you can apply warm, wet washcloths. These help bring the stye to a head.

Caution: Do not squeeze the stye or pop the head. It can spread bacteria to the eye.

There are over-the-counter remedies that can help, such as Similasan. Avoid any that contain mercuric oxide, which can irritate the eye.

CORNEAL ABRASIONS

A scratch on the cornea—usually caused by dust or other debris—can make the eye feel scratchy. Patients often have the sensation that something is stuck under the eyelid even when the debris is gone.

Most corneal abrasions heal within a few days. To relieve the pain, you can take aspirin (not acetaminophen, which does not help with inflammation). See your doctor if the discomfort is severe or doesn't get better within twenty-four to forty-eight hours.

Natural care: Any sterile saline

solution can help, and sleeping does too. Also, keep the area around the lids clean to reduce the chance of bacteria getting into the eye.

PTERYGIUM

This is a triangular-shaped growth that forms on the white of the eye—it usually is flat and yellowish with blood vessels going through it. People who spend a lot of time in the sun, such as farmers or surfers, tend to get it. Other risk factors include dust and living in a hot, dry climate. A pterygium (the *p* is silent) doesn't need to be removed unless it spreads onto the cornea and interferes with vision.

Natural care: Try to stay inside when the wind is blowing. Avoid smoky environments. Reducing environmental irritants can slow or stop further growth.

Also important: Always wear a brimmed hat when you're out on sunny days. Also, wear sunglasses that block 100 percent of UV radiation—close-fitting wraparound styles are best.

› Jeffrey R. Anshel, OD, optometrist and founder of Corporate Vision Consulting, Carlsbad, California. He is president and founding director of the Ocular Nutrition Society and author of *Smart Medicine for Your Eyes: A Guide to Natural, Effective and Safe Relief of Common Eye Disorders.* CVConsulting.com.

Caffeine: All-Natural Solution for Dry Eyes

Gritty, scratchy eyes that burn—that's the norm for the four million Americans who suffer from dry-eye syndrome. But research shows that a certain substance—high amounts of which are found in a very popular beverage—helps add moisture to dry eyes from the inside out. Here's what to sip on to find relief.

ONE STIMULATING SUBSTANCE

Earlier studies had shown that just 13 percent of caffeine users had dry eyes while 17 percent of people who didn't drink beverages containing caffeine suffered from the problem. So Japanese researchers set out to examine caffeine's impact on tear volume.

Dry-eye syndrome can vary greatly in severity, so to keep measurements standard, researchers decided to study healthy adults who did not have dry-eye syndrome. To prepare for the study, subjects did not have any caffeine for six days before each of the two test sessions. At the first test session, subjects randomly took either a placebo pill or a caffeine pill with the amount of caffeine depending on body weight. Six days later, at the second test session, subjects took the opposite. In each session, subjects didn't know which kind of pill they were taking. Researchers measured tear volume one hour and two hours after subjects consumed the caffeine and the placebo.

Findings: Tear volume was 30 percent higher, on average, after both one and two hours when subjects had ingested the caffeine versus the placebo. Future studies hopefully will explore how long this tear volume increase will last.

HOW MUCH CAFFEINE TO CONSUME

If you suffer from dry-eye syndrome, consider consuming caffeine each day while continuing to use whatever dry-eye treatment you normally use (such as eyedrops), and see if it helps. However, pregnant and nursing women, people with GERD, peptic ulcers, or heart conditions, and those using certain drugs and supplements, such as certain antidepressants, antipsychotics, anticoagulants, and muscle relaxants, should check with their doctors before consuming caffeine, because it could lead to unwanted side effects or adverse interactions.

How much caffeine? If you want to approximate the amount taken by the people in the study, follow these guidelines. If you weigh:

- 90 pounds or less, 200 mg of caffeine per day.
- 91 to 128 pounds, 300 mg of caffeine per day.
- 129 to 165 pounds, 400 mg of caffeine per day.
- 166 to 205 pounds, 500 mg of caffeine per day.
- 206 pounds or more, 600 mg of caffeine per day.

You can take caffeine in pill form. Caffeine is also, as you know, easy to get through many beverages. Just remember that amounts vary depending on the brand and/or how the drink is made. Coffee, of course, is king with 95 to 200 mg per eight-ounce cup. But you can also drink black tea (14 to 61 mg per eight-ounce cup) or green tea (24 to 40 mg per eight-ounce cup), for example. Plenty of other foods and beverages contain caffeine, such as soda, iced tea, energy drinks, and chocolate, but they can be loaded with sugar and calories.

Study subjects took their designated caffeine amounts all at once rather than spacing it out, but see what makes your peepers feel best. Since it's unclear exactly how long the effect might last, you may want to time your consumption around day-to-day activities that heavily involve your eyes. For instance, have it an hour or two before completing a major computer task or watching a movie.

If the caffeine causes insomnia, try consuming it before midafternoon. If that doesn't help, or if it gives you the jitters or makes you overly anxious, then the benefits might not outweigh the side effects. Keep in mind that everybody responds to caffeine differently—one person might feel shaky after half a cup of coffee, while another might need five cups to feel alert throughout the day.

Whether you choose to consume caffeine or not, remember that dry-eye syndrome can lead to serious health problems, such as impaired vision or infection. So ask your ophthalmologist how often you should make appointments to keep tabs on the condition of your eyes.

› Reiko Arita, MD, PhD, clinical researcher, department of ophthalmology, University of Tokyo School of Medicine, Japan. Her study was published in *Ophthalmology*.

Quick Fixes for Eye Ailments

PINK EYE

Here's a quick fix for pink eye, worth trying before calling your doctor. Place your thumb and index finger just below the bridge of the nose, where the pads of eyeglasses would rest. Gently massage the area. Then soak a clean washcloth in warm water, wring it out, and place it over one eye for ten minutes. Repeat with the other eye. Do this three or four times a day.

These steps can unblock tear ducts so that the body clears up a minor infection itself. Results should be noticeable within a few hours. If the condition does not improve by then, call your doctor.

> Ken Haller, Jr., MD, associate professor of pediatrics, Saint Louis University School of Medicine, St. Louis.

PUFFY EYES

If you slept in after a night of tossing and turning (or too much late-night partying), your eyes might look like fat little balloons. You probably don't have a whole hour to let them deflate before the day begins, so here's what to do.

Wet two chamomile tea bags with tepid water (you don't need to steep in boiling water), and place one on each of your closed eyelids. Relax that way for fifteen minutes. Whistle or talk to yourself to keep from falling back to sleep!

> Joan Wilen and Lydia Wilen, health investigators and folk-remedy experts based in New York City who have spent decades collecting "cures from

the cupboard." They are authors of *Bottom Line's Treasury of Home Remedies & Natural Cures, Bottom Line's Household Magic,* and *Bottom Line's Secret Food Cures.*

ITCHY, SORE, AND TIRED EYES

Congratulations! You finished that project at work that made you look at the computer screen for hours on end. But now your eyes are itchy, sore, and just plain tired. Here's a quick fix that will help your whole body relax.

Cut two thin slices of a raw red potato, and place them on your closed eyelids for at least twenty minutes. Red potatoes have a kicked-up portion of anti-inflammatory properties, but other potatoes will make your eyes feel better too.

> Joan Wilen and Lydia Wilen, health investigators and folk-remedy experts based in New York City who have spent decades collecting "cures from the cupboard." They are authors of *Bottom Line's Treasury of Home Remedies & Natural Cures, Bottom Line's Household Magic,* and *Bottom Line's Secret Food Cures.*

How to Stop an Annoying Eyelid Twitch

There can be many *different* reasons for eyelid twitches, and the way to get them to stop is to address the actual cause. In some rare cases, an eyelid twitch could be a sign of an underlying condition, such as multiple sclerosis, Parkinson's disease, or Sjögren's syndrome, an autoimmune disorder that causes dryness throughout the body and destroys tear glands.

It is also possible to get twitching from everyday dry eyes, pink eye, or as a side effect from medication, such as antihistamines, some antidepressants, and epilepsy drugs.

However, too much stress is the biggest cause of eyelid twitching. Coming up with a plan to address the factors contributing to stress is key. Some great stress-reducing tools include meditation, acupuncture, and regular exercise. You may also need to get more sleep and/or cut down on alcohol and caffeine.

Magnesium citrate can help with eyelid twitches too. I usually recommend a 150-mg magnesium citrate supplement taken once or twice a day for two to four weeks. (Check first with your doctor if you have heart or kidney disease or take medication.) Magnesium will help relax muscles while you treat the underlying cause of the twitching. Magnesium deficiency itself can also lead to eyelid twitching.

Consult your doctor if the twitching persists.

› Samantha Brody, ND, LAc, naturopathic physician, licensed acupuncturist, and founder, Evergreen Health Center, Portland, Oregon. DrSamantha.com.

Feet

Strengthen Feet to Reduce Pain and Stiffness

Our poor feet just don't get what they need to be healthy and happy. And you know who pays the price, don't you? Modern life is hard on our feet. An astonishing 25 percent of the body's bones are in the feet, and every one of them has a job to do.

We actually weaken our feet by wearing shoes. Encasing them this way diminishes their natural strength and abilities.

Walking on artificially flat surfaces does further damage, since the foot is deprived of the natural workout it is supposed to get from varying natural terrain. The result of all this is that we're no longer really using our feet. By midlife, most of us have lost not only muscle strength, but also the fine motor skills that our feet need to properly support us. We end up using the ankle muscles instead, and in a vicious cycle, this further weakens foot muscles.

TEST YOUR FEET

Here is an easy way to test your foot muscle strength. Try to raise your big toe, by itself, and then the second toe with it. It sounds easier than it is—few are able to do more than lift the big toe slightly off the floor. When the foot is being used properly, however, all toes should retain their ability to move independently from the other four.

WALK THIS WAY

Foot problems start in your feet. Your posture and style of walking play a role too. You may never have noticed it, but if you are like many folks, you're likely walking with your feet slightly turned out, duck-fashion. This interferes with how the muscles and ligaments in the feet, knees, and hips are supposed to work. Your feet should point straight ahead in the direction you are walking.

Try this: Find straight lines on the floor (a tile joint or wood slat works well), and line up the outside edges of both feet. Keeping that alignment, walk forward. As you try to adapt to this new gait, you may initially feel like you've become pigeon-toed and knock-kneed, but if you stay with it, you'll soon notice how your hips are engaged and rotating smoothly. It all feels quite facile and natural.

STRAIGHTEN UP

When standing and walking, many people tuck their pelvises under, creating weak abdominal muscles. Wearing elevated heels (men's shoes too) further amplifies this effect. Coupled with the turned-out duck-walking style, this posture puts too much weight on the front of the feet, which is what creates bunions. Instead, the weight should be back over the heels and spread among four contact points.

Try this: Picture your foot as a rectangle with four corners. Now consciously distribute your weight equally to the inside of the heel, the outside of the heel, the ball of the foot, and just below the pinkie toe.

Here's an exercise that can help you identify a forward-thrusting pelvis and poor weight placement. Stand barefoot and move your hips back until they are over your ankles. When you do this correctly, you should be able to lift all ten toes off the floor. Do this near a chair or wall in case you need support. Once you learn what this centered position feels like, try to achieve it regularly.

WHAT TO WEAR?

I advise walking shoeless often. When footwear is required, select heels that are as flat as possible. An elevation of even an inch or so puts too much weight on the ball of the foot—it's like walking downhill. In fact, I recommend shoes that draw your weight back, onto the heels. Arch supports may be helpful for people with very high or very low arches, but regular use weakens foot muscles.

I am ardently against flip-flops—they force the wearer to scrunch the toes, which can cause hammer toes and also makes proper weight distribution (those four proper contact points) impossible. Neither do I favor the new types of workout shoes that rock the foot and purposely throw off the body's balance to make leg muscles work harder—including FitFlops and MBTs. The shape of the sole creates an unnatural gait pattern that can harm the feet, knees, hips, and spine.

You can probably imagine how I feel

about high heels. For dress-up occasions, I suggest women bring heels to put on at the last minute. If you wear them regularly, visit the chiropractor or a naturopathic physician to get some special attention for your feet and sacroiliac joints, which will help to minimize the damage.

EASY STEPS TO FEEL-GOOD FEET

The real path to pain-free feet, however, involves giving them tender, loving care in the form of regular exercises that stretch, balance, and strengthen their muscles, tendons, and ligaments. Start by simply spreading and lifting your toes as often as possible. Here are some other easy exercises:

- **Toe lifts.** While standing, lift your big toe alone, followed in succession by each of the remaining toes. Repeat in the opposite direction, big toe last.
- **Toe tucks.** Stand with one foot flat on the floor and the other pointed slightly behind you, toes tucked under so that the tops of your toes are resting on the floor. This stretches your upper foot. (This won't be easy or comfortable at first.)
- **Arch support.** Stand erect, shift your weight to the outside of one of your soles, and lift that foot's ball and toes. Slowly lower the ball of the foot without letting your arch

collapse, and then relax your toes back to the ground.
- **Toe spacers.** Available at nail-care salons, online, and in many stores, they fit between your toes and spread them. They may feel odd at first but then are soothing. If you use them fairly often, such as while reading or watching TV, your toes will eventually relearn their normal spreading motion.
- **Barefoot walking.** Do this as often as you can.

Here are some fast fixes for feet that hurt:

- **For instant relief of aching feet, run your foot repeatedly over a tennis ball.** Start while you are in a seated position, and then slowly stand, increasing the weight on your foot.
- **Elevating tired, sore feet feels great,** as does wrapping them in a warm, wet towel.
- **A gentle foot massage** or a session with a well-trained reflexologist does wonders for the heart and sole.

....

> Katy Bowman, MS, director, Restorative Exercise Institute, Ventura, California. RestorativeExercise.com.

....

Strengthen Your Ankles

I*t's best to keep your* ankles strong and flexible so you can avoid problems such as ankle arthritis and sprains.

Try doing "alphabet" exercises at least three times a week. Pretend you are holding a pen between your first and second toe. Using only your foot, not the entire leg, draw the letters of the alphabet in the air, making exaggerated motions.

This takes only a few minutes, you can do it at your desk or while watching TV, and you can have fun with it, writing in script, in print, with great flourish, and other ways you can think of to change your "handwriting" while also strengthening your ankle joints.

› David I. Zaret, MD, orthopedic surgeon in Long Island, New York.

How to Choose the Right Athletic Shoes

W*hen you work out or* play a sport, your shoes affect your performance—and your risk for injury.

Key: Choose sport-specific footwear.

Examples: Tennis shoes have side support and flexible soles for fast changes in direction, running shoes give maximum shock absorption, and walking shoes need low heels that bevel inward so feet roll easily through the stride. Here are some additional tips:

* **Learn your foot type.** Ask a podiatrist or athletic trainer or visit a shoe store that offers computerized foot-type analysis.

   Wide feet: A too-narrow shoe leads to shin splints, so if even wide-size women's shoes feel tight, try men's shoes.

   High arches: Look for a shoe with a thick, shock-absorbent heel, such as a gel heel or air bladder.

   For feet that roll inward: You need a deep heel cup and wide midfoot base.

   For feet that roll outward: Choose a somewhat rigid shoe.

* **Check a shoe's flexibility by bending and twisting it.** It's too flexible (and thus can lead to ankle sprains) if it bends at midsole instead of the ball, flattens at the heel cup, or wraps like a towel when twisted. A shoe that's hard to bend or twist is too rigid (except for cycling) and may cause shin splints.

* **Know when to purchase a new pair.** Wear and tear affect a shoe's ability to support and protect. Replace sports shoes after they've taken about five hundred miles' worth of steps. If you're

a walker or runner, that's easy to calculate. Otherwise, replace shoes when treads and heels are visibly worn.

› Vahan Agbabian, clinical instructor and rehabilitation specialist, MedSport sports medicine program, University of Michigan Health System, Ann Arbor.

DIY Achilles Tendonitis Relief

Even though the Achilles tendon, located in the back of the heel, is the strongest and largest in the body, it's still among the most vulnerable, and when it hurts, it can hurt a lot. Symptoms include pain above the heel or in the back of the leg.

Inflammation of the tendon, known as Achilles tendonitis, usually is due to overuse. The tendon gets weaker and susceptible to injuries with age. If you overwork the tendon—say, by spending a few hours on the dance floor or the basketball court—the fibers can develop small tears and get inflamed. It typically takes at least three months for it to heal completely. In the meantime, don't engage in high-impact exercises such as running, and switch to low-impact activities such as biking or swimming. Here are some more tips:

- **Start with ice.** Ice is one of the best ways to reduce inflammation and help the tendon heal. When you first feel pain at the back of the heel, apply an ice pack for up to twenty minutes. Keep applying ice throughout the day, and keep the heel elevated as much as possible for a few days. You can further reduce inflammation by taking aspirin or ibuprofen.

- **Try heel lifts.** These are thin wedges that slip into your shoes. Raising the heel as little as one-eighth of an inch reduces stress and helps the tendon heal quicker. Use lifts in both shoes so that your body is balanced. I like Spenco RX Heel Cushions and AliMed Heel Lifts. Both are available online and in pharmacies and some stores.

Important: If you can't stand up on your toes even for a second, there's a good chance that the tendon has ruptured (completely torn). Surgery is the only treatment for a ruptured Achilles tendon.

› Johanna S. Youner, DPM, podiatrist and cosmetic foot surgeon in private practice and attending physician at New York Downtown Hospital, both in New York City. She is a spokesperson for the American Podiatric Medical Association, a delegate of the New York State Podiatric Medical Association, and a fellow of the American College of Foot and Ankle Surgeons. HealthyFeetNY.net.

Surprising Fixes for Bunions

A bunion is a bony bump that develops over the joint at the base of your big toe. Too-tight shoes are commonly the culprit, but bunions may also be inherited or can occur if you have arthritis.

Besides causing pain, bunions can create tingling from nerve compression. Orthotics and ice can help alleviate pain, and steroid injections can ease joint inflammation. But these treatments won't get rid of the bunion. If you do opt for surgery, a bunionectomy can be effective (a small incision is made so that the bunion can be removed and the big toe straightened). Most individuals are back on their feet within three days, but full recovery can take up to eight weeks. Swelling may last for six months.

Surprising fix: Before resorting to surgery, start by loosening your shoelaces and/or buying slightly larger shoes. Your bunion may be taking up space in your shoes and compressing the nerves.

To ease pain in the big-toe joint, bunion sufferers should wear rigid shoes that provide extra support to the painful joint. (When shopping for a shoe, try to twist the sole. If you can twist it, put it back.)

Good brands for men: Rockport Dressports, Ecco, and Allen Edmonds.

Good brands for women: Munro, Ariat, and BeautiFeel. Avoid flip-flops—they provide no support, which worsens bunions.

In addition, consider wearing a night splint (available at drugstores and online), which can help stretch and straighten the joint.

Good product: The PediFix Nighttime Bunion Regulator.

....

› Johanna S. Youner, DPM, podiatrist and cosmetic foot surgeon in private practice and attending physician at New York Downtown Hospital, both in New York City. She is a spokesperson for the American Podiatric Medical Association, a delegate of the New York State Podiatric Medical Association, and a fellow of the American College of Foot and Ankle Surgeons. HealthyFeetNY.net.

....

Foot Cramp Relief

One minute, you're fine, and the next, yelp! You have a cramp in your foot that's so painful, you don't know what to do with yourself. (If you're like me, you start hopping up and down on it in hopes of making it stop!) Sometimes foot cramps can wake you when you're asleep or even strike in the middle of a workout. They can also occur when you're just sitting—for instance, when driving or simply relaxing on the couch. No matter when they happen, they disrupt whatever you're doing.

Fortunately, there are several things you can do to ease a foot cramp when it's happening, and a few natural solutions can help to prevent them too (if you get them regularly).

A foot cramp is a sudden contraction of a muscle or muscles. This sudden contraction or spasm causes the pain. Several things can cause your feet to cramp up, including dehydration or a dietary imbalance. Even a bad case of anxiety, which leads to shallow breathing and a reduction in oxygen going to the muscles, can cause cramping.

WHAT TO DO IN THE MIDDLE OF A CRAMP

Give your foot a massage. For many people, the first reaction to a foot cramp is to massage the area of the foot that is cramping. This is smart!

You can use a hard or soft touch, whatever works best for you. You also might want to try doing acupressure—namely, pressing with your fingers on one of three points that correspond to your feet. These acupressure points include the spot between your upper lip and nose, the base of your calf muscle (on the leg where you have the cramp), and the top of the foot between the big toe and second toe (on the foot where you have the cramp). Press firmly on any of these spots and hold for one minute, then release. If the first point doesn't provide relief, try the others.

Stretch and flex. When a foot cramp strikes, try doing a stretching exercise. With your leg extended in front of you (either in a sitting or standing position), point the toes up to the sky and then straight ahead. Do this movement for about a minute. It helps to get blood flowing to ease the cramp.

Apply a heating pad. Put a heating pad on your foot where the cramp is. Make it comfortably warm but never so hot that you might burn yourself. In most cases, the pain will disappear in a few minutes, although it's best to hold the pad on the foot for ten minutes to be sure it's gone. If the pain doesn't subside after ten minutes, remove the heating pad and wait twenty minutes, then apply it again.

Drink apple cider vinegar or pickle juice or eat mustard. These foods contain vinegar, which consists of acetic acid. This acid helps the body make acetylcholine, which is a neurotransmitter that helps our muscles work. The more acetylcholine you have, the better your muscles function. Try dissolving two teaspoons of apple cider vinegar in honey, or consume about three teaspoons of pickle juice or mustard (any type). These vinegar remedies work so well that athletes are known to pick up mustard packets from fast-food restaurants in order to get fast relief from cramps.

Sip some tea. If stress and anxiety are causing your foot to cramp, drinking a cup of chamomile tea, which relaxes the body, can help. Another option is cramp bark tea, which is available at health-food stores. It contains valeric acid, a muscle relaxant, and is known to relieve cramps of all kinds.

Take Magnesia phosphorica. This homeopathic remedy contains magnesium, a mineral that helps relax muscles. Have the remedy on hand so that you can take it when the cramp occurs. Follow label instructions.

HOW TO PREVENT CRAMPS (IF YOU GET THEM REGULARLY)

Drink tonic water. *This common* carbonated beverage contains quinine, which is known to be a muscle relaxant. People who are prone to foot cramps can drink one twelve-ounce can or bottle of tonic water daily to prevent cramping. Tonic water contains only small amounts of quinine, but quinine can interact with medications. Check with your doctor first before using tonic water regularly.

Eat bananas. An imbalance of electrolytes, either because of excessive sweating or a dietary imbalance, can affect your muscle function. Getting too little potassium or too much sodium can make you vulnerable to cramps. To help bring electrolytes into balance, try eating a banana every day. Bananas contain potassium, which can help offset excess sodium.

Drink up. Dehydration is a common cause of cramps of any kind. You can become dehydrated if you consume too much sodium or sweat a lot. Increase the amount of water you drink daily—aim for eight eight-ounce glasses. If you have trouble downing that much plain water, increase your intake by jazzing up your water with slices of fruit, or drink herbal tea—that counts too!

› Johanna S. Youner, DPM, podiatrist and cosmetic foot surgeon in private practice and attending physician at New York Downtown Hospital, both in New York City. She is a spokesperson for the American Podiatric Medical Association, a delegate of the New York State Podiatric Medical Association, and a fellow of the American College of Foot and Ankle Surgeons. HealthyFeetNY.net.

Fixing Hammertoes

With this condition, one of your toes becomes permanently bent at the middle joint due to pressure on the toes' muscles and ligaments.

Hammertoes are mainly caused by shoes with a low toe box in which the toe joint presses into the top of the shoe. Arthritis, toe injuries, and a family history of hammertoes also increase risk. Traditional treatments include padding the hammertoe with a silicone or gel pad.

Stretching exercises also may be useful.

What to do: Take hold of the tip of the toe and gently pull it out straight. Hold for five seconds. Repeat the exercise three times a day.

If these measures are not effective, a surgeon can make a small incision to straighten the tendon associated with the hammertoe and/or remove some of the affected bone.

Surprising fix: It sounds obvious, but the best solution is to look for a shoe with a roomy toe box and a heel of an inch to an inch-and-a-half—the range that supports your foot's natural curve. Contrary to what many people think, flats and very low heels do not give the most natural foot position.

If wearing different shoes doesn't give you adequate relief, an injection of a hyaluronic acid gel filler commonly used to help smooth wrinkles, such as Juvéderm Ultra 4 or Restylane, works well for reducing the pain of a hammertoe.

What happens: This ten-minute office procedure begins with an injection of lidocaine to numb the affected area. An injection of hyaluronic acid is then administered at the bony top of the bent toe. Hyaluronic acid for hammertoes is not covered by insurance—treatment for one hammertoe usually requires one syringe, which costs $700 to $1,000. The effect generally lasts for six to nine months.

> Johanna S. Youner, DPM, podiatrist and cosmetic foot surgeon in private practice and attending physician at New York Downtown Hospital, both in New York City. She is a spokesperson for the American Podiatric Medical Association, a delegate of the New York State Podiatric Medical Association, and a fellow of the American College of Foot and Ankle Surgeons. HealthyFeetNY.net.

How to Treat Swollen Feet

Are your feet swollen? Are your ankles puffy? Here's some information about when it's normal, when it's not, and what to do about it.

What happens: Your body usually maintains a precise fluid balance. It holds on to fluids when you need them, and it excretes fluids when you have too much. Anything that disrupts this balance can cause fluids to accumulate.

The fluids usually go downhill. Fluid in the feet or lower legs has to push its way upward, against gravity. If your veins aren't as robust as they should be or if you're sedentary and your leg muscles aren't flexing against the veins, the fluid tends to pool and cause swelling. This is called peripheral edema.

Self-test: Press a finger on your foot/ankle. If the area stays indented for more than a few seconds, you probably have some degree of peripheral edema.

A dangerous sign: Mild swelling that comes and goes usually is harmless. But see your doctor if you have swelling much of the time, especially if you also have shortness of breath or high blood pressure. Swelling can be caused by heart or kidney damage, liver problems, or damage to the veins.

Red flag: Painful swelling that occurs in one leg, foot, or ankle. It's a classic sign of a blood clot. A clot that forms in one of the deep veins in the legs, a condition known as deep-vein thrombosis, is potentially deadly. Get to an emergency room immediately.

Here are some of the common causes of swelling:

+ **Too much salt.** Your body has a natural defense against excessive salt—it retains fluids to dilute it.

People who are sensitive to salt or whose kidneys are unable to excrete it efficiently may notice foot or leg swelling after eating a single high-salt meal.

+ **Medications.** Swelling is a side effect of many drugs. These include the hormones in oral contraceptives, some antidepressants and blood pressure medications, and even the common painkiller naproxen (like Aleve and Naprosyn, among others).

+ **Overweight.** Pressure from extra weight can make it harder for blood to move uphill. Also, people who are overweight tend to develop other health problems, including diabetes and heart disease, that interfere with circulation.

+ **Prolonged standing or sitting.** Fluid tends to pool.

To reduce swelling: Lose weight, limit salt, and keep your feet moving, particularly during plane flights or car trips. Flexing the feet and ankles causes muscles to press against veins, which prevents blood from pooling. And don't cross your legs. It puts pressure on the veins, making it harder for fluids to circulate. Here are a few other things to try:

+ **Raise your legs.** Once or twice a day, lie down and prop your legs against a wall or on a chair or a stack of pillows. It's makes it easier for blood to exit the legs and return to the heart. For sleeping, raise the bottom of your bed by putting each bottom bed leg on a brick or book.

- **Wear compression stockings.** The over-the-counter stockings sold at pharmacies exert enough pressure to "firm up" the veins and improve blood flow. I recommend them for waitresses, police officers, and other people who are on their feet all day.
- **Drink more water.** It flushes excess sodium from the body.

> Johanna S. Youner, DPM, podiatrist and cosmetic foot surgeon in private practice and attending physician at New York Downtown Hospital, both in New York City. She is a spokesperson for the American Podiatric Medical Association, a delegate of the New York State Podiatric Medical Association, and a fellow of the American College of Foot and Ankle Surgeons. HealthyFeetNY.net.

Home Remedies for Foot Ailments

INGROWN TOENAIL: CITRUSY FIX

An ingrown toenail can happen when the nail is pushed down into the skin of the toe, usually from poorly fitting shoes or lack of a proper trimming. This can cause redness, swelling, and a lot of pain!

Here's how to fix it: At bedtime, put a slim wedge of lemon on the problem toenail, keeping it in place with a Band-Aid and covering it with a sock. Sleep that way, and by morning, the acid in the lemon should have softened the nail enough so that you can ease it away from the skin and trim it. The right way to trim the nail is to cut it straight across, not down at the sides, and not shorter than the toe (which promotes growing into the skin).

CALLUSES: OVERNIGHT CURE

Are painful calluses (patches of thick skin that form on the soles of feet) keeping you home and off your feet instead of out and about?

Here's how to get rid of them overnight: Cut an onion crosswise into two big slices—use an onion large enough to cover the callused area. Let the two onion slices soak in wine vinegar (red or white) for four hours, then take the onion (one slice for each foot or wherever needed) and apply them to the calluses. Bind them in place with plastic wrap, put on socks, and leave them on overnight. The next morning, you should be able to gently scrape away the calluses (the edge of a metal nail file should do the trick). Be sure to wash and rinse your feet thoroughly to get rid of the onion/vinegar smell.

CORNS: SLICK SOLUTION

The difference between an oak tree and a tight shoe is that one makes acorns, the other makes corns ache. Corny jokes aside, corns—calluses that form on the tops or sides of toes—are not a terribly serious condition, but you'll be more comfortable if you stop wearing those shoes that made the corn.

After you do that, try this remedy: Rub castor oil on the corn twice a day, and it will gradually peel off, leaving you with soft, smooth skin. Or, every night, put one small piece of fresh lemon peel on the corn (the inside of the peel on your skin). Wrap a bandage around it to keep it in place until morning. In a few days, the corn should be gone.

ACHY FEET: SOOTHING SOAK

Were you on your feet all day and now your dogs are barking? Or maybe there's some weird ache around your ankles or shin area, and you need a little natural soothing.

To dissolve foot pain after too much time on your feet, add one cup of apple cider vinegar to a basin (or two plastic shoe boxes) filled halfway with lukewarm water. Then soak your feet for at least fifteen minutes. The aches and pains should melt away.

› Joan Wilen and Lydia Wilen, health investigators and folk-remedy experts based in New York City who have spent decades collecting "cures from the cupboard." They are authors of *Bottom Line's Treasury of Home Remedies & Natural Cures*, *Bottom Line's Household Magic*, and *Bottom Line's Secret Food Cures*.

Exercise Away Your Plantar Fasciitis

Lots of people experience pain at the underside of the foot or the heel (known as plantar fasciitis) and run to the podiatrist for treatment. This seems to make sense. After all, the pain is in the foot, and a podiatrist treats feet.

The problem with this logic is that in most cases, the cause of heel pain is not in the foot at all. How could that be? The body works like a chain. Gravity pushes down on you as you perform your daily activities. Muscles throughout the body must respond together to allow you to move pain-free. The foot happens to be the last point at which force is going through the body to get to the floor, so all the muscles *above* the foot play a role in how the forces run through it.

THE ANATOMY OF HEEL PAIN

Ultimately, gravity's force should run through the middle of the foot. When standing, you should feel like there is equal pressure at the inside of the foot and the outside. For this to occur, the pelvis must be maintained at a level position. The gluteus medius muscle sits at the side of the pelvis and is responsible for keeping the pelvis level even when single leg standing (as you do when walking). When this muscle weakens, the weight of the body on the inside of the leg causes you to start to tilt inward. This affects your ability to bear weight through the middle of the foot, moving the force toward the inside of the foot.

The arch of the foot exists at the inside. Excessive force developing at the inside of the foot from the weakness of the gluteus medius stresses the muscles that support the arch. Once strained, the muscles can no longer support the arch, and it flattens. A tissue called the plantar fascia attaches from the balls of the feet to the heel. When the arch breaks down, the distance between the balls of the feet and the heel increases. The plantar fascia becomes overstretched and begins to emit pain at its attachment to the heel.

THE RIGHT EXERCISES FOR RELIEF

To resolve foot pain from plantar fasciitis, you must strengthen the hip muscles (gluteus medius) and the ankle support muscles (the anterior and posterior tibialis muscles). Here are three exercises that do just that. All you need are a resistance band and ankle weights. Perform them three times a week. For each exercise, do three sets of ten repetitions with a one-minute break between sets. Continually increase the resistance used until the muscles involved are strong enough to perform your functional activities without straining and free from pain.

Hip Abduction (Gluteus Medius)

Lie on your side with the knee of the bottom leg bent and the top leg straight and in a continuous line from the torso. (If the leg were angled in front of the torso, you would use a different muscle.) Raise the top leg off the supporting leg until your leg is parallel with the floor. When doing this, try to turn the leg in slightly so the heel is the first part of the foot that is moving. This puts the gluteus medius in the optimal position as you raise your leg. Once your leg reaches parallel to the floor, begin to lower back onto the supporting leg. Start without ankle weights, but add them over time as you gain strength.

Dorsiflexion (Anterior Tibialis)

Secure a resistance band under a sturdy table, or knot one end and put the knot behind a closed door. Sit on the floor, and extend your weak leg, keeping your knee bent. Slip the end of the resistance band over your foot so that it is supported on the front of the foot in the midfoot region. Start with the ankle angled about thirty degrees forward. Next, flex your foot, pulling it toward you about ten degrees beyond perpendicular. Return to the start position.

Inversion (Posterior Tibialis)

Secure a resistance band as described above. Sit in a chair placed parallel to the door or table. Place the resistance band around the instep of the foot and sit with your working leg at a ninety-degree angle so that your heel is under the knee. Keeping your heel touching the ground, raise the rest of your foot, and place the toes outside the line of the ankle. Pull the toes inward until they are inside the line of the ankle. (A small portion of the sole of the foot will be exposed at the end of the range.) Return to the start position.

....

› Mitchell Yass, DPT, creator of the Yass Method, which uniquely diagnoses and treats the cause of chronic pain through the interpretation of the body's presentation of symptoms. Dr. Yass is the author of two books, *Overpower Pain: The Strength Training Program That Stops Pain Without Drugs or Surgery,* and *The Pain Cure Rx: The Yass Method for Resolving the Cause of Chronic Pain.* Additionally, Dr. Yass starred in the PBS special "The Pain Prescription." MitchellYass.com.

....

Plantar Fasciitis Self-Defense

These strategies can help prevent a recurrence in people who have beaten plantar fasciitis and, better yet, help avoid the problem in the first place.

Wear proper shoes. They should not be too thin (the ever-popular flip-flops are not a good choice, nor are lightweight ballet slippers) but rather should provide good arch support and shock absorbency. Heels can actually be helpful (women, take heed), though they should be no higher than three inches. It's also a good idea to vary the height of your heels daily.

Replace athletic shoes often. Be aware that wear first appears on the inside of the shoe, so know that you can be losing important support even if your sole looks fine. Buy supportive shoes. Use the fold test, meaning if a shoe folds or bends more than just a little, look for a different pair.

Stretch your feet regularly. Walk around on your tiptoes for five minutes, three times a week, or walk around your bed on your toes several times each night before you go to sleep. Also stretch your calf muscles and Achilles tendons before you get out of bed in the morning.

Maintain a normal weight. There has been a rapid increase in cases of plantar fasciitis, which correlates neatly with increasing obesity rates in this country.

Put your feet up. Moments of relaxation throughout the day go far for both your feet and state of mind. Elevate both, whenever you can.

....

› Arnold S. Ravick, DPM, spokesperson for the American Podiatric Medical Association and in private practice in Washington, DC.

....

Real Relief for Neuropathy Without Meds

Nerve damage can be both myste-rious and maddening. It's myste-rious, because about one-third of those with neuropathy never discover what's causing the pain, tingling, and numbness. It's maddening, because damaged nerves recover slowly—if they recover at all. Even when an underlying cause of neuropathy is identified (diabetes, for example, is a big one) and corrected, the symptoms may persist for months, years, or a lifetime.

MORE THAN PAIN

About one in every fifteen American adults has experienced some form of neuropathy, also known as peripheral neuropathy. The symptoms vary widely—from sharp, shooting pains that feel like jolts of electricity, to burning sensations, tingling, numbness, muscle fatigue, and/or a lack of muscle strength in the feet. Symptoms typically start first in both feet, then slowly move up the legs and to the hands. Nerves that control functions such as sweat, blood pressure, digestion, and bladder control can be affected as well.

There are hundreds of different causes of neuropathy. Diabetes, mentioned above, accounts for about one-third of all cases. Elevated blood sugar damages nerve cells and blood vessels and can cause numbness and other symptoms.

Other common causes of neuropathy: Heavy alcohol use, rheumatoid arthritis, vitamin deficiencies (including vitamin B-12), and certain medications, especially some chemotherapy drugs.

Important finding: One-third to one-half of patients with neuropathies of unknown origin have inherited neuropathies—that is, they're genetically susceptible to nerve damage, even in the absence of a specific disease/injury, according to research conducted at the Mayo Clinic.

A few medications are FDA-approved for neuropathy, but the side effects may be more uncomfortable than the condition itself. Fortunately, there are some surprisingly effective nondrug therapies.

NATURAL TREATMENTS

It can be a challenge for doctors (usually neurologists) to identify what is responsible for neuropathies. But it's worth making the effort, because treating the cause early can stop ongoing damage and potentially allow injured nerves to regenerate. When nerves repair, there may be some increased sensitivity, but this is usually temporary.

When the cause of neuropathy can't be identified, the symptoms can still be treated. If your symptoms make you very uncomfortable, there are medications that can help. The drugs that have been FDA-approved for neuropathic pain include pregabalin, also often used for seizures, and duloxetine, also used for depression. Pregabalin can cause drowsiness and weight gain, and duloxetine can cause drowsiness as well as sweating in a small number of people. Gabapentin and tricyclic antidepressants, such as amitriptyline and nortriptyline, are used off-label for neuropathy. Gabapentin is similar to pregabalin, with the same side effects, and the antidepressants can cause sedation, dry mouth, and, in high doses, arrhythmias.

My advice: If you'd describe your symptoms as uncomfortable and annoying—*but not debilitating*—you might want to start with nondrug treatments. They probably won't eliminate the discomfort altogether, but they can make it easier to tolerate. Plus, if you do decide to use medication, these treatments may enable you to take it for a shorter time and/or at a lower dose. Try one or more of the following at a time.

Vibrating footbath. Most patients will first notice tingling, numbness, or other symptoms in the feet. Soaking your feet in a warm-water vibrating footbath (available in department stores, pharmacies, and online) for fifteen to twenty minutes dilates blood vessels and increases circulation in the affected area. More important, the vibrations are detected and transmitted by large-diameter sensory nerve fibers. Because of their large size, these fibers transmit signals very quickly. The sensations of vibration reach the spinal cord *before* the pain signals from damaged nerves, which blunts the discomfort.

The pain relief is temporary but reliable. You can soak your feet as often as you wish throughout the day.

Helpful: Soak your feet just before bed—the pain relief you get will help you fall asleep more easily.

For discomfort in other parts of the

body, you can get similar relief from a whirlpool bath or a pulsating showerhead.

Important: Some people with neuropathy are unable to sense temperatures and can burn their feet in too-hot water. Test the temperature with your hand first (or have someone else test it).

Menthol cream. The smooth muscles in arterial walls are lined with receptors that react to menthol. When you rub an affected area with menthol cream (such as BENGAY), the blood vessels dilate, create warmth, and reduce discomfort. Creams labeled "menthol" or "methyl salicylate" have the same effects. These creams can be used long-term as needed.

Transcutaneous electrical nerve stimulation (TENS). This therapy delivers low levels of electric current to the surface of the skin. It's thought that the current stimulates nerves and sends signals to the brain that block the discomfort from damaged nerves.

How well do the devices work? The research is mixed. In 2010, a meta-analysis of TENS in patients with diabetic neuropathies found that the treatment led to a decrease in pain scores. Other studies, however, have shown little or no benefit.

Battery-powered TENS units cost about thirty dollars for low-end models. The treatment is largely without side effects, and some people have good

results. Treatments are typically done for thirty minutes at a time and can be repeated as needed throughout the day. Treatments should not be done on skin that is irritated.

My advice: If you want to try TENS at home, start using it under the direction of a physical therapist so that he/she can suggest the appropriate settings and amount of time for treatment.

Percutaneous electrical nerve stimulation (PENS). *Percutaneous* means that the electric current is delivered under the skin, using short needles. Studies have shown that the treatments, done in rehabilitation/physical therapy offices, decrease pain, improve sleep, and may allow patients to use smaller doses of painkilling medication. After each treatment, the pain relief can potentially last for weeks or longer.

The treatments take about thirty minutes per session and are generally repeated three times a week, until the patient achieves the desired amount and duration of pain relief. The risks are minimal, although you might have mild bruising or a little bleeding. Infection is possible but unlikely. Most patients have little or no pain during the treatments. PENS is not advised for those with pacemakers and should not be done on areas of irritated skin. The treatments might or might not be covered by insurance—be sure to ask.

Self-massage. Firmly rubbing and/or kneading the uncomfortable area is another way to block pain signals. You don't need to learn sophisticated massage techniques, but you (or a loved one) must use enough pressure to stimulate the big nerves that carry the pressure sensations. A too-light touch won't be helpful.

Caution: If you have a history of deep vein thrombosis, ask your doctor before massaging your legs.

Relaxation techniques. Stress and anxiety do not cause neuropathy, but patients who are tense may feel pain more intensely. A multiyear study found that patients with chronic pain who completed a mindfulness/stress-reduction program reported significantly less pain—and the improvement lasted for up to three years.

Helpful: Meditation, yoga, and other relaxation techniques. Most large medical centers offer programs in anxiety/stress management. Excellent guided meditations are also available on YouTube.

....

> Janice F. Wiesman, MD, FAAN, associate clinical professor of neurology at New York University School of Medicine in New York City and adjunct assistant professor of neurology at Boston University School of Medicine. She is author of *Peripheral Neuropathy: What It Is and What You Can Do to Feel Better.*

....

10

First Aid and Quick Cures

Your First Aid Kit: Ten Natural Medicines for Every Home

Most Americans make a mad dash to the nearest drugstore if an acute illness, such as sore throat or diarrhea, or a minor injury, such as muscle strain, needs attention. But that's not always necessary. It's easy to keep a few well-chosen natural medicines on hand to treat most minor ailments. At my home, we keep rubbing alcohol, 3 percent hydrogen peroxide, adhesive bandages, gauze, and medical tape for basic first aid. Here are the natural medicines (available at health-food stores) that I keep at home (unless I've indicated otherwise, follow manufacturers' recommendations for dosing):

1. **T-Relief.** *Use for:* Sprain, muscle strain, or pain after surgery or dental procedures. This homeopathic anti-inflammatory/analgesic (topical or oral) contains a variety of plant medicines, including arnica.

2. **Rescue Remedy.** *Use for:* Emotional stress, anxiety, and worry. This Bach flower remedy contains essences of five plants, including impatiens and clematis. Use four drops on the tongue as needed, up to five times daily.

3. **Calendula spray.** *Use for:* Skin injuries—cuts, abrasions, insect bites, and burns. Used topically, tincture of calendula flowers acts as a mild antiseptic and anti-inflammatory.

4. **Echinacea tincture.** *Use for:* Cold, flu, or sore throat. At the onset of illness, take sixty drops in one to two ounces of water every four waking hours. Continue for two to five days.

5. **Cough formula.** *Use for:* Dry cough and sore throat. Use a tincture formula

that contains the herbs elecampane, marshmallow, osha, cherry bark, fennel, and licorice mixed in a honey base. This remedy moistens the throat and reduces the frequency of coughs.

6. **Charcoal.** *Use for:* Acute diarrhea. Take two tablets every two to three waking hours.

    Caution: Charcoal should not be taken with medication—it can block the drug's absorption.

7. **Aloe plant.** *Use for:* Burns. Immediately after a burn, cut off a small piece from the tip of an aloe leaf (I keep an aloe plant in my kitchen), slice it open, and place the moist inner gel directly on your burn to reduce pain. (If you prefer to buy aloe gel, be sure to refrigerate it.)

8. **Peppermint leaf.** *Use for:* Fever, nausea, gas, and sore throat. To make peppermint tea, steep loose-leaf peppermint tea or tea bags covered for at least five minutes in boiled water. Drink one to four cups daily.

9. **Epsom salts.** *Use for:* Sore muscles or tension headaches. Rich in magnesium, which helps relax muscles, Epsom salts (two cups) can be used in a bath.

10. **Homeopathic flu remedies.** *Use for:* Flu. Take at the first signs.

    My favorite homeopathic flu

remedies: Muco Coccinum by UnDA and Oscillococcinum by Boiron.

For safety and optimal effectiveness, keep all medicines, including natural ones, in a cool, dry place that is out of the reach of children, and check the expiration dates of your products.

....

› Jamison Starbuck, ND, naturopathic physician in family practice and a guest lecturer at the University of Montana, both in Missoula. She is past president of the American Association of Naturopathic Physicians. Starbuck is a columnist for the *Bottom Line Health Insider* and hosts *Dr. Starbuck's Health Tips for Kids* on Montana Public Radio. DrJamisonStarbuck.com.

....

Seventeen Natural Remedies You Always Have with You

Here are seventeen remedies for common health problems that all have one thing in common—you always have these simple remedies with you!

Dry mouth. When it's important for you to seem calm and sound confident, don't let your dry mouth get in the way. Gently chew on your tongue. Within about thirty seconds, you will manufacture all the saliva you need to end this uncomfortable condition. If people notice, they will just think that you're chewing gum or sucking a candy.

Burned fingertips. If you get a minor burn on your fingertips, simply hold your earlobe—it's an acupressure point. Place your thumb on the back of the lobe and the burned fingertips on the front of the lobe. Stay that way for one minute. It works like magic to relieve the pain.

Hiccups. Here are *two* remedies:

+ Pretend that your finger is a mustache. Place it under your nose, and press in hard for thirty seconds. That should do it, but if not…
+ Take a deep breath. Without letting any air out, swallow. Breathe in a little bit more, then swallow. Keep inhaling and swallowing until you absolutely can't inhale or swallow anymore. Then, in a controlled way, slowly exhale.

Motion sickness. Pull out and pinch the skin in the middle of your inner wrist, about one inch from your palm. Keep pulling and pinching, alternating wrists, until you feel better. It shouldn't take too long.

Leg cramps. The second you get a cramp in your leg, "acupinch" it away. Use your thumb and your index finger to pinch your philtrum—the skin between your nose and upper lip. Pinch it for about twenty seconds until the pain and the cramp disappear.

Stomachache. This remedy came to us from an Asian massage therapist. If you are having stomach discomfort, massage the acupressure points at the sides of your knees, just below the kneecaps. This will relieve your stomachache.

Warts. First thing each morning, dab some of your own spittle on the wart (but do *not* lick the wart). "First thing" means before you brush your teeth. We don't know why it works—it just does.

Hemorrhoids. Edgar Cayce, who is often called the father of holistic medicine, recommended this exercise for the treatment of hemorrhoids:

+ Stand with your feet about six inches apart, hands at sides.
+ Then raise your hands up to the ceiling, and if balance isn't a problem for you, gradually rise up on your toes at the same time.
+ Bend forward, and bring your hands as close to the floor as you can get them.
+ Go back to the first position, and do it again.

Perform this exercise for two or three minutes twice every day, one hour after breakfast and one hour after dinner, until your hemorrhoids are relieved.

Choking cough. When you're not actually choking on something but you just are coughing as though you are, raise your hands as high as you can, and the choking cough will stop.

Tension headache. Tense all the muscles in your face, neck, jaw, scalp, and shoulders. Hold that tension for at least thirty seconds. Then, suddenly, relax completely, letting go of all the tension and your headache along with it.

Gas. Try this yoga pose called the wind-relieving pose. Lie on your back with your legs and arms extended. As you exhale, draw both knees to your chest. Clasp your hands around them. While holding only your right knee with both hands, release your left leg and extend it along the floor. Hold this pose for one minute. Draw your left knee back in toward your chest, and clasp your hands around both knees again. Then while holding only your left knee, release your right leg and extend it along the floor. Hold this pose for up to a minute. Finally, draw both knees to your chest. Then, with an exhalation, release and extend both legs.

Fatigue. If you are having a hard time staying awake or paying attention, here are *five* energizing strategies. Try the one that is doable in your situation.

+ A Chinese theory is that "tiredness" collects on the insides of your elbows and the backs of your knees. Wake up your body by slap-slap-slapping those areas.
+ Run in place for about two minutes.
+ Energy lines directly connected to internal organs and body functions run through your earlobes. Use your thumbs and index fingers to rub your earlobes for about fifteen seconds. This should wake up your entire nervous system.
+ This visualization exercise will help you overcome drowsiness. Sit back, close your eyes, and let all the air out of your lungs. Imagine a bright blue-white energizing light entering and filling your entire body as you inhale slowly through your nostrils. Then open your eyes. You will feel refreshed.
+ Boost your energy by belting out a few bars of a favorite cheerful song. Inhale deeply as you sing to bring more energizing oxygen into your lungs and increase circulation in your body.

› Joan Wilen and Lydia Wilen, health investigators and folk-remedy experts based in New York City who have spent decades collecting "cures from the cupboard." They are authors of *Bottom Line's Treasury of Home Remedies & Natural Cures*, *Bottom Line's Household Magic*, and *Bottom Line's Secret Food Cures*.

Home Remedies for Headaches

Next time your head starts to ache, instead of popping a pain pill, try a natural remedy. Science cannot explain why these alternative approaches work, but they have stood the test of time, have no side effects, and often work faster than drugs.

Caution: If headaches recur regularly or are severe, seek professional medical help.

Most of the categories below include several options. Try one or more remedies to see which work best for you. Products are sold in health-food stores.

- **Try acupressure.** Clip a clothespin to the earlobe that is closest to your headache and leave on for one minute.
- **Stick out your tongue about one-half inch, and bite down as hard as you comfortably can.** Continue for five minutes.
- **Ask your partner or a friend to slowly move one thumb down the right side of your back,** heading from your shoulder blade toward your waist and stopping to exert steady pressure for one minute on any tender spots.
- **Try aromatherapy.** Rub a dab of rosemary or peppermint essential oil (properly diluted in a carrier oil) on your forehead, temples, and behind the ears, and inhale the fumes from the open bottle four times.

  Caution: Never place undiluted essential oil directly on the skin.
- **Crumple a fresh, clean mint leaf, roll it up, and gently insert it into one nostril** (leaving a bit sticking out for easy removal). Remove after two to three minutes.
- **Boil one cup of water mixed with one cup of apple cider vinegar.** Remove from heat, then drape a towel over your head to trap steam, and bend over the pot. Breathe deeply through your nose for five minutes.
- **Use a compress.** Dip a white cotton scarf in distilled white vinegar and wring it out, then tie it around your forehead as tightly as possible without causing discomfort. Leave in place for fifteen to thirty minutes.
- **Eat certain foods.** Eat an apple, a cup of strawberries, a handful of raw almonds (chew thoroughly), one teaspoon of gomasio (Japanese sesame salt), or one teaspoon of honey mixed with one-half teaspoon of garlic juice.
- **Drink a cup of chamomile tea.**
- **Put your hands in hot water.** Fill a sink with water that is as hot as you can tolerate, and dunk your hands for one minute.

+ **Fill a bathtub ankle-high with very cold water.** Dress warmly but leave feet bare, then walk around in the tub until feet start to feel warm (from one to a maximum of three minutes). Get out, dry your feet, slip under the bedcovers, and relax.

....

> Joan Wilen and Lydia Wilen, health investigators and folk-remedy experts based in New York City who have spent decades collecting "cures from the cupboard." They are authors of *Bottom Line's Treasury of Home Remedies & Natural Cures*, *Bottom Line's Household Magic*, and *Bottom Line's Secret Food Cures*.

....

Best Itch Control for Bug Bites

Drugstores *are stocked with creams* and capsules that promise relief from the annoying itch and pain of bug bites, and the internet suggests some off-the-wall ideas—deodorant, transparent tape, or nail polish anyone? There are tons of options!

What really works? Here is my proven protocol, which involves two over-the-counter remedies and two natural treatments.

First and foremost, when you get a bite, try not to scratch the heck out of it.

(If you already have, then skip steps 1 and 2 below, and go straight to the subsection: "For Irritated Skin.") Scratching the bite can make it hurt more later, and it can break the skin, which raises the risk for infection.

Step 1: After you wash the bite with soap and warm water and dry it off, the first thing that you want to do is to blunt the pain and itchiness as fast as possible. The moment you notice a bug bite— within seconds, even—apply a dime-sized amount of an over-the-counter antihistamine cream that contains diphenhydramine, such as Benadryl. Choose this type of cream—rather than calamine lotion or hydrocortisone cream—because it helps your body deal with the initial, traumatic histamine response to the bite. You can buy a one-ounce tube for about seven dollars at any drugstore.

Step 2: Once you've reduced the severity of the pain and itchiness, try to get rid of the agent in the bite that's causing the pain and itchiness. That's where one of my favorite natural products comes in—lye soap. You can buy a three-ounce bar for about five dollars.

The alkaline properties of the soap neutralize and break down the bug's stinging saliva, which means that the bite is less likely to be itchy and painful in the hours and days that follow.

About ten to fifteen minutes after you apply the antihistamine cream, wash the affected area with lye soap two times in a row with warm water, and then dry the area. Next, rinse the bar to get it wet and rub it onto your hand until it forms a rich, stiff lather. Wipe that lather onto the affected area. When the lather hardens after a few minutes, wash it off. Try this routine once a day—more often if the pain or itchiness is severe—and stop using the Benadryl after that initial treatment.

FOR IRRITATED SKIN

When you've been scratching at a bite, don't use the antihistamine or the lye soap, because they might irritate skin that's aggravated or broken. Here are two alternatives.

If the skin is scratched only a little, use Aveeno Active Naturals Moisturizing Bar. Rub the bar with just enough water to create a thick paste. Rub the paste gently into the skin over and around the bite, and let it dry before washing it off. The Aveeno bar is almost as effective as the lye soap in helping remove the bug's stinging saliva, but it's more gentle on the skin. You can buy the bar for about three dollars.

If the skin is broken, dab on a dime-sized amount of antibiotic cream, such as Neosporin, to keep the bite from becoming infected. You can buy a half-ounce tube for about seven dollars at any drugstore. Then cover it with a bandage to prevent further scratching and/or infection. Wait until the skin has healed over to apply any of the products listed above.

> › Andrew L. Rubman, ND, medical director of Southbury Clinic for Traditional Medicines in Southbury, Connecticut. He is a founding member of the American Association of Naturopathic Physicians. His blog, *Nature Doc's Patient Diary*, is published on BottomLineInc.com. SouthburyClinic.com.

Natural Treatments for Itching and Common Rashes

The causes of itching are so varied that there is at least one associated with nearly every letter of the alphabet—starting with allergies, bug bites, contact dermatitis (from such things as soap or chlorine), drug reactions (antibiotics and painkillers are common culprits), eczema, fungus, gallbladder disease, and hives. Exposure to poison ivy, oak, or sumac is another common cause. Unfortunately, the instinctive desire to scratch an itch can exacerbate the underlying problem. Many people scratch their skin raw in an effort to get relief. Natural medicines that gently—yet effectively—treat the most common causes of itching are much better options.

Chamomile tea. For itching due to insect bites, eczema, hives, or poison ivy, oak, or sumac, use two tea bags per twelve ounces of water and let it steep for six minutes. Soak sterile gauze or clean cotton cloth in the tea, and apply compresses for fifteen minutes to the itchy area several times per day.

Calendula and comfrey salve. These plants are common ingredients in topical salves that often include vitamins A and E in an olive oil base. This salve works best for dry, scaly rashes that result from contact dermatitis, fungus, or eczema. For a moist, itchy rash with oozing clear or yellow fluid (such as that caused by insect bites or poison ivy, oak, or sumac), use a tea or tincture preparation of calendula only. Apply the tea in a compress or pour or spray it on the area.

Oatmeal. It is best for itching caused by hives or insect bites.

What to do: Fill a muslin or cotton bag with one cup of raw, rolled oats. Attach the bag to the spout of your bathtub and let the water flow through the bag as you fill a tub with warm (not hot) water. Lie in the oatmeal water for twenty to thirty minutes several times a day until the itch is gone. An oatmeal bath product, such as Aveeno, also can be used. For poison ivy, oak, or sumac, use a compress of the oatmeal water.

Grindelia spp (gumweed). This is my favorite remedy for itching caused by poison ivy, oak, or sumac. Wash the plant oil from the skin with soap and water, then apply a lotion or tincture of grindelia three times daily for several days.

White vinegar. Itching caused by sunburn, bug bites, or yeast responds well to white vinegar. Dilute vinegar with an equal amount of water, and test a small area first to make sure the vinegar solution does not sting. Dab it on the skin, or apply it with a compress. If tolerated, the diluted vinegar can be applied to itchy areas several times a day.

Water. It's surprising how often simply drinking one-half ounce of water per pound of body weight daily can heal troublesome dry, itchy skin, which can result from inadequate hydration.

If itching is accompanied by a fever, or if you notice skin discoloration or red or purple streaking near a bite, or if you have confused your medications, are urinating frequently, are having shortness of breath, or are in significant pain, see your doctor. These could be signs of an infection, a reaction to medication, or a medication overdose.

....

› Jamison Starbuck, ND, naturopathic physician in family practice and a guest lecturer at the University of Montana, both in Missoula. She is past president of the American Association of Naturopathic Physicians. Starbuck is a columnist for the *Bottom Line Health Insider* and hosts *Dr. Starbuck's Health Tips for Kids* on Montana Public Radio. DrJamisonStarbuck.com.

Muscle Cramp Relief

As a kid, I loved the funny sound of "charley horse." Somewhere along the line, I learned that the term may have originated from a baseball pitcher who played in the late 1800s—Charley "Old Hoss" Radbourne evidently suffered from excruciating muscle cramps while playing baseball. Nowadays, I know how painful a muscle cramp can be, and as a naturopathic physician, I disagree with my medical doctor colleagues who believe that a muscle cramp is just one of those things you must learn to live with. The truth is, muscle cramps usually result from one of three causes—dehydration, muscle overuse, or mineral deficiency. Here's how to protect yourself.

Get enough fluids. If you don't get enough fluids, your risk for muscle cramps increases, especially while exercising. Soda, juice, coffee, diet drinks, and even sweetened electrolyte-replacement beverages are no substitute for plain water.

For adequate hydration: I recommend drinking one-half ounce of water per pound of body weight per day. (Do talk to your doctor before significantly changing your daily water intake.) So, if you weigh 150 pounds, you should drink seventy-five ounces. It's wise to increase your total daily water intake by sixteen to thirty-two ounces if you are doing vigorous exercise (such as hiking, biking, or running), are out in hot weather (above 80°F), are pregnant (a risk factor for muscle cramps), are flying long distances (through two or more time zones), or if you are starting a new project, such as gardening or house painting, involving physical activity that stresses the muscles in new ways.

Stretch your muscles properly. Sometimes we can't avoid overusing our muscles. But we can stretch. This should be done before overusing your muscles, but if you forget, then do so afterward and again before bed.

What to do: Immediately after vigorous activity, spend ten minutes elongating the muscles you used, especially those of the thigh, calf, and lower back, which are most likely to suddenly spasm. For example, try forward bends (bend from the waist to touch the floor, if possible; use a table edge for support if you feel unsteady) and calf stretches (put your hands on the wall while standing about three feet away from it, then lean in, elongating the calf muscles).

Get the right minerals. Inadequate blood levels of such minerals as magnesium, potassium, and sodium will increase your risk for muscle spasms. Most people get plenty of sodium in their diets but lose much of it when they perspire during exercise and/or are out in hot weather. Potassium and magnesium in vegetables, whole grains, beans, nuts, seeds, and fresh fruit are most readily available for absorption. However, if you suffer from muscle spasms, talk to your doctor about taking daily mineral supplements of potassium and magnesium to ensure adequate levels. Be sure to consult your doctor first if you have kidney or heart disease or take any type of medication.

Try homeopathy. The homeopathic remedies Magnesia phosphorica (6x) and Kalium phosphoricum (6x), taken together, often relieve muscle cramps. The remedies, manufactured by Hyland's/Standard Homeopathic, are available in stores selling natural medicines. Dissolve two pellets of each remedy (four pellets total) under the tongue. Repeat the same dose every ten minutes for up to one hour until the pain is gone.

› Jamison Starbuck, ND, naturopathic physician in family practice and a guest lecturer at the University of Montana, both in Missoula. She is past president of the American Association of Naturopathic Physicians. Starbuck is a columnist for the *Bottom Line Health Insider* and hosts *Dr. Starbuck's Health Tips for Kids* on Montana Public Radio. DrJamisonStarbuck.com.

Natural Pain Busters for Your Aching Head

When something hurts, you want to feel better quickly. Often, that means reaching for an over-the-counter or prescription drug. But there are natural pain stoppers that offer the same relief—without the risks.

Aspirin and ibuprofen can both cause intestinal bleeding, acetaminophen can lead to liver damage, and powerful prescription pain relievers, such as acetaminophen with hydrocodone and acetaminophen with codeine, may make you drowsy and can be addictive.

Despite the dangers, these medications are valuable for treating occasional severe (long-lasting) or acute (sudden but stopping abruptly) pain. But for many chronic conditions that need ongoing relief, such as osteoarthritis, natural pain stoppers work just as well with a much lower risk for side effects.

Caution: Severe pain, or mild pain

that gets suddenly worse, can be a sign of a serious injury or other medical problem. Seek medical attention immediately.

HOW TO USE NATURAL REMEDIES

For each common pain problem discussed here, I give more than one treatment. You may have more success with or simply prefer a particular treatment. If something has worked for you in the past, start there. If you don't get much relief from a treatment, try another option. If you get only partial improvement, try adding another supplement. Because natural remedies have a very low risk for serious side effects, it's usually safe to use them in combination with prescription or nonprescription medications, such as for high blood pressure, and over the long run, they can help reduce the need for these drugs entirely. Check with your doctor before starting a natural regimen or changing your drug regimen.

Natural remedies also work well in combination with pain-relieving body work, such as chiropractic, physical therapy, and acupuncture.

HELP A HEADACHE

Migraines and other headaches are often set off by food sensitivities—most commonly, to red wine, caffeine, chocolate, and food additives, such as monosodium glutamate. Other triggers, such as lack of sleep or hormonal fluctuations, can also leave you with headache pain.

Best: Pay attention to patterns and avoid your triggers.

Fortunately, headaches are usually very responsive to natural remedies.

Mild (tension) headaches. First, try acupressure. This ancient Chinese technique uses gentle pressure and light massage on specific points. In traditional Chinese medicine, chi (*chee*) is the vital energy of all living things. Your chi flows along twelve meridians that run through your body and nourish your tissues. Each meridian is associated with a particular organ, such as the liver or gallbladder. Along each meridian are specific points, designated by numbers, that are the spots where the flow of chi can be affected.

For headaches, the standard acupressure points are:

- **Gallbladder 20**—the small indentation below the base of the skull, in the space between the two vertical neck muscles. Push gently for ten to fifteen seconds, wait ten seconds, then repeat five to ten times.
- **Large intestine 4**—located in the webbing between the thumb and index finger. Push gently for ten to fifteen seconds (as described above).

Do this on one hand, then switch to the other.

+ **Yuyao**—the indentation in the middle of each eyebrow (straight up from the pupil). Push gently for ten to fifteen seconds (as described above) on both points simultaneously.

If you don't feel relief within several minutes after trying a particular pressure point, move on to a different one.

Another option for mild headaches: A cup of peppermint tea or a dab of peppermint oil on the temples can banish a mild headache quickly.

Note: Peppermint essential oil is highly concentrated—don't take it internally.

To brew peppermint tea, make an infusion using one to two teaspoons dried peppermint leaves in eight ounces of boiling water. Let steep for five minutes. You may find relief after one cup. Drink as much and as often as necessary.

Migraine headaches. The herb feverfew has been used effectively for centuries to treat migraines. Take a feverfew capsule standardized to contain 300 micrograms (mcg) of the active ingredient parthenolide every thirty minutes, starting at the onset of symptoms. Take a maximum of four doses daily or until you feel relief.

Prevention: Take a feverfew capsule standardized to contain 300 to 400 mcg of parthenolide or thirty drops of a standardized tincture, either in a few ounces of water or directly on your tongue, every day. In about three months, you should notice dramatically fewer migraines and/or less severe symptoms.

Note: Feverfew may thin blood, so consult your doctor if you are taking a blood thinner, such as warfarin.

White willow bark has anti-inflammatory and blood-thinning benefits similar to those of aspirin, but unlike aspirin, it doesn't appear to damage the stomach lining. For centuries, the bark of the white willow (*Salix alba*), a tree found in Europe and Asia, was noted for its pain-relieving qualities. Its active ingredient is salicin, which the body converts to salicylic acid, a close cousin to aspirin (acetylsalicylic acid).

Dose: Take 120 mg daily of white willow bark extract capsules. If this amount does not reduce pain, try 240 mg.

Note: Avoid this if you have an aspirin allergy and for one week before undergoing surgery. White willow bark is a blood thinner, so take it only while being monitored by a physician if you take blood-thinning medication.

Any of these supplements can be used alone or in combination. Natural pain stoppers can be effective alternatives to drugs, but pain is also your body's way of telling you that something is wrong. If your pain is very sudden or severe and/or accompanied by other symptoms—such as weakness, nausea, redness and swelling in the painful area, shortness of breath, or fever—get medical attention immediately.

> Mark A. Stengler, NMD, naturopathic doctor and founder of the Stengler Center for Integrative Medicine in Encinitas, California. He is author and coauthor of numerous books, including *The Natural Physician's Healing Therapies* and *Bottom Line's Prescription for Natural Cures*, and is the author of the newsletter *Health Revelations*. MarkStengler.com.

Bouncing Back from Food Poisoning

So you had a great time at an outdoor cookout. The barbecued chicken was delicious, and you even had seconds of the potato salad. But now you're struck with a queasy, sick feeling. As you rush off to the bathroom, a sinking realization takes hold—you have food poisoning.

If you've ever had this extremely uncomfortable condition, the symptoms are unmistakable: nausea, stomach pain, and loose bowel movements that come fast and furious every half hour or so. As the

infecting organisms invade your intestines, it gets even worse. You're likely to start vomiting, have a mild fever and ongoing abdominal cramps, and just feel lousy.

Natural medicine can shorten an episode of food poisoning from three to four days to a day or two and dramatically reduce the severity of symptoms. Here are my favorite methods:*

+ **Take activated charcoal.** At the first sign of food poisoning, take two capsules of activated charcoal and repeat every four waking hours until your symptoms are gone. Activated charcoal can be purchased from a natural-food store. Inside your system, toxins attach to the surface of the activated charcoal and are drawn out of the stomach and intestines.

+ **Use antiseptic herbs.** Oregon grape root, uva ursi, and gingerroot will help kill the organism causing your food poisoning. You can use any of these herbs individually or buy a tincture that contains all three of them for the greatest benefit.

   Typical adult dose: Sixty drops (about one-quarter teaspoon) in one ounce of water every four waking hours for up to three days.

* Check with your doctor before using herbal therapies.

- **Try carob powder.** Unsweetened carob powder, available in bulk at most natural-food grocers, has a binding effect and will ease diarrhea. I usually prescribe it along with slippery elm powder, an herb that soothes the digestive tract and helps reduce abdominal pain. Add two teaspoons of carob powder and two teaspoons of slippery elm powder to one-quarter cup of unsweetened apple-sauce. Eat the mixture slowly throughout the day. Repeat daily until symptoms are gone.

- **Drink clear liquids.** If you limit your diet to mostly clear liquids, you can reduce diarrhea by slowing down the activity of your gut.

  Good choices: Vegetable broth; peppermint, chamomile, and/or raspberry leaf herbal teas; and plain water.

  Also helpful: Try rice water. Cook one cup of brown or white rice in four cups of water, strain off the liquid, and drink six ounces several times a day. This gives you starch, which slows diarrhea, without taxing your gut to digest the rice. Avoid dairy products, meat, eggs, and beans—these foods are hard to digest when the body is fighting a bug and will worsen your symptoms.

Caution: Seek prompt medical attention if you experience diarrhea for more than three days. Also see a doctor if you have a fever above 101.5°F, blood in the stool or in vomit, severe abdominal pain, lack of urination, or more than one episode of difficulty swallowing, vision changes, fainting, or dizziness. These can be signs that infection has spread throughout your body.

› Jamison Starbuck, ND, naturopathic physician in family practice and a guest lecturer at the University of Montana, both in Missoula. She is past president of the American Association of Naturopathic Physicians. Starbuck is a columnist for the *Bottom Line Health Insider* and hosts *Dr. Starbuck's Health Tips for Kids* on Montana Public Radio. DrJamisonStarbuck.com.

How to Survive an Asthma Attack Without an Inhaler

If you have asthma, then you know how scary it can be when you have an attack and have trouble breathing for anywhere from a few minutes to a few days, depending on its severity.

So you're probably careful to keep your rescue inhaler with you at all times—in case of an emergency.

But what happens if an attack starts

and you discover that your inhaler is empty or you don't actually have it?

How can you lessen the severity of an asthma attack and/or stop it altogether without your trusty inhaler?

DO YOU NEED TO GO TO THE ER?

First off, quickly determine whether you're in immediate danger. If you have a peak-flow meter—a device that measures how much air you can expel from your lungs and that many asthmatics keep around the house—use it. If you're less than 25 percent off your normal mark, go on to the following steps, but if your number is off by more, get to an emergency room, because this indicates that there is a serious problem—one that could be life-threatening. If you don't have a peak-flow meter, then think about your symptoms. For example, if your lips or fingernails turn blue, you can't stop coughing, you feel soreness or tightness around the ribs, you feel like you're having a panic attack, or you're so exhausted from the effort of breathing that you can't finish a short sentence or stand up, then you need help fast—get to an ER.

HOW TO BREATHE EASIER

If you're not in immediate danger, try these tricks below. Some of these techniques may help within minutes, while others

may take a few hours to kick in, but since it's possible for an attack to last for days, try all of them to play it safe. During a typical asthma attack, the airways are constricted, muscles all over your body become tense, and your body produces extra mucus—all those things make it harder to breathe. You know your body best, so if you try all these tips but your attack still gets worse, go to a hospital.

Change your location. Asthma is typically triggered by an irritant—either an allergen or toxin—that inflames the airways. So remove yourself from the environment that contains the trigger (if you know what it is) as fast as you can. If you're reacting to dust, pets, mold, or smoke, for example, get away from it, or at the very least, breathe through a sleeve, a scarf, or your jacket collar to reduce your exposure.

Tell someone. Talking to someone may reduce your anxiety, and that's especially helpful, because anxiety can make your asthma attack worse. Also, if your asthma attack becomes more severe later on, you may need a ride to the hospital, so it's always good to keep someone else in the loop.

Sip hot coffee or nonherbal tea. Have one or two cups right away (but no more than that in one sitting, or your heart rate might spike too high—this is true among all people, not just asthmatics). Caffeine is metabolized into theophylline, which is also a drug that's used to prevent and treat asthma by relaxing the airways and decreasing the lungs' response to irritants. Getting caffeine from any source (a soda, an energy drink, a supplement, etc.) will likely help, but tea and coffee have other compounds that act similarly to caffeine (plus, liquids—especially hot liquids—help loosen mucus), so getting your caffeine in this form is best.

Practice breathing exercises. Many people panic when they have an asthma attack and start breathing quickly, but that only restricts the amount of oxygen that the lungs get. In other words, it makes the attack worse. So breathe in through your nose to the count of four and then out to the count of six. Pursing your lips as you exhale will help slow the exhalation and keep the airways open longer. Continue breathing this way for as long as you need.

Press on some acupressure points. The front parts of your inner shoulders (just above the armpits) and the outer edges of the creases of your elbows (when your elbows are bent) are "lung points." Pressing on one area at a time for a few consecutive minutes may relax muscles that have tightened up.

Steam things up. Take a hot shower or stay in the bathroom with the hot water running from the showerhead or tub or sink faucet. Steam or warm moisture is better than cold moisture, because it loosens mucus, so using a cool-air humidifier, although helpful, is not ideal.

Ask your doctor about taking magnesium and vitamin C. Taking 500 mg of magnesium and 1,000 mg of vitamin C during an asthma attack may help if you're an adult. (Children ages ten to seventeen should take half the doses, and children between the ages of five and nine should take one-third of the doses.) Magnesium is a bronchodilator that relaxes the breathing tubes, and vitamin C has a slight antihistamine effect.

Take medications. The prescription corticosteroid prednisone, available in pill form, is used only for acute problems, such as during an attack, because it helps reduce inflammation, so if your doctor has already prescribed it to you and you have it on hand, use it. This medication will not work as quickly as an inhaler, but it may prevent the problem from getting out of hand if you're having a lengthy attack. Just call your doctor, and let him or her know that you're taking it, so that he or she can supervise your dosing.

Also consider taking an over-the-counter decongestant (such as pseudoephedrine) and/or an expectorant (such as guaifenesin) or a drug that's a combination of the two, because these loosen mucus and make coughs more productive so you can rid your body of more phlegm.

> Richard Firshein, DO, board-certified in family medicine and certified medical acupuncturist and founder and director of the Firshein Center for Integrative Medicine, New York City. He is author of *Reversing Asthma: Breathe Easier with This Revolutionary New Program.* FirsheinCenter.com.

> C. Norman Shealy, MD, PhD, founding president of the American Holistic Medical Association and a leading expert in the use of holistic and integrative medicine. He is the author of numerous books, including *The Healing Remedies Sourcebook and Living Bliss: Major Discoveries Along the Holistic Path.* NormShealy.com.

Ease a Toothache

Few things are more painful than a toothache, and it always seems to erupt on weekends or late at night, when you can't get to a dentist. Here's something to try until you can see a dentist.

Cinnamon oil. Dip a cotton ball in the oil and apply it to the painful area. The oil often curbs pain almost instantly. It's also an antimicrobial that kills oral bacteria and can reduce inflammation and swelling.

If cinnamon oil doesn't help after five to ten minutes, add crushed garlic. Like cinnamon, it's a natural antibiotic with analgesic properties. If it doesn't hurt too much, you can chew a whole clove, using the tooth (or teeth) that is aching. Or you can crush a clove and apply the pulp to the area that's hurting.

Look Younger

How to Look Ten Years Younger in Seconds

In our mind's eye, *most* of us imagine ourselves still young and in our prime. But one look in the mirror can quickly bring us back to reality. Although we've all earned every wrinkle, age spot, and sag while experiencing life to the fullest, we all yearn to look a little (or a lot) younger.

Well, we can—and we can do it without much effort, expense, or *Real Housewives*–like scary plastic surgery. Some of these suggestions take just minutes, and others take almost no time at all, yet they can take as much as ten years off a woman's appearance.

Here are some youth-restoring options for when you have only 1.3 seconds to spare:

- **Project your "love glow."** A study from Syracuse University shows that falling in love takes only one-fifth of a second! Remember how new love could light you up from the inside, projecting youth and vitality? OK, maybe it's not possible to fall in love just now. But you can think a loving thought and give a big smile, which will bring a youthful sparkle to your face.

- **Check your posture.** Nothing reads old like slumping. For an instantly improved figure, stand up straight, raise your chin, throw those shoulders back, and pull in your tummy.

- **Do a facial exercise.** Open your mouth and eyes wide, then scrunch up your face, then release. This gets the blood flowing, putting roses in your cheeks.

- **Brighten your eyes.** Use two drops of homeopathic Similasan eyedrops in each eye every three hours, as needed. This remedy, which is generally safe for everyone, reduces redness and soothes dryness and irritation.

+ **De-stress with instant aromatherapy.** The scent of lavender makes you feel—and look—more relaxed and rejuvenated. Lightly spritz yourself with a lavender product designed for use on the skin, such as Aura Cacia Lavender Harvest Aromatherapy Mist ($7.99 for four ounces at www.AuraCacia.com), or rub a drop of lavender essential oil onto the pulse point on your wrist, or swirl four drops of lavender oil into your bathwater.

+ **Dash on the right lipstick—a light-colored one.** Dark lipstick seems old-ladyish and actually emphasizes tiny lip lines.

+ **Take a pass on heavy makeup.** Pancake foundation and too-bright blush look unnatural and make wrinkles more noticeable.

Heres' what to try when you have three minutes:

+ **Exfoliate your face.** Getting rid of dead cells with a facial scrub makes your complexion glow.

   Natural option: Combine a spoonful of ground oatmeal with enough honey to make a paste, then gently rub it onto your clean face. Rinse.

+ **Use contrast hydrotherapy.** To rinse your face, use two splashes of medium-hot water followed by two splashes of cold water. The hot/cold contrast increases circulation and tones skin.

   Next: Moisten a cotton ball with a natural astringent, such as rose water, aloe vera juice, or green tea, and stroke it across your face to remove lingering residue and restore the skin's proper pH.

+ **Combat sun damage.** Smooth a dab of vitamin C serum over your face—its antioxidants protect against ultraviolet rays and environmental toxins.

+ **Counteract saggy eyelids.** Curling your eyelashes is a simple beauty technique that makes eyes appear larger.

+ **Eat some blueberries.** Berries won't restore youthful comeliness instantly, of course, but they take just a moment to eat, and their vitamin C and bioflavonoids promote skin health and strengthen connective tissues.

If you can indulge yourself for ten minutes:

+ **Make your hair shine.** Rosemary essential oil gives tresses an extra sheen and a scent that's light and clean.

It is particularly helpful for dry, brittle, or frizzy hair.

After shampooing: Add a few drops of rosemary oil to your conditioner, work through your hair for a few minutes, then rinse, or towel-dry your hair, rub a dab of rosemary oil between your palms, and stroke it onto your damp hair. Then style as usual. Repeat after each shampoo (as I do to keep my long hair frizz-free despite the Hawaiian humidity) or as often as desired.

+ **Clear up blemishes.** Even if pimples remind you of being a teen, they don't make you look any younger.

The fix: Use your fingertips to spread honey over your face, avoiding the eye area. Leave on for five minutes, rinse off with water, then cleanse your face as usual. For people prone to acne, this works like a charm if used every day.

+ **Give yourself a steam facial.** Steam cleans pores, boosts circulation, and promotes a rosy complexion.

Method: Fill a sink or bowl with steaming hot water. If desired, add a few drops of stimulating peppermint essential oil and/or anti-inflammatory lavender essential oil. Drape a towel over your head to trap the steam. Then bend over the water for several minutes, keeping eyes closed and taking care not to burn yourself.

+ **Ease eye puffiness.** Dampen cotton balls with diluted witch hazel, then lie down with eyes closed and place the cotton balls over your eyes for five minutes (be careful not to let the witch hazel get into your eyes). Witch hazel contains catechol tannin, which reduces puffiness by constricting tiny capillaries just below the skin's surface.

+ **Do some quickie aerobics.** Just ten minutes of dancing or brisk walking increases circulation and reduces puffiness in the face, hands, ankles, and elsewhere.

+ **Drink a cleansing shake.** I put many of my patients on a "magic smoothie." It is chock-full of vital nutrients and supports regular elimination, promoting the health and vitality of the whole body. And the healthier you are, the more youthful you tend to look.

To prepare two servings: In a blender, combine one cup of chopped parsley or spinach, one chopped carrot, one-half chopped, peeled cucumber, one-half chopped, peeled apple, one banana, one-half cup blueberries, one heaping tablespoon of whey or rice protein powder, and two cups of water. Blend well. Enjoy immediately or refrigerate and drink later in the day.

> Laurie Steelsmith, ND, LAc, a licensed naturopathic physician and acupuncturist and medical director of Steelsmith Natural Health Center, Honolulu. She is the coauthor of *Natural Choices for Women's Health* and *Great Sex, Naturally*. DrSteelsmith.com.

How to Make a Bruise Go Away Faster

Tomorrow's forecast calls for a beautiful spring day—perfect to go sleeveless—but you have that unsightly arm bruise!

What to do: Spread a thin layer of blackstrap molasses on a piece of brown paper (grocery bag) and apply the molasses side to the bruise. Then bind it in place with medical tape and leave it there for a few hours. Your skin color should go from black and blue to looking much more normal—maybe even free and clear!

> Joan Wilen and Lydia Wilen, health investigators and folk-remedy experts based in New York City who have spent decades collecting "cures from the cupboard." They are authors of *Bottom Line's Treasury of Home Remedies & Natural Cures*, *Bottom Line's Household Magic*, and *Bottom Line's Secret Food Cures*.

The Secret to Keeping Spider Veins Away

Nobody wants to see spider veins—those tiny, twisty, red or blue blood vessels—spring up on her legs or face, or anywhere else, for that matter.

To the rescue: Rutin, an antioxidant flavonoid naturally found in buckwheat, citrus fruits, apple peels, and black tea. Supplementing with 500 mg of rutin daily (continuing indefinitely) helps prevent spider veins, possibly by reducing inflammation.

Taking rutin won't get rid of existing spider veins. For that, you'll need treatment from a dermatologist (for instance, injections of a sclerosing solution to close the blood vessels, making them fade away). However, the supplements can lower your risk for recurrence once spider veins have been treated. Rutin supplements are sold over the counter in health-food stores and online. Having recommended rutin to hundreds of adult patients over more than fifteen years, I have had no reports of allergic reaction or adverse side effects.

Additional prevention strategy: Heat promotes spider vein formation, so avoid sitting with your legs near a radiator or fireplace. If you want to soak in a hot bath or Jacuzzi, put your legs up on the edge of the tub, out of the water.

› Karen Burke, MD, PhD, assistant clinical professor of dermatology and research scientist at Mount Sinai Medical Center in New York City. She has a private practice for dermatology and dermatologic surgery, also in New York City.

Do-It-Yourself Face-Lift

If you've got facial wrinkles that you would like to reduce but you don't want to get Botox injections or a surgical face-lift, there's a do-it-yourself option that's far less invasive and far less expensive. With a technique known as facial acupressure (similar to acupuncture but performed without needles), you can take up to five to ten years off your appearance—and perhaps even improve your overall health in the process.

Sound far-fetched? I have treated hundreds of patients who were contemplating face-lifts but found success with acupressure.

Bonus: Unlike Botox or surgery, acupressure won't give you a tight, frozen, or pulled-back appearance. The results are softer and more natural.

WHY ACUPRESSURE?

Acupressure is based on a Chinese healing technique that involves pressing or kneading key points on the body to stimulate energy flow, known as qi or chi (pronounced *chee*), through invisible pathways called meridians. It can be used to relax or tone muscles, boost circulation, and even improve digestion.

The conventional view: From the Western medical perspective, wrinkles are formed by changes in the skin's composition, thickness, and elasticity as well as continuous muscle activity. For example, forehead wrinkles may appear after years of furrowing your eyebrows or squinting. As a result, the skin covering the muscle creases, eventually creating a wrinkle.

Chinese medicine has a different perspective. For example, specific meridians (that correspond to organ systems, such as those for the liver and gallbladder) are believed to affect certain body parts, but they don't always seem to correlate. For instance, a meridian located at the junction between your thumb and index finger corresponds to the head—rubbing that area can reduce headaches and, yes, wrinkles.

DO-IT-YOURSELF ROUTINES

To help reduce wrinkles and puffiness, use the following routines each day until you are satisfied with the results and then as needed.

Forehead Wrinkles

Begin at the top of your right foot, in the junction between your big and second toes. (This point is called liver 3.) Using medium to firm (but not painful) pressure, massage the point in a clockwise circle ten times. (If you have arthritic fingers, use your knuckle instead.) Repeat on left foot.

Next, move to the back side of your right hand between your right thumb and index finger (large intestine 4). In a clockwise circular motion, massage this point for ten rotations. Repeat on the left hand.

Then, move to the back of your neck. Place both thumbs where your spine meets the base of your skull and move them two inches to either side until they each land in an indentation (gallbladder 20). Massage clockwise with firm pressure for ten rotations.

Lastly, move to your face. Place the pad of each index finger a half inch above the center of each eyebrow (gallbladder 14). Massage with medium pressure in ten clockwise (right to left) circles.

Repeat the entire sequence three times in a single session each day. For deeper wrinkles, do the sequence several times throughout the day. You should notice a reduction in forehead wrinkles within twenty days.

Under-Eye Puffiness (Due to Age or Allergies)

Place your index finger two inches above the inside of your right ankle between the bone and muscle (spleen 6). Do ten clockwise rotations using medium to firm pressure. Repeat on the left leg. Next, move to the back of your right hand (large intestine 4), as described earlier, and perform ten clockwise rotations. Repeat on the left hand.

Then, with your arm at your side, bend your left elbow to make a ninety-degree angle. Pinpoint the area located at the outside edge of the elbow crease, between the bend and the bone (large intestine 11). Use your index finger to massage ten times in a clockwise rotation using medium to firm pressure. Repeat on your right elbow.

Lastly, move to your face. Place your right index finger just to the side of your right nostril. Move the finger laterally to a spot directly underneath the center of your eye, in your sinus area (stomach 3). Press in and slightly upward, performing ten clockwise rotations. Repeat on the left side.

Do the entire sequence three times daily. You should notice a reduction in puffiness under your eyes after a few days.

> Shellie Goldstein, LAc, licensed acupuncturist, esthetician, and certified Chinese herbologist

who maintains a private practice in New York City and Amagansett, New York. One of the first acupuncturists to work in hospitals and health-care facilities in New York state, Goldstein is the author of *Your Best Face Now: Look Younger in 20 Days with the Do-It-Yourself Acupressure Facelift.* HamptonsAcupuncture.com.

discoloration should be evaluated by a dermatologist to rule out skin cancer.

› Joan Wilen and Lydia Wilen, health investigators and folk-remedy experts based in New York City who have spent decades collecting "cures from the cupboard." They are authors of *Bottom Line's Treasury of Home Remedies & Natural Cures,* *Bottom Line's Household Magic,* and *Bottom Line's Secret Food Cures.*

Age-Spot Eraser

Flat *brown spots on your* face and hands, often called age spots or liver spots, develop on fair-skinned folk around middle age or older. They are caused by an accumulation of pigment in the skin. True age spots are harmless, but if you don't love how they look, here's a natural remedy to make them disappear. Squeeze a grated onion through cheesecloth so that you have one teaspoon of onion juice. Mix it with two teaspoons of white vinegar, and massage the brown spots with this liquid until it's pretty much absorbed into the skin. Do this daily—twice a day, if possible—until you no longer see spots before your eyes.

Keep in mind that these brown spots, usually caused by sun exposure or a nutrition deficiency, took years to form, so it may take a few months for this remedy to work.

Caution: Any suspicious mark or skin

Banish Morning Wrinkles

Is *your face creased with* wrinkles when you wake up?

Cosmetic pencils and creams sold as line erasers are widely available and will help improve the appearance of these wrinkles for an hour or so. But that's only a temporary solution.

These facial creases—which are caused by sleeping with your face pressed into your pillow—eventually will become permanent if the skin is folded the same way every night over a long period. The best way to prevent these lines altogether is to sleep on your back.

Helpful: Buy a U-shaped cushion—often sold to make airline travel more comfortable—and sleep with the back of your neck nestled into it. This should help to keep your face crease-free.

> Neal B. Schultz, MD, assistant clinical professor of dermatology at Mount Sinai School of Medicine and owner of Park Avenue Skin Care center, both in New York City. He also is the founder of www.DermTV.com and author of *It's Not Just About Wrinkles: A Park Avenue Dermatologist's Program for Beautiful Skin—in Just Four Minutes a Day*. NealSchultzMD.com.

Cold-Weather Skin Care

Winter is lizard-skin season—when skin turns dry, scaly, itchy, and flaky. But don't blame the cold weather.

The real culprits are low humidity outdoors and dry, heated air indoors, which draws moisture out of the inner layers of skin. In addition, normal shedding of skin cells slows with age because cells become less active, so you end up with visible layers of dead, scaly skin. These tips can help:

- **Shorten your shower.** Though it seems counterintuitive, excess water dries out skin by breaking down its natural oils. The hotter the water, the worse it is.

  Best: Use lukewarm water, and limit showers to no more than five minutes.

- **Take an Epsom salt bath.** Epsom salts contain magnesium, which helps slough off dead skin cells. Once or twice a week, add one to two cups of Epsom salts to a tubful of lukewarm water and soak for ten to fifteen minutes.

- **Use cleansing lotion, not soap.** Soap is alkaline and can strip skin of moisture.

  For face and body: Try Cetaphil Gentle Skin Cleanser or Purpose Gentle Cleansing Wash.

- **Exfoliate—gently.** Use a loofah in the shower or bath to manually remove dead skin cells from your body. Allow the loofah to dry completely after each use to minimize bacteria. On your face, use a mildly abrasive facial exfoliating cream, such as Dermalogica Daily Microfoliant (800-345-2761, www.Dermalogica.com). I recommend exfoliating no more than twice weekly to avoid irritating the skin.

- **Slather on a body moisturizer** with a high oil-to-water ratio. Choose a brand that feels rich and slick, such as Éminence Honeydew Body Lotion (888-747-6342, www.EminenceOrganics.com). Apply liberally while skin is still damp from your shower or bath. Reapply at least once more per day, first dampening skin with a wet washcloth.

- **Spritz your face with water.** Do this before applying makeup and again before bed. Follow with moisturizer, such as Cetaphil Daily Facial Moisturizer.

◆ **Avoid irritating laundry products.** Use detergent that has no bleach or fragrances, such as All Free Clear or Cheer Free. Never use dryer sheets—even the unscented ones leave tiny irritating fibers on clothes.

› Brandith Irwin, MD, board-certified dermatologist and internist and director of the Madison Skin & Laser Center in Seattle. She has been a guest medical expert on *The Oprah Winfrey Show* and is author of *The Surgery-Free Makeover: All You Really Need to Know for Great Skin and a Younger Face.* SkinTour.com.

For the Smoothest Skin, What Matters Most Is What You Put in Your Mouth

Lots of women spend big bucks on facial creams and other lotions and potions that promise to minimize crow's feet, lip creases, and other wrinkles.

Problem: Research shows that your skin would benefit more if you focused on what you put in your mouth rather than in your cosmetics case.

The same metabolic factors that contribute to chronic illnesses such as

heart disease and diabetes also can damage the skin's cellular structures, leading to wrinkling. Those factors are highly influenced by the nutrients we ingest. Here's what really keeps skin looking young.

ANTIWRINKLE FOODS

Among the chief metabolic factors that harm skin (as well as other body tissues) are chronic inflammation, oxidation (a kind of biological rust), and high blood sugar. Certain foods help prevent such damage; other foods make it worse.

Evidence: Australian researchers studied the skin of 453 seniors and, in an article in the *Journal of the American College of Nutrition*, posed the question, "Skin Wrinkling: Can Food Make a Difference?" Their answer, an emphatic yes, identified specific foods and food groups associated with the least and the most wrinkling.

Wrinkle preventers include eggs, fish, fruits (especially apples, cherries, melons, and pears), legumes (especially fava beans and lima beans), low-fat dairy foods (skim milk, low-fat yogurt), olive oil and other monounsaturated fats (avocados, nuts), tea, vegetables (especially dark leafy greens and asparagus, celery, eggplant, garlic, and onions), and whole-grain breads and cereals. These foods are high in antioxidant vitamins and phytochemicals that protect skin.

Wrinkle promoters include butter and margarine, cakes and pastries, high-fat dairy foods (whole milk, ice cream), potatoes, red meat (particularly processed meats), and soft drinks (the study did not distinguish between sugar-sweetened and diet soda). Researchers found that these foods were associated with a high degree of photoaging (sun damage).

Another nutritional factor that ages skin is the advanced glycation end products—with the apt acronym AGE. Collagen and elastin are fibrous proteins that help maintain the skin's firm, supple structure. AGEs are sugar molecules that bind with collagen and elastin, weakening and warping those fibers. AGEs also inactivate enzymes that protect against UV rays.

To reduce AGEs in your skin, try these tips:

+ **Avoid sugar.** The number-one dietary source of damaging AGEs is sugar—so cut down on candy, cookies, ice cream, and other sugary foods.

+ **Cook right.** When certain food is cooked using high heat (above 375°F) and no water—for instance, oven-roasted, baked, grilled, or fried—AGEs form. All foods can form AGEs, even vegetables, though the highest levels occur when protein and

carbohydrates are combined, such as in baked goods made with eggs and flour.

    Best: Steam, boil, stew, use a slow cooker, or roast at 350°F or lower.

+ **Add spice.** Turmeric, garlic, cinnamon, and ginger inhibit AGEs' ability to bind with collagen and elastin, so use these liberally. You'll add flavor to your food and subtract years from your skin.

SKIN-SMOOTHING SUPPLEMENTS

Even if you are conscientious about your diet, it can be hard to get sufficient amounts of the most powerful skin-protecting nutrients from food alone. That's why I recommended taking any or all of the following supplements daily (with your doctor's OK), continuing indefinitely.

    Multivitamin/mineral. Choose a brand that includes 100 percent of the recommended daily value for vitamin A, which helps prevent dryness; vitamin C, vitamin E, and selenium, essential for the manufacture and function of collagen; and zinc, which protects against the sun's damaging UV rays.

    Fish oil. This is rich in omega-3 fatty acids that shield skin from UV rays, protect against oxidation, and improve skin elasticity. Take a daily fish oil supplement that supplies 1,000 to 2,000 mg of eicosapentaenoic acid (EPA), the omega-3 that best protects collagen.

Gamma-linolenic acid (GLA). This fatty acid enhances EPA's skin-saving effects.

Dosage: 250 to 500 mg of GLA from borage oil or evening primrose oil, taken along with your fish oil.

Probiotics. These friendly intestinal bacteria not only support digestive health, they also combat inflammation and oxidation throughout the body—including in the skin. Probiotics help prevent certain harmful substances from passing through the gut wall and entering the bloodstream, where they could provoke a systemic inflammatory response and contribute to oxidative stress. I recommended Align Probiotic Supplement from Procter & Gamble or UltraFlora Intensive Care from Metagenics, which in clinical trials have proven to be effective at lowering inflammation and oxidative stress. Follow dosage guidelines on labels.

Cocoa. An intriguing study showed how much cocoa's antioxidant flavanols help the skin. Every day, one group of women drank 3.4 ounces of water mixed with high-flavanol cocoa powder, and another group drank a low-flavanol cocoa mixture.

After twelve weeks: Compared with the low-flavanol group, the high-flavanol group's skin had, on average, 25 percent less reddening from UV exposure, 30 percent less roughness, and 43 percent less

scaling. Their skin also was significantly more moist and firm and had 100 percent better blood circulation.

Daily options: Mix two tablespoons of unsweetened cocoa powder (not Dutch process) with a smoothie, yogurt, or glass of water, or take a cocoa bean supplement.

> Alan C. Logan, ND, board-certified naturopathic physician, invited faculty member in Harvard's School of Continuing Medical Education in Boston, and author or coauthor of four books, including *Your Skin, Younger* and *The Clear Skin Diet.* DrLogan.com.

Eat Chicken Soup and Other Secrets to Healthier Skin

You don't need to buy lotions and creams at the drugstore or department store to reduce wrinkles, prevent breakouts, add color and moisture to your skin, and/or reduce the uncomfortable and unappealing effects of problems such as oily skin, eczema, psoriasis, and rosacea.

Not only are lotions and creams usually pricey, but they often are laced with potentially toxic and harsh chemicals such as parabens and formaldehyde that have been associated with hormonal disruption and cancer.

Even if you feel attached to your favorite brand of skin lotion, it might be time to give it up, because there's a safer and cheaper alternative—and it doesn't involve anything external.

You can improve your skin naturally—from the inside out—by consuming certain foods and supplements.

CHICKEN SOUP—THE WRINKLE POTION

Simmer a quartered chicken (skin, bones, and all) with some onion, celery, carrots, and a bay leaf for two hours in enough water to cover the contents. Leave the pot uncovered for the full two hours, which will allow for evaporation and concentrate the liquid. The poultry and vegetables will give up their flavor and nutrients to the remaining water, and after you remove the solids, you'll be left with a broth rich in hyaluronic acid (HA)—the same substance that we make in our own bodies that provides skin with fullness, volume, and plumpness. As we grow older, our bodies produce less HA, which causes our skin to wrinkle and sag, so consuming extra HA may help. Organic and free-range chickens tend to produce more HA than traditionally raised chickens because their diets are healthier and they're allowed to exercise more. Make a big pot of this concentrated chicken broth, and then freeze half and refrigerate half upon cooling. Have a warmed cup every evening before dinner, spiced with a pinch of sea salt and fresh ground pepper for extra flavor. Feel free to adjust the recipe with your own choice of herbs and spices, and you'll still get the benefit. Chicken broth that you buy in a supermarket is just not the same, because valuable compounds in the chicken skin and bones don't make their way into store-bought broths and bouillon cubes. If you find that this soup isn't helping your skin enough, ask your doctor about taking extra HA in supplement form.

ADD COLOR AND MOISTURE

For great skin, be sure to consume enough of vitamins A, D, and E and the mineral zinc. Many people don't meet the recommended daily requirements. And that's too bad, because they can help protect your skin from the aging and cancerous effects of the sun's UV rays and from damaging environmental irritants, such as exhaust fumes and smog that can make skin dry and dull. Foods high in vitamin A include sweet potatoes, carrots, and dark, leafy greens; foods high in vitamin D include salmon, mushrooms, and fortified milk; foods high in vitamin E include sunflower seeds, almonds, and peanuts; and foods high in zinc include oysters, low-fat roast beef, and lentils. Also, colorful fruits and vegetables are filled with carotenoids, organic pigments that can add color to your skin, giving you a literally healthy glow. The amount of foods that you should consume depends on how deficient you are. If you eat lots of the foods mentioned above and don't notice any results within a few months, ask your doctor whether it's a good idea to take daily supplements containing vitamins A, D, and E and zinc, as well as a supplement complex that contains mixed carotenes and other carotenoids including lutein, lycopene, and zeaxanthin.

PREVENT BREAKOUTS

Plenty of adults get pimples. The best natural defense is nuts and seeds, which are packed with antioxidants and omega-3 fatty acids that calm systemic and facial inflammation and therefore reduce the frequency and severity of outbreaks.

Antipimple dose: A one-ounce serving per day of almonds, Brazil nuts, walnuts, pecans, or sunflower seeds. Try the foods first, and if the effect isn't strong enough within a few months, talk to your doctor about taking both antioxidant and omega-3 supplements, which might amplify the effect. Your health-care provider can help you figure out how much you need. If you have a peanut allergy, try algae-sourced omega-3s and food-grade coconut oil for antioxidants. Note that those with a severe preexisting allergy should consult their doctors before introducing any new substance.

RELIEF FOR OILY SKIN, ECZEMA, PSORIASIS, AND ROSACEA

The skin problems listed above are sometimes signs of poor digestive health. And one key to healthy digestion is making sure that there's enough good bacteria in your gut. As we grow older, the army of beneficial bacteria that normally crowds out the bad bacteria declines, so it doesn't hurt to call for backup, so to speak, in the form of probiotic supplementation. Eat a healthful diet—whole foods, not processed—because that creates the best environment for healthful bacteria. But probiotics contained in foods, such as yogurts, don't build up as well as those found in supplements. Ask your doctor about taking a supplement containing both *Lactobacillus* and *Bifidobacterium*, which may help restore a proper balance of bacteria in your intestine and lead to healthier, better-feeling, better-looking skin.

....

› Andrew L. Rubman, ND, medical director of Southbury Clinic for Traditional Medicines in Southbury, Connecticut. He is a founding member of the American Association of Naturopathic Physicians. His blog, *Nature Doc's Patient Diary*, is published on BottomLineInc.com. SouthburyClinic.com.

DIY Body Lotions for All Your Skin Ailments

When it comes to treating common conditions such as dry skin, sunburn, bug bites, rosacea, eczema, and even wrinkles, using oils that you already have on hand or making your own lotions from them can provide great relief. Besides working very well, they often are far less expensive than lotions that you would buy in the store. The oils are available at supermarkets, health-food stores, and drugstores. Below are tips on how to use them to make your skin look and feel better.

For dry winter skin: A nickel-sized amount of evening primrose oil, pressed from the seeds of the evening primrose plant, is great for moisturizing the face in cold weather due to its gamma-linolenic acid (a beneficial fatty acid), and you can use even more if you would like to cover your whole body. It doesn't feel heavy like many lotions do, but it still prevents chapping from windburn and becomes invisible when the skin absorbs it. You can apply it in the morning or at night or both times, if needed. Do not use evening primrose oil if you are pregnant, because of a possible risk for early uterine contractions. However, data on this is controversial, so consult your doctor.

For sunburn and bug bites (including spider bites!): Any type of olive oil can work very well for relieving the discomfort of sunburns and bug bites, because it reduces skin inflammation. That calms the skin, which makes it itch and hurt less, and accelerates healing. Use only the amount of oil that you need to lightly cover the affected area, and gently massage it into the skin once a day. If the scent of olive oil reminds you a bit too much of dinner, make your own scented oil.

My favorite: Pour olive oil into a jar containing dried organic chamomile flower buds. Use enough to submerge the buds. The buds are available online and in many health-food stores. Then seal the jar and let it sit for a month in a dark, dry place. Before using the oil, strain out the flower buds, and you will be left with a chamomile-scented oil to use on your skin.

For rosacea: To reduce the severity of flare-ups that leave your cheeks and nose glowing red, you can try evening primrose oil (mentioned above) or hazelnut oil. You can't cure rosacea (no one knows how to do that), but due to their astringent properties, both oils cleanse and repair damaged skin; prevent dehydration; reduce inflammation, redness, and swelling; and stimulate skin regrowth. Put a few drops directly onto the face before bed each night and gently massage them into your skin. Do not mix the two oils. Instead, alternate them each day. (And talk to your doctor before using evening primrose oil if you're pregnant.)

To relieve eczema: Many people with eczema find that they can soothe the redness, itching, and soreness with plain avocado oil. For the dry, flaky skin that eczema brings, avocado oil can be mixed with brown sugar and used as a gentle scrub. It not only helps moisturize and calm the irritation, but because brown sugar is coarse (but not too abrasive) and contains a form of natural glycolic acid, it exfoliates, so it also helps eliminate the flaking that is part of this condition. Any oil would moisturize, but avocado oil is particularly helpful for eczema patients because it is unusually thick and better protects the skin from dehydration.

To use: Make a mixture by adding just enough avocado oil to granulated brown sugar to create a grainy paste. You can make a batch that will keep in the refrigerator or in a dark, dry, cool place for several months. Apply to the dry portions of your skin using a gentle, circular massage for a few minutes two to three times per week.

Then rinse the skin with lukewarm water and pat dry with a towel.

Important: Never scrub over open wounds. Avoid those areas until they are completely closed. And if the scrub is too irritating for your skin, then use less brown sugar, use the scrub less often or less vigorously, or stop using the scrub altogether.

To reduce fine wrinkles: Rubbing a nickel-sized amount of evening primrose oil on your face in the morning and/or evening may help. It is high in antioxidants, which help protect and repair damaged cells that lead to wrinkles, so it may smooth out your skin. (Talk to your doctor before using it if pregnant.)

For almost all of these skin conditions, the oils will provide immediate relief, except when it comes to smoothing out wrinkles, which could require daily use for a month, so be patient!

› Aimee Masi, MA, licensed medical aesthetician, department of plastic surgery, Loyola University Medical Center, Maywood, Illinois.

Homemade Face Masks

REPAIR SUN-ABUSED SKIN
Soften the leathery look of skin that has had too much sun with this centuries-old beauty mask formula. Mix two

tablespoons of raw honey with two table-spoons of flour. Add enough milk (two to three tablespoons) to make the mixture the consistency of toothpaste. Be sure your face and neck are clean and your hair is out of the way. Smooth the paste on your face and neck. Stay clear of the delicate skin around your eyes. Leave the paste on for a half hour, then rinse it off with tepid water and pat dry. Do this once or twice a week, and wear a hat when you go out in the sun, please!

MILK FACE MASK: FRENCH SECRET FOR GETTING RID OF WRINKLES

This is the secret formula for wrinkle-free skin from a French beauty we know. (She never seems to age!) French women are the envy of women worldwide when it comes to beautiful skin!

Combine and bring to a boil one cup of whole milk, two teaspoons of lemon juice, and one tablespoon of brandy. Remove from heat. While the mixture is still warm (not hot!), paint it on your face and neck with a pastry brush. (Yes, you will feel like a delectable pastry.) When it is thoroughly dry, wash off the residue with warm water and pat dry with a freshly laundered towel. Do this three times a week for beautiful skin and fewer wrinkles.

THE ANTIWRINKLE MASK THAT COSTS NOTHING (ALMOST)

An easy, inexpensive wrinkle mask calls for one teaspoon of honey and two tablespoons of heavy whipping cream. Mix them together vigorously. Dip your fingertips in the mixture and, with a gentle massaging action, apply it to your face and neck, wherever wrinkles and lines reside. Leave it on for at least a half hour. You'll feel it tighten on your face as it becomes a mask. When you're ready, splash it off with tepid water. Do this daily for naturally beautiful skin.

SKIN-TIGHTENING TONIC

Skin experts often advise using an astringent skin tonic to help clean skin and refine pores. We have an easy, inexpensive tonic with rave reviews! One source described it as "the cleansing acid that cuts through residue film and clears the way for a healthful complexion." And still another said, "This formula is, by far, the simplest natural healer for tired skin. It gives you the glow of fresh-faced youth." With endorsements like that, what are you waiting for?

Mix one tablespoon of apple cider vinegar with one tablespoon of just-boiled water. As soon as the liquid is cool enough, apply it to the face with cotton balls. Do not get it near your eyes. No need to rinse…unless you can't stand the smell. (Lydia tried this skin tonic. Her eyes were a little teary from the strong fumes of the diluted vinegar, and for about ten minutes, she smelled like coleslaw. But after that, the smell was completely gone, and her skin felt smooth and tight.)

Use this treatment to freshen your skin at least every other day—or whenever you have a craving for that deli smell.

FIRMING FRUIT FACIAL FOR SUPERHEALTHY SKIN

The best time to apply a face mask is just before going to sleep, when your skin remains makeup free for at least six to eight hours. Also, try to apply the mask right after you've taken a bath or shower or after you've gently steamed your face so that your pores are open and ready for a healthy treat.

Here's an all-natural mask that will make your skin look great. In a blender, purée one cup of fresh pineapple and one-half cup of fresh (slightly green) papaya. Put the pureed fruit in a bowl, and mix in two tablespoons of honey. Apply it to your just-washed face and neck but not on the delicate area right around your eyes. Leave it on for five minutes—not more—and rinse with cool water.

This once-a-week natural alpha hydroxy acid facial can boost the production of collagen (making your face firmer), slough off dead skin cells, even out skin tone, and make tiny lines less noticeable. The enzymes in pineapple (bromelain) and papaya (papain) do most of the work, while the honey acts as a natural antibiotic, gently healing blemishes.

BANISH BROWN SPOTS WITH BEANS

No, you don't have to eat more beans to get rid of age spots. This is a topical remedy that calls for chickpeas, also known as garbanzo beans. If you don't want to cook dry beans, you can use precooked canned chickpeas. Mash about one-third cup chickpeas, and add a little water. Smear the paste on your brown spots (on your hands, arms, or face), and leave it there until it dries and starts crumbling off. Then wash it off completely. Do this every evening for two months. (Those age spots took a long time to form, so it'll take a bit of time to fade them naturally.)

› Joan Wilen and Lydia Wilen, health investigators and folk-remedy experts based in New York City who have spent decades collecting "cures from the cupboard." They are authors of *Bottom Line's Treasury of Home Remedies & Natural Cures*, *Bottom Line's Household Magic*, and *Bottom Line's Secret Food Cures*.

Homemade Eye Cures

WRINKLE ERASER

Some wrinkles bring character and wisdom to our faces, and some…well… If you don't love those wrinkles that can look like whiskers around your eyes, and you don't want to splurge on plastic surgery, here's what to do. With your fingertips, apply two or three drops of castor oil on the delicate area around the eyes to reduce eye wrinkles. Do this every night just before you go to bed, and remove any residue in the morning with your usual face wash. You should see fewer lines in about a month or so (after which you can oil up just a few nights a week). Castor oil is a natural emollient that will make your skin soft and supple.

NO MORE DARK UNDER-EYE CIRCLES

If you had a night of too much alcohol and not enough sleep, you might wake up with dark circles under your eyes. Those raccoon rings could also be from allergies, general irritation, or just getting old. If you've checked out your rings with the doctor and he/she says that there's nothing majorly wrong with you, try these remedies.

If you have access to fresh figs, try cutting one in half and placing the halves under your eyes with the moist fig insides against your skin. You should, of course, lie down and relax for fifteen to thirty minutes while you do this. OK, fig face, time to get up and gently rinse the sticky stuff off with tepid water. Dab on some peanut oil or olive oil to give the thin eye skin a subtle, healthful glow.

When figs are not in season, grate an unwaxed cucumber or a small scrubbed (preferably red) potato. Put the gratings on two gauze pads (or cheesecloth, anything that will allow some seepage), lie down, and place the pads, gauze-side down, under your eyes. Rinse your face with cool water, and dab on some peanut or olive oil.

> › Joan Wilen and Lydia Wilen, health investigators and folk-remedy experts based in New York City who have spent decades collecting "cures from the cupboard." They are authors of *Bottom Line's Treasury of Home Remedies & Natural Cures*, *Bottom Line's Household Magic*, and *Bottom Line's Secret Food Cures*.

Natural Cures for Cold Sores

Caused by a herpes virus, cold sores can be unsightly and painful.

Solutions: L-lysine, 1,000 mg, taken three times daily between meals at the first sign of the tingling/burning that precedes an outbreak. It's an amino acid that aids in tissue repair and can help cold sores heal more quickly.

Avoid foods that are high in the amino acid L-arginine, such as peanuts, almonds, whole wheat, and chocolate. L-arginine makes it easier for the virus to thrive.

Also helpful: Apply lemon balm cream to the area four times daily at the first sign of an outbreak. One double-blind study found that people who did this had less discomfort and fewer blisters during outbreaks than those who used a placebo.

› Mark A. Stengler, NMD, naturopathic doctor and founder of the Stengler Center for Integrative Medicine in Encinitas, California. He is author and coauthor of numerous books, including *The Natural Physician's Healing Therapies* and *Bottom Line's Prescription for Natural Cures*, and is the author of the newsletter *Health Revelations.* MarkStengler.com.

Natural Remedies for Thinning Hair

If you are concerned about the common problem of alopecia (hair loss), first see your doctor to find out whether there's an underlying medical problem, such as a thyroid disorder, that needs treating. But if no such problem is found, don't be too quick to turn to conventional hair-loss treatments, because these can be problematic.

For instance: Topical medications can cause itching and increased facial or body hair. There's limited evidence for the effectiveness of laser therapy, and costly hair-replacement surgery isn't appropriate for diffuse thinning throughout the scalp, the type of hair loss women often experience.

Fortunately, there are other options. The following natural therapies have a long tradition of use. Safe and economical, they offer do-it-yourself alternatives to conventional hair-loss treatment. (All products mentioned below are sold at health-food stores and online.)

SCALP CIRCULATION BOOSTERS

For many women, the key to reversing hair loss is to increase blood flow in the scalp. Try any or all of the following for six weeks. If you notice improvement, continue indefinitely or for as long as needed.

Massage with rosemary oil. Rosemary oil works by widening tiny blood vessels in the scalp, thus stimulating hair follicles and helping promote hair growth. Massaging the scalp with your fingertips also promotes improved circulation.

Directions: Dilute rosemary oil with an equal amount of almond oil. This is important—rosemary oil by itself may be too strong and can irritate skin. Every evening (or every other evening, if you prefer), use your fingertips to massage a few drops of oil into your scalp, particularly where hair is thinning. Leave on overnight, and wash off in the morning.

Rinse hair with nettle tea. Nettle promotes hair growth not only by improving circulation, but also by reducing inflammation.

To prepare: Mix one-half tablespoon of dried nettle with one cup of water. Bring to a boil, reduce heat, cover, and simmer for thirty minutes. Remove from heat. Let sit, covered, for fifteen minutes. Strain through cheesecloth. Cool before using. Apply to hair, massaging into scalp for several minutes. Leave on for fifteen minutes, then shampoo.

Easier: Steep two nettle tea bags in very hot water for ten minutes. Cool, then apply as described above.

Good brand: Traditional Medicinals Organic Nettle Leaf tea bags (800-543-4372, www.TraditionalMedicinals.com).

Drink herbal tea. Consuming certain herbal teas can improve sluggish circulation from the inside out, which can stimulate hair growth. Choose either or both of the following teas and drink a total of three cups per day.

- **Hawthorn.** Steep a heaping teaspoon of dried hawthorn berries in one cup of very hot water for five to ten minutes, then strain. If you prefer, take hawthorn in supplement form as an extract of either dried berries or flowers and leaves at a dosage of 300 mg twice daily.
- **Ginger.** Add several slices of fresh ginger to one cup of water and boil for five minutes, then remove the ginger.

HAIR-SAVING STRESS BUSTERS

Emotional ordeals can provoke numerous physical reactions, including hair loss. To help manage stress, practice a daily relaxation technique (such as deep breathing) and follow a whole-foods-based diet that emphasizes fruits and vegetables and minimizes red meat and alcohol. Also try the following tips.

Supplement with B vitamins. The various B vitamins are needed to convert food to energy and help cells grow, but physical or emotional stress can deplete these key nutrients. Take a daily supplement of a B-complex formulation. Follow the dosage guidelines on the label and continue indefinitely.

Try an herbal adaptogen. Adaptogenic herbs have been used for thousands of years to increase the body's resistance to stress, trauma, anxiety, and fatigue. Their mechanism is not well understood, but they are thought to work in part by balancing hormones. Choose one of ashwagandha (also called withania), rhodiola, or Siberian ginseng (not regular ginseng, which is too strong). Select a product labeled "standardized" (indicating that the brand uses consistent amounts of the active ingredient), and follow the dosage instructions on the label. If you experience headaches, discontinue use. Otherwise, continue daily for one month. If you notice improvement, stay with it for another month, then give your body a two-week break. If you do not notice improvement after one month, try one of the other adaptogens listed above.

> David Hoffmann, clinical medical herbalist based in Sonoma County, California, fellow of Britain's National Institute of Medical Herbalists, advisory board member of the American Botanical Council, and founding member and past president of the American Herbalists Guild. He teaches at the California School of Herbal Studies in Forestville, is a visiting faculty member at Bastyr University in Kenmore, Washington, and is the author of seventeen books, including *Herbal Prescriptions After 50*.

Ten Tricks to Look Ten Years Younger

Most of us want to look as youthful and vital on the outside as we feel on the inside. But without realizing it, we may be appearing older than we need to.

Here are ten simple things you can do that will make you look younger.

CLOTHING AND ACCESSORIES

Cut back on the black. Wearing all black is certainly stylish, but as you age, it can make dark circles under the eyes and facial wrinkles appear even more pronounced. It's better to wear bright colors, which instead convey a sense of youth and vibrancy. You don't have to cover yourself from head to toe in loud colors to accomplish this. Just add a dash of color, ideally near the face or neck where it will draw people's attention up toward your eyes. People are more likely to consider you as an individual—and less likely to judge you based on your age—if they make eye contact with you. A brightly colored scarf or necklace is a good choice for women; a brightly colored tie, pocket square, or polo shirt works for men.

Alternative: If you prefer to wear muted colors, not bright ones, at least replace black garments with navy, cranberry, charcoal, brown, and olive.

Stop wearing worn garments. Teens and twentysomethings can get away with wearing threadbare or vintage clothing. But when older people wear past-its-prime clothing, it makes them seem old and past their prime too. Once an item of clothing goes out of style or starts to show wear, it's time to stop wearing it, at least in public.

Buy clothes that fit the body you have today. Some people are so used to wearing clothes of a certain size that they go right on purchasing that size even as they age and their bodies change shape. Other people intentionally buy baggy clothing because they think it will hide the physical imperfections that inevitably come with age. In reality, wearing clothes that do not fit properly only calls additional attention to physical imperfections.

When you try on clothes in a store, take your usual size along with one size larger and one size smaller into the fitting room, then purchase whichever fits best, regardless of what size you thought you were. If you're not great at gauging fit, shop with a friend who knows a lot about clothes, or ask a store employee for assistance.

Also: Women should get a bra fitting—and purchase new bras if necessary—at least once a year. Women's bra sizes often change as they age.

Take a look at your eyeglasses. These days, wire-frame glasses seem old and dated, which can make their wearers seem old and dated too. Consider switching to more fashionable plastic frames, either black or colored. If that doesn't fit your personality, switch to rimless glasses.

Also: If you wear bifocals (or trifocals), try switching to progressive lenses. These serve the same purpose but without that line across the lens that often is associated with old age.

Avoid being too "matchy." Carrying a handbag that matches one's shoes was once considered stylish. These days, it is associated with older women. Young women tend to prefer a more casual, unmatched look. If you own sweater sets, break them up.

Skip the turtleneck. Some people think wearing a turtleneck will hide the sagging neck that often comes with age. But turtlenecks actually call attention to the portion of the saggy neck and jowls that still can be seen.

Instead, women should consider wearing V-necked or scoop-necked shirts that visually extend the length of the neck, then add a brightly colored necklace, scarf, or high-collared jacket. Men should opt for collared shirts.

SKIN AND BODY

Apply sunscreen to your hands. You probably already know that using sunscreen regularly on your face can help you look younger. The moisture in the sunscreen gives older, dry skin a moist, younger look, and the UV protection limits age spots and other skin damage that is associated with age.

Also, sunscreen prevents a deep-tan look, which appears old and out-of-touch in today's skin cancer-conscious society. A light tan is fine; too dark is dated.

What many people do not consider is that sunscreen should be applied to the backs of the hands in addition to the face. Wrinkled, dry, heavily tanned, or age-spotted hands can make people appear old even if the skin on their faces still looks young. Spots on the hands are one of the first signs of aging.

Men who are losing their hair or are already bald should apply sunscreen to the scalp, or they can wear a baseball cap or a straw fedora, which are stylish and youthful options. Sunburn, flaking, or overall redness will draw attention to your head and make you look old.

Helpful: Research suggests that broad spectrum sunscreens that protect against UVA light, in addition to the UVB associated with sunburns, are particularly effective in combating the aging effects of the sun.

Also: Stay hydrated. Drinking eight eight-ounce glasses of water each day can help your skin maintain the moist, dewy glow that is associated with youth.

Strong arm yourself. Toned arm muscles can help you look younger, but which muscles you should target varies by gender. Consider working with a trainer to learn the best exercises for you.

Women: Sagging biceps and triceps in the upper arm can make women look old. Exercising with dumbbells is the best way to tone these. Start with very light dumbbells if necessary—even two-pound weights can make a difference. Do bicep curls, hammer curls, and tricep exercises several times a week.

Men: Broad shoulders help men continue to look young and powerful as they age. Bench presses and/or push-ups help here.

Stand up straight. Hunching over makes people seem old and wizened. Sitting or standing with your back straight and your shoulders back conveys an air of youthful strength and confidence.

Tip: If you find it difficult to maintain proper posture, take a Pilates class. Pilates is an exercise regimen that focuses on core strength, which is crucial for good posture.

Trim facial hair. Women should be on the lookout for long, stray hairs and pluck them.

Having a beard doesn't make a man look old—even if the beard is gray—but having an unkempt beard does. Trim your beard at least once a week, and shave your neck and around the other edges of the beard every day.

Also: Trim nose hair, ear hair, and bushy eyebrows frequently. Excess hair in these areas doesn't just look sloppy; it is associated with old age. Ask your barber to trim your eyebrows when you get a haircut if you're not confident in your ability to trim your own brows properly.

› Lauren Rothman, style and trend expert who has appeared on *Entertainment Tonight*, CNN, *E! News*, and *ABC News*, among other news outlets. She is a style consultant for individuals and corporations in the greater Washington, DC, area and author of *Style Bible: What to Wear to Work*. StyleAuteur.com.

Eleven Things That Make You Look Older

As you get older, wardrobe and style choices that worked when you were younger may no longer be serving you well. This goes for both men and women. Without knowing it, you may be looking older than you are. This could cause others to treat you as older and potentially hold you back from employment opportunities and advancements. This also can

make you feel like you are not up to your game or comfortable in your skin. When you are not style confident, you are less body confident, which makes you feel less life confident.

Helpful: Seek out style mentors—people who look elegant and modern without chasing youth-oriented trends. Observe them carefully, and adapt elements of their style to your own. TV newscasters make good style mentors, because they are required to look contemporary while also projecting dignity and authority.

Give yourself a good, hard look, and ask yourself whether you are looking older than your actual age with any of these common signals.

1. **Sneakers for everyday wear.** Your feet should be comfortable, but sneakers outside the gym just look sloppy and careless. Young people get away with it—but there are more stylish options when you're older. These include loafers or driving moccasins for men and low-heeled pumps with cushioned soles for women. Wedge-soled shoes are a comfortable alternative to high heels.

2. **Baggy pants.** Although young men may look trendy in loose-fitting jeans, this style screams old on anyone else.

For women, the rear end tends to flatten with age, causing pants to fit loosely in the rear. And front-pleated pants for women generally are unflattering and unstylish.

Better: Spend the time to find pants that fit well, or figure a tailor into your wardrobe budget. Baggy is dowdy, but overly tight makes you look heavier. Well-fitting clothes make you look slimmer and younger.

3. **Boring colors.** Skin tone gets duller with age, so the colors you wear should bring light to your face. If you are a woman who has worn black for years, it may be too harsh for you now. Brown makes men fade into the woodwork.

Better: Stand in front of a mirror, and experiment with colors that you never thought you could wear. You may be surprised at what flatters you. Avoid neon brights, which make older skin look sallow, but be open to the rest of the color spectrum. Try contemporary patterns and prints. For neutrals, gray and navy are softer alternatives to black for women, and any shade of blue is a good bet for men.

4. **Boring glasses and jewelry.** Men and women should have some fun with glasses. It's a great way to update your look and make it more modern. Tell your optician what you're looking for, or bring a stylish friend with you.

As for jewelry for women, wearing a large piece of fab faux jewelry (earrings, necklace, ring) or multiple bracelets adds great style and youth to your look.

5. **Stiff or one-tone hair.** An overly styled helmet of hair looks old-fashioned. Hair that's a solid block of color looks unnatural and harsh.

Better: Whether hair is short or shoulder-length, women need layers around the face for softness. As for color, opt for subtle highlights in front and a slightly darker tone toward the back.

Keep in mind that gray hair can be beautiful, modern, and sexy. You need a plan to go gray though, which means a flattering cut and using hair products that enhance the gray. Ask your stylist for recommendations. Also, if your hair is a dull gray, consider getting silver highlights around your face to bring light and energy to your hair.

Men who dye their hair should allow a bit of gray at the temples—it looks more natural than monochrome hair. But avoid a comb-over or a toupee. A man who attempts to hide a receding hairline isn't fooling anyone—he just looks insecure.

Better: Treat your thinning hair as a badge of honor. Either keep it neatly trimmed or shave your head.

6. **Missing (or bushy) eyebrows.** Women's eyebrows tend to disappear with age. Men's are more likely to grow wild.

Better: Women should use eyebrow pencil, powder, or both to fill in fading brows. Visit a high-end cosmetics counter, and ask the stylist to show you how. You may need to try several products to find out what works best. Men, make sure that your barber or hair stylist trims your eyebrows regularly.

Also: Women tend not to notice increased facial hair (especially stray hairs) on the chin and upper lip, a result of hormonal change. Pluck!

7. **Deeply tanned skin.** Baby boomers grew up actively developing suntans using baby oil and sun reflectors. Now, pale is the norm. A dark tan not only dates you, it increases your risk for skin cancer and worsens wrinkling.

Better: Wear a hat and sunscreen to shield your skin from sun damage.

8. **Less-than-white teeth.** Yellowing teeth add decades to your appearance. Everyone's teeth get yellower with age, but with so many teeth-whitening products available, there is no excuse to live with off-color teeth.

Better: Ask your dentist which whitening technique he/she recommends based on the condition of your teeth—over-the-counter whitening strips, bleaching in the dentist's office, or a custom bleaching kit you can use at home.

9. **Women: Nude or beige hose.** Nude stockings on women look hopelessly out-of-date. Bare legs are the norm now for young women, but they are not a good option for older women who have dark veins.

Better: In winter, wear dark stockings or opaque tights. In summer, use spray-on tanner for a light tan, or wear nude fishnet stockings or slacks or capris.

10. **Poor-fitting bra.** Get a bra that fits. Most women don't know that bra size changes as your body does. Giving your breasts a lift will make you look younger and trimmer.

11. **Excess makeup.** Thick foundation, heavy eyeliner, bright blusher, and red lipstick all add years to your face.

Better: Use a moisturizing (not matte) foundation, and dab it only where needed to even out skin tone. To add color to cheeks, use a small amount of tinted moisturizer, bronzer, or cream blush. Use liquid eyeliner in soft shades such as deep blue or brown, and blend it well. For lips, choose soft pinks and mauves, depending on your skin tone.

Bottom line: The idea is to have fun putting yourself together. That inner spark and personal style will show that you are getting better with age.

....

› Kim Johnson Gross, cocreator of the *Chic Simple* book series and author of *What to Wear for the Rest of Your Life* and *Chic Simple Dress Smart: Men.* Based in New York City, she is a former Ford model and has been fashion editor at *Town & Country* and *Esquire* magazines and a columnist for *More* and *InStyle.* KimJohnsonGross.com.

....

12

Mood

Natural Mood Elevators

Ads for antidepressants make it seem as though the most logical solution for a case of the blues is to seek a prescription. Pharmaceutical drugs may be helpful—even necessary—for people with severe depression, but for others, there are natural solutions that may work even better, with less risk of adverse side effects. Dietary supplements and lifestyle changes can be used to naturally lift your spirits.

"I think that a lot of our modern-day fatigue and depression has to do with the fact that we're totally separated from nature," says Eric Yarnell, ND, core faculty member in the department of botanical medicine at Bastyr University and author of *Clinical Botanical Medicine*. "People don't eat well, and they watch huge amounts of television and don't spend much time relating to people or the outdoors." He believes that eating plenty of whole, unprocessed foods and getting regular exercise are the first steps to take in attempting to boost your mood and energy level. "Also, I tell people to turn off their televisions," he says, noting that replacing TV with even fifteen minutes of daily outdoor activity and sunlight will help, as will getting enough sleep.

SUPPLEMENTS THAT HELP
Eating whole foods with little or no added sugar, exercising (even a bit), and getting some moderate sun exposure are all highly effective ways to beat the blues and lift the spirits. Some people, however, still feel like there are times when they need a more controllable lift, and for them, Dr. Yarnell says there are natural supplements that really do help. Research supports three in particular—St. John's wort (*Hypericum*

perforatum), golden root (*Rhodiola rosea*), and eleuthero (*Eleutherococcus senticosus*).

St. John's wort. A meta-analysis published in the *British Medical Journal* in 1996 reviewed twenty-three trials on St. John's wort involving more than 1,700 patients, with researchers reporting it was more effective than a placebo at treating mild to moderately severe cases of depression. "The evidence is very strong that St. John's wort is an effective natural antidepressant for people whose depression is mild," says Mark Blumenthal, founder and executive director of the nonprofit American Botanical Council. This distinction is an important one, he notes. You might recall that the reputation of St. John's wort was sullied by a 2001 study published in the *Journal of the American Medical Association*, calling it ineffective. Blumenthal explained that this particular study had examined a group of patients that included those who had already been unresponsive to treatment with a conventional antidepressant drug, so their depression was quite severe.

Caveats for people interested in using St. John's wort to elevate their mood: Those with severe depression should seek medical advice to ensure proper treatment and monitoring. Also, cautions Blumenthal, "St. John's wort interacts with a whole suite of conventional

pharmaceutical drugs, so you must check with your health care provider about any possible interactions before taking it." Your prescriber will quite likely recommend preparations standardized to contain 0.3 percent hypericin, a naturally occurring compound in St. John's wort to which manufacturers standardize their extracts for quality control purposes. And if you are scheduled to have elective surgery, make sure you discontinue this supplement ahead of time.

Rhodiola/golden root. In Europe, *Rhodiola rosea* or *R. rosea*, the best known and most studied of different species of rhodiola (also called golden root), has a long history of being used to treat chronic fatigue, especially in Sweden and Russia. One interesting study tested the effect of 170 mg of *R. rosea* root extract on fifty-six physicians who were on stressful night-call duty. *R. rosea* brought about a statistically significant reduction in general fatigue for the first two weeks, but the positive effect seemed to fade by six weeks, suggesting it might be a good short-term solution that is helpful for acute stressful conditions but not for chronic stress. An experienced naturopath can provide advice on what's the best dosage in your case.

As for depression, a clinical trial found that *R. rosea* can also work as an antidepressant and mood elevator. In this Swedish study, *R. rosea* extract was found to not only help reduce symptoms of depression in patients with mild to moderate depression, but also to enhance their cognitive and sexual function, as well as mental and physical performance under stress.

Eleuthero. There is some debate about eleuthero, also known as Siberian ginseng (although it is no longer marketed under that name in the United States). Blumenthal is not enthusiastic about eleuthero, calling it "not great" for fatigue, but Dr. Yarnell believes it's effective, doesn't have significant adverse effects, and works "to balance people's systems." One clinical study evaluated ninety-six adults who had complained of fatigue for at least six months. They were given four capsules per day of eleuthero. While some reported their fatigue lessened considerably, the results were not statistically significant, though two subgroups in the population—those with longstanding fatigue and those with less severe fatigue—experienced some effect from the treatment after two months.

ASK YOUR DOCTOR

Natural supplements aren't necessarily risk-free, so it is vitally important to seek supervision by a physician experienced in their use, advice that rings as true when talking about moods as with physical ailments. You may find these products can be very beneficial and produce less adverse effects than pharmaceutical products, but use them responsibly.

› Mark Blumenthal, founder and executive director, American Botanical Council, and editor, *HerbalGram.* ABC.HerbalGram.org.

› Eric Yarnell, ND, core faculty member, department of botanical medicine, Bastyr University, and in private practice. He is author of *Clinical Botanical Medicine.*

Herbs That Help Fight Stress and Anxiety

*C*hamomile tea is a gentle relaxant that has traditionally been used as a "nerve tonic." Other herbs have similar effects. One of my favorites is passionflower. Despite the name, passionflower is more relaxing than arousing. It increases brain levels of gamma-aminobutyric acid (GABA), a neurotransmitter that dampens activity in the part of the brain that controls emotions, making you feel more relaxed. In one study, participants drank either passionflower tea or a placebo tea before going to bed.

Those who drank passionflower tea slept better and were more likely to wake up feeling refreshed and alert.

How to use it: Steep one teaspoon of dried passionflower in three ounces of just-boiled water. Drink it two to three times daily when you're stressed. Or take passionflower capsules or tinctures, following the label directions.

....

› Mark A. Stengler, NMD, naturopathic doctor and founder of the Stengler Center for Integrative Medicine in Encinitas, California. He is author and coauthor of numerous books, including *The Natural Physician's Healing Therapies* and *Bottom Line's Prescription for Natural Cures*, and is the author of the newsletter *Health Revelations.* MarkStengler.com.

....

Feeling Lonely Can Lead to Health Problems, Including Dementia

L oneliness is a miserable feeling, and generic advice such as joining a hiking club or a senior center may not help. The key to relieving your own loneliness is to understand it. Why are *you* lonely?

It's an important question to answer, because loneliness has been linked to a variety of health problems, such as weakened immunity and hardening of the arteries. Research also suggests that the dangers associated with loneliness are on par with those related to obesity and cigarette smoking.

Latest development: Loneliness is now considered a risk factor for Alzheimer's disease according to a study published in the *Archives of General Psychiatry.* Although the exact link between loneliness and the brain is unknown, some experts hypothesize that loneliness provokes a chronic stress reaction that promotes inflammation, which accumulating evidence suggests may contribute to Alzheimer's disease, the most common cause of dementia.

Here are some tips on how to fight loneliness and its associated health risks.

BEING ALONE VS. BEING LONELY

Many people choose to live by themselves and are perfectly content. Conversely, you can be lonely without being alone. Many lonely people are married, and some even have lots of friends.

So what is this thing called loneliness? It can include feeling that you lack companionship, feeling left out, and feeling isolated. You can even be lonely without knowing it. You can have one of these feelings and not recognize it as loneliness, in the same way that some depressed people do not identify their negative moods and lethargy as depression.

WHAT CAUSES LONELINESS?

Some people may be more vulnerable to feeling lonely because of their personalities. But other times, people are in situations that promote loneliness. For example, maybe they need to stay home due to an illness and miss seeing others, or perhaps they are living in a rural area where it's difficult to connect with others, and they crave more daily contact with people.

Loneliness also increases with age. In one study, 43 percent of seniors reported feeling lonely. There are two main reasons for this:

- **Relationships frequently dwindle with age.** Upon retirement, your career-long social network may crumble, friends and family may move away, or a beloved life partner may die.
- **Our ageist, youth-centered culture tends to ignore the wisdom and experience that aging provides.** The elderly are often stigmatized as a burden on society. It's easy to believe that your life no longer has a purpose when you feel unacknowledged by a world in which you once played a productive role.

EASING LONELINESS

There's no one-size-fits-all remedy for loneliness. But if you ask yourself the important question—*Why am I lonely?*—you may discover a solution that works for you. The following suggestions often help people pinpoint the cause of their loneliness and allow them to overcome it.

If you feel that you lack companionship:

- **Connect with more people.** Connecting with people who share your strong interest in something may help fill that void. Try joining a book group if you love to read or an activist group if you are passionate about politics. Consider volunteering to tutor children or serve meals at a shelter. Beneficial connections can happen one-on-one or in groups. Some people find that getting a pet is helpful.

Unfortunately, the loneliness of social isolation may have deep roots. Even if you are lonely for companionship, you may find it difficult or unpleasant to connect with others, particularly if the problem is long-standing. Dig down to find out why.

Some people never developed the social skills that foster friendships, and some hold maladaptive beliefs about themselves (a sense of inferiority or superiority, for example) or about others (such as mistrust). If this is the case, self-reflection and therapy can help.

+ **Put technology to work.** Computer, tablet, or smartphone applications like Skype and FaceTime allow you to talk with—and see—friends and family who aren't nearby. The apps are free (once you own the device).

If you're uncomfortable with technology, consider taking a free class at a public library or senior center. Check SeniorNet (SeniorNet.org), a nonprofit company that offers in-person classes across the country specially designed for older adults.

Useful: The AARP-sponsored website Connect2Affect.org offers valuable information and an interactive guide to local resources, such as job opportunities, volunteer programs, and tax preparation services. Also, SeniorCenterWithoutWalls.org enables isolated seniors to participate in groups via phone or computer.

Important: Social media, such as Facebook, provides a measure of connectedness but shouldn't displace real-life contact.

If you feel left out:

+ **Deepen your relationships.** Taking steps to deepen your friendships—by revealing more about yourself and listening and responding wholeheartedly to what your friends have to say—may bring the warmth of true connection into your life. Here too a therapist can help by giving you the tools you need to deepen your relationships.

Is it your relationship with your life partner that needs more intimacy? If your marriage leaves you lonely, you and your spouse may benefit from couples counseling.

If you feel physically isolated:

+ **Overcome barriers.** Mundane difficulties can cut you off from others. Transportation is often an issue for older people who have mobility problems or don't drive. Local agencies for the aging can provide help, as can the website Connect2Affect.org (mentioned above).

Consider using a task-sharing service where people trade skills for what they need. For example, you help someone with balancing her checkbook, and she gives you a ride to the supermarket.

Websites to try: SwapRight.com or Simbi.com. You could also take a taxi or use Uber if you cannot get a ride otherwise.

Maybe your diminished hearing or vision makes you reluctant to socialize. If that's the case, talk to your doctor about ways to improve your hearing or sight.

› Carla Perissinotto, MD, associate professor of geriatrics at the University of California at San Francisco. Dr. Perissinotto's research into the association between loneliness and health was published in *Archives of Internal Medicine.*

Use Mindfulness to Overcome Depression and Loneliness

Most people who experience depression—or even just a bout of the blues—try to fix it with an antidepressant or something else to make them feel better.

A different but highly effective "approach: Do not try to fix the uncomfortable feelings. That's a key aspect of *mindfulness*—which involves paying special attention to what's going on in our minds and bodies in a nonjudgmental way. With this approach, many people who have battled depression or sadness have experienced significant improvement in their symptoms.

For anyone who has ever suffered the pain of depression or low moods, this approach may sound wrongheaded. But the truth is it works. Of course, there are instances in which antidepressants may be needed. However, when people stop taking the drugs, depression often returns.

Important finding: People with a history of depression who used mindfulness in an organized program had half as many recurrences as people not on the program.

Here's what you need to know to use mindfulness to cope with sadness or depression.*

THE OLD WAY DOESN'T WORK

Most people don't realize that it's not the sad thoughts and feelings that cause us to spiral downward. It's what we do about them that matters. Two of the most common coping mechanisms to get out of a bad mood—trying to think our way out of a problem or trying to avoid painful feelings—actually trap us in the darkness.

Why thinking doesn't help. We are accustomed to believing that we can think our way out of any problem. So it's only natural to regard a dark mood as a problem to be solved. When we're in

* Consult a doctor before trying this approach if you have experienced suicidal thoughts or your depression interferes with your ability to perform daily activities.

this dreary state, we might ask ourselves questions such as *Why do I feel this way? How can I change my life? What should I be doing differently?* We believe that if we think hard enough, we'll find a solution.

But the opposite is true. Dwelling on how bad you feel, on the distance between the way things are and the way things should be, just reinforces your mood. Your mind begins running in an endless circle— and it seems as though there is no way out.

Why ignoring feelings doesn't help. We often think that if we ignore painful feelings, they will go away. When we try to push away these strong emotions, they rebound, stronger than ever. Think about it this way: if someone told you not to think about a white bear, guess what you would do. You couldn't help but think about a white bear or how you shouldn't think about it. Suppressing thoughts or feelings doesn't work.

WHAT TO DO INSTEAD

The practice of mindfulness enables you to look at your thoughts and feelings in a different way. Instead of dwelling on how bad you feel and struggling to do something about it, you simply *experience* what's going on.

Mindfulness encourages you to be aware of your emotions, thoughts, and bodily sensations without judging or interpreting them. You watch them, identify them, and acknowledge them instead of lingering over each one.

To get an idea of what mindfulness feels like, apply it to an ordinary activity that you do every day. While washing the dishes, for instance, notice how the warm water feels on your hands, how your hands and arms feel as you turn a dish over and rinse it off. Make washing dishes the full focus of your attention, not a task to get past. If your mind wanders, bring your focus back to the dishes. What you've done is to bring physical sensations into the realm of mindfulness.

Next, take thoughts and feelings into the realm of mindfulness. Being aware of your thoughts and feelings without reacting to them is the key to keeping negative emotions from cascading. This can be particularly challenging, which is why it's helpful to begin as though thoughts are sounds that you are simply listening to.

Here's how: While sitting quietly, let your attention shift to your hearing. Open your mind to sounds from all directions, near and far, subtle as well as obvious sounds. Be aware of these auditory sensations without thinking about where they're coming from or what they mean. Note the way they appear and fade. When you realize that your attention has drifted, note where it has gone and gently come back to the sounds.

After trying this a few times with sounds, shift your awareness to your thoughts. Let your mind "hear" them as if they were coming from outside, noting how they arise, linger, and move on.

Helpful: Imagine your thoughts projected on a screen at the movies, or see them as clouds passing across a clear sky. When a thought provokes strong emotions or physical feelings, notice this as well but only notice it, without trying to draw any conclusions from it.

Acknowledge if a feeling is particularly unpleasant. Does it cause any physical sensations or discomfort? Instead of ignoring the thought or the discomfort because it's unpleasant and you don't want to deal with it, sit with it for a little while. This can be difficult to do.

Helpful: Notice your thought patterns. If you are feeling like this—*I'll never be happy again* or *I feel like a failure*—you can say to yourself, *There's that "never-be-happy-ever" feeling again.*

How often to practice: It is recommended that you set aside thirty minutes every day to practice mindfulness. You can do this in a variety of ways—lying on the floor comfortably and focusing on your breathing, or walking and focusing on how your legs and arms feel as they move.

Even incorporating mindfulness for just five minutes at a time into routine daily activities—such as showering, brushing your teeth, or taking out the garbage—can help. The point is to be able to focus on what you are doing when you are doing it.

When you practice mindfulness regularly, it makes it easier to use the technique when you need it most—when you are upset because you are stuck in traffic, are in the middle of a heated argument, or begin to feel a bout of depression coming on.

› Zindel V. Segal, PhD, Cameron Wilson Chair in Depression Studies, University of Toronto, Ontario, Canada, and head of the Cognitive Behavioral Therapy Unit at the university's Centre for Addiction and Mental Health. He is coauthor of *The Mindful Way Through Depression: Freeing Yourself from Chronic Unhappiness.* MBCT.co.uk.

Foods and Supplements That Boost Mood

What we eat can affect our mood, making us feel happier. A number of people who suffer from depression, for example, improve significantly when they eat less (or eliminate) processed/sugary foods and consume more complex carbohydrates, such as grains and vegetables.

A healthy diet may reduce brain inflammation, important for improving neuron (brain cell) functions and reducing anxiety and depression. Here are some important dietary changes that can improve mood.

OMEGA-3 FATTY ACIDS

Population studies clearly show that people with a high intake of omega-3 fatty acids have a lower incidence of depression. The membranes that surround brain cells contain significant amounts of fatty acids. When more of these fats consist of omega-3s, the membranes become more flexible and porous—important for absorbing nutrients and receiving/transmitting chemical signals, vital in boosting mood.

Recommended: Eat two or three fish meals a week. Cold-water fish, such as sardines, mackerel, and herring, are the best food sources of omega-3s. If you don't like fish, try a supplement of 3,000 mg of omega-3 fatty acids, divided into two daily doses. Choose a supplement that provides 180 mg EPA and 120 mg DHA per 1,000-mg capsule.

DIETARY FIBER

Constipation is a common symptom— and possibly a cause—of the blues. People who don't eat enough fiber have smaller, less frequent bowel movements. This means that toxins that are present in the stools can get reabsorbed into the body. This can trigger depression and other mood changes.

Recommended: At least 30 g of fiber daily—more is probably better. People who mainly eat plant foods automatically get enough fiber. If your diet is short on fiber, add four to five tablespoons of unprocessed oat bran to your morning cereal or smoothie.

Red flag: Having three or fewer bowel movements a week. This is not normal. You should be having one or more bowel movements a day. If you're not, you probably need to consume more fiber (and water too).

MULTISUPPLEMENT

Everyone who is feeling down should take a daily multisupplement. The majority of Americans are deficient in one or more of the essential micronutrients, including selenium, magnesium, and B vitamins.

Why it matters: A deficiency of even one nutrient can impair the body's ability to utilize other nutrients. Nutritional deficiencies are a common cause of low energy as well as depressed mood.

One study found that people who consumed less than the recommended daily amount of selenium had significant mood improvements when they took supplements.

Magnesium is particularly important for mood because it's used for the production of serotonin, the neurotransmitter that increases when people take prescription antidepressants.

Recommended: Start with a daily supplement that provides all the key vitamins and minerals. You also might want to take a separate B-complex supplement, because B vitamins are vital to the metabolism of cells—in particular, the cells of the nervous system.

SAMe

S-adenosylmethionine (SAMe) releases a methyl molecule in the body that is necessary for the production of dopamine and serotonin. A review of scientific studies found that SAMe relieves symptoms of depression significantly better than a placebo and sometimes as well as prescription drugs. SAMe is far less likely than medications to cause significant side effects.

Recommended: I usually advise patients with depression to start with dietary changes, stress-reduction techniques, exercise, and sometimes talk therapy. If these aren't effective, it's helpful to take SAMe for several weeks or months or, in those with chronic depression, sometimes indefinitely.

The starting dose usually is 200 mg at morning and noontime. The amount can be slightly increased after several weeks if the initial dose isn't effective. If you feel agitated, you'll want to decrease the dose.

TRYPTOPHAN/5-HTP

If other approaches don't work, I may recommend tryptophan, an amino acid. Both tryptophan and the more easily available 5-HTP (into which tryptophan is converted) increase the body's production of serotonin. Tryptophan was largely banned in the early 1990s following contamination at a manufacturing plant. The supplement itself is entirely safe.

Both tryptophan and 5-HTP make it easier to fall asleep—important because insomnia and/or disturbed sleep are common in those with depression.

Recommended: Take 500 mg of tryptophan at bedtime. If tryptophan is not available, take 50 to 100 mg of 5-HTP twice daily.

PROBIOTICS

Healthy adults have trillions of beneficial intestinal bacteria known as probiotics. These organisms facilitate the production of energy within cells, promote the synthesis of B vitamins and other nutrients, and improve digestive health. Many people with depression have lower-than-expected levels of probiotic organisms.

Recommended: One to two capsules daily of a supplement that provides two to three billion organisms. Look for a combination supplement that includes acidophilus and bifidophilus organisms.

FOOD SENSITIVITIES CAN CAUSE DEPRESSION

An important factor in some people's depression is a sensitivity to one or more foods. I believe that food sensitivity is far more pervasive and far more often a cause of or contributor to depression than we know.

Food sensitivity can be caused by the passage of large, reaction-stimulating protein molecules out of an intestine that has been made "leaky." Infections and antibiotics and other drugs may be responsible for these leaky guts, but there may be dietary causes as well, including consumption of refined and processed foods. As large protein molecules pass across the gut into the bloodstream, they are believed to provoke defensive reactions in nearly every system in the body.

This immune reaction can cause depression and may produce a variety of physical symptoms as well, including fatigue.

Many people are sensitive to gluten, a protein found in wheat and some other grains. Other problem foods may include milk, eggs, citrus, and soy.

If you suspect that your depression might be linked to diet, you can try an elimination diet using these tips:

- **Completely eliminate possible food culprits from your diet.** Begin by saying no to gluten, milk and other dairy products, eggs, soy, and sugar. Keep a diary. Every day, note any symptoms, how you're feeling, and whether your energy has increased or decreased.

- **After three weeks, reintroduce the foods one at a time.** For example, eat a slice or two of wheat bread at dinner. See how you feel the next day. If your mood doesn't change, then you probably aren't sensitive to that food. Wait a week, and reintroduce another food.

....

› James S. Gordon, MD, founder and director, Center for Mind-Body Medicine, Washington, DC, clinical professor, departments of psychiatry and family medicine, Georgetown University School of Medicine, and former chair, White House Commission on Complementary and Alternative Medicine Policy. He is author of *Unstuck: Your Guide to the Seven-Stage Journey Out of Depression.* JamesGordonMD.com.

....

Exercise Can Work Better Than Drugs for Low Moods

Exercise really is nature's antidepressant. Several studies have shown that working out is just as effective, if not more so, than medication when it comes to treating mild-to-moderate depression. Exercise also can help reduce the amount of medication needed to treat severe cases of depression and even prevent depression in some people.

A Norwegian study that tracked about thirty-nine thousand people for two years found that those who reported doing moderate-to-high physical activity, including daily brisk walks for more than thirty minutes, scored significantly lower on depression and anxiety tests compared with nonexercisers.

There are many effective antidepressant drugs, but they are frequently accompanied by bothersome side effects, including sexual dysfunction, nausea, fatigue, and weight gain. And while most of these drugs can take a month to work, a single exercise session can trigger an immediate lift in mood, and consistent aerobic exercise will make an even more lasting positive impact.

What to do: The key is to boost your heart rate high enough to trigger the release of endorphins, feel-good chemicals that elicit a state of relaxed calm. Spend thirty to forty-five minutes at a level of exertion where carrying on a conversation is quite difficult due to panting. Do this three to five days a week, to benefit.

You also may want to try exercising outdoors. A study published in *Environmental Science & Technology* found that outdoor exercise produces stronger feelings of revitalization, a bigger boost of energy, and a greater reduction in depression and anger than exercising indoors.

Strength training also is effective in treating depression—lifting weights releases endorphins and builds a sense of empowerment. For a strength-training program, ask your doctor to recommend a physical therapist or personal trainer.

If it's difficult to motivate yourself to exercise when you're depressed, relying on a personal trainer—or a "workout buddy"—can help.*

---

*   Be sure to check with your doctor before starting any fitness program. If your condition is severe, he/she may initially want you to use exercise as an adjunct to medication, not as a replacement. Never stop taking a prescribed drug without talking to your doctor. Caution: With this or any workout, seek immediate medical attention if you experience chest pain, shortness of breath, nausea, blurred vision, or significant bone or muscle pain while exercising.

> Jordan D. Metzl, MD, sports medicine physician, Hospital for Special Surgery, New York City. The author of *The Exercise Cure: A Doctor's All-Natural, No-Pill Prescription for Better Health & Longer Life,* Dr. Metzl maintains practices in New York City and Greenwich, Connecticut, and is a medical columnist for *Triathlete* magazine. He has run in thirty-three marathons and finished 12 Ironman competitions (and is still going).

The Healing Powers of Meditation and Yoga

Everyone feels down at times, and if you've ever experienced the pervasive, persistent, profound sadness that characterizes depression, you know how debilitating this condition can be.

Doctors try to help, but often treatment falls short. Therapists may not be available 24/7, and antidepressant medication can cause unacceptable side effects or fail to bring sufficient relief. The good news is that there are additional safe, effective options—namely, meditation and yoga.

According to Kelly McGonigal, PhD, an instructor of yoga, meditation, and psychology at Stanford University, who has extensive experience in this area, certain meditation and yoga techniques have been shown to be particularly effective in restoring energy, enthusiasm, focus, and self-esteem to people who are down or depressed, and you can practice them almost any time. You have absolutely nothing to lose and so very much to gain.

RECONNECT TO LIFE

Among the most effective mood-elevating meditation techniques are those that focus on the breath. In Sanskrit, *prana* means not only "breath," but also "energy" and "life force." Reconnecting with your breath helps you reconnect to life. Practice one or both of the following techniques daily, breathing slowly and deeply throughout.

Breath-focus meditation trains you to guide your mind, helping you disengage from depressed or destructive thoughts. Sit or lie comfortably in a safe, secure place. Breathe in a relaxed, natural way (without trying to breathe especially deeply or otherwise alter your breathing), observing the natural cycle of inhaling and exhaling. Then focus on silently counting your breaths in cycles from one to ten. After your tenth exhalation (or if you lose track of your count), begin again at one.

Alternative: Repeat a calming mantra in your mind, such as, *Now I inhale. Now I exhale.* If your mind wanders, don't berate yourself—simply return your attention to your breath. Continue for five to fifteen minutes.

Sun breath is a "moving meditation" that helps restore energy. Sit or stand with arms at your sides. Inhale through your nose, and lift your gaze skyward as you slowly raise your arms on either side of your body (elbows straight and palms up) until they are overhead. Then, exhaling and lowering your gaze, slowly bring your arms down (palms facing down). Repeat for ten breaths.

MOOD-ENHANCING YOGA POSES

Different yoga poses alleviate depression in different ways, so before each yoga session, assess your energy level and mood, then choose the order in which to do the three types of poses below. When you are feeling anxious or wired, start with standing poses, which are more active. If you are feeling drained, start with restorative poses.

If you are new to yoga, try the simple poses described below. If you have experience with yoga, also do the more advanced poses suggested. Practice for twenty minutes per day, remembering to breathe slowly and deeply.

+ **Standing poses** help shift a depressed mind-set. These provide momentary experiences of inner strength and courage—emotions a depressed person has not felt in a while—and so serve as reminders that there is hope.

Yoga novices: Try the tree pose. Stand with your right hand on a counter for support. Keeping your right leg straight, bend your left knee, and place the sole of your left foot on the inside of your right leg, just above or below the right knee. If you can keep your balance, place your palms together in prayer position in front of your heart. Hold for fifteen to thirty seconds. Repeat on the other side.

More advanced: Warrior 1 and warrior 2 poses.

+ **Backbends** challenge the physical expression of depression by lifting a dropped gaze, straightening a slumped spine, opening the chest, and relaxing tension in the belly. When you have embodied depression for a long time, experiencing its physical opposite can be powerfully healing.

Novices: Try the bridge pose. Lie on your back, knees bent, feet flat on the floor and shoulder-width apart, arms on the floor at your sides. Lift your buttocks, lower back, and middle back off the floor, supporting your weight on your feet, arms, and upper back. Gaze skyward and hold for fifteen to thirty seconds, then lower yourself to the floor. Repeat.

More advanced: Locust, camel, and upward bow poses.

+ **Restorative poses** help the body relax deeply. A depressed person might feel exhausted yet have few opportunities to truly rest. Restorative poses are especially healing if you use supportive props, such as pillows and blankets.

Novices: Try the supported relaxation pose, a modification of the traditional *savasana* pose that uses a folded towel, a rolled-up towel, and a blanket as props. Lie flat on your back, the folded towel under your head, the rolled-up towel under your slightly bent knees, feet shoulder-width apart, arms at your sides, and the blanket over your body. Relax completely. Hold the pose for five minutes.

More advanced: Child's pose and legs-up-the-wall pose.

> Kelly McGonigal, PhD, instructor of yoga, meditation, and psychology, Stanford University, Stanford, California. She is also author of *Yoga for Pain Relief: Simple Practices to Calm Your Mind and Heal Your Chronic Pain* and former editor-in-chief of the *International Journal of Yoga Therapy.* KellyMcGonigal.com.

Down and Depressed? Acupuncture Can Help

Mention acupuncture and many people think of therapy for physical aches and pains, but what if the problem is the persistent inner ache of sadness? The ancient healing technique of acupuncture also is used as a complementary treatment for various types of depression, including the notoriously tricky bipolar disorder (manic-depressive disorder), in which patients cycle between deep depression and manic episodes.

Though Western-style research studies on the topic are somewhat limited, clinical trials have reported significant findings. For instance, there is evidence for acupuncture's effectiveness in treating the following:

+ **Major depression.** A study published in *Psychological Science* found that 70 percent of women with mild to moderate depression who underwent twelve acupuncture sessions experienced at least a 50 percent reduction in symptoms—results comparable to the success rates of antidepressant medication but without the drugs' risk for side effects. Other studies have shown greater improvement in patients treated with acupuncture alone or with acupuncture plus antidepressants than in patients treated with antidepressants alone.

+ **Bipolar disorder.** In two studies from Purdue University, all bipolar patients who received eight to twelve weeks of acupuncture sessions (in addition to their usual medication) showed improvement in their symptoms. This was true regardless of whether they entered the study during a phase of depression or a phase of mania.

+ **Depression during pregnancy.** In a study published in the *Journal of Affective Disorders*, 69 percent of pregnant participants got significant relief after twelve sessions of acupuncture in which depressive symptoms were specifically addressed. In a control group that received massage therapy instead of acupuncture, only 32 percent of patients improved. A similar study in *Obstetrics & Gynecology* reported comparable results.

According to Daisy Dong, LAc, OMD, a licensed acupuncturist and herbalist in private practice in Denver and a professor at Southwest Acupuncture College, for patients with various types of depression, acupuncture treatment generally brings increased energy, greater calmness, reduced anxiety, more positive thoughts and fewer negative ones, and improved sleep. For bipolar patients, acupuncture also helps to stabilize moods. When performed by a qualified professional, acupuncture has no adverse effects other than perhaps mild temporary discomfort at the needle sites. In contrast, antidepressant medications carry a risk for side effects including nausea, weight gain, fatigue, and sexual problems. In bipolar patients, drugs must be very carefully managed to avoid triggering mania, and during pregnancy, there are concerns about potential negative effects of drugs on the fetus.

If you decide to give acupuncture a try: The first visit generally takes about an hour, with subsequent sessions lasting thirty to forty-five minutes depending on the complexity of the case. Depression patients typically receive one or two treatments per week. Some people notice improvement after the first treatment, but for many people, it takes several treatments before results are seen, and sustained improvement generally requires about ten sessions.

Acupuncture treatment for depression costs the same as acupuncture for other ailments—about $60 to $120 per session, depending on your location and the individual practitioner. Some health insurance policies cover acupuncture, so check your plan.

If you are taking medication for depression or bipolar disorder: It is very important that you not simply stop taking the drugs on your own even if you start feeling better after beginning acupuncture. Depending on your condition, you may indeed be able to reduce or even discontinue your medication, but this must be done under the supervision of your prescribing physician.

To find a qualified acupuncturist: Ask your doctor or mental health professional for a referral, talk to friends who have used acupuncture, or check the online databases of the American Association of Acupuncture and Oriental Medicine or the National Certification Commission for Acupuncture and Oriental Medicine.

> Daisy Dong, LAc, OMD, chief acupuncturist, Center for Integrative Medicine, University of Colorado Hospital, Aurora, and professor, Southwest Acupuncture College, Boulder. Her private practice, Colorado Boulevard Acupuncture, is based at Colorado Boulevard Chiropractic Centers in Denver. Dr. Dong received her medical degree from the Beijing College of Traditional Chinese Medicine, where she practiced and taught for twenty-six years.

Light Therapy: Not Just for Wintertime Blues

The short days of winter can leave you feeling blah and out of sorts. For many, mood-lifting light therapy—which basically consists of sitting in front of a special light-emitting device called a light box each morning—will chase away the wintertime blues.

But there is research that shows that light therapy relieves not only wintertime seasonal affective disorder (SAD), but also nonseasonal depression.

In a study in *Archives of General Psychiatry*, one group of seniors (age sixty and up) with depression were exposed to the bright light of a light box for one hour daily for three weeks; the control group got a "sham" treatment with dim light. The bright-light group showed significantly greater improvement in mood and sleep quality (poor sleep often accompanies depression), lower levels of the stress hormone cortisol, and more normal levels of melatonin, a hormone that helps regulate circadian rhythms and sleep-wake cycles by rising in the evening and falling in the morning. In fact, light therapy was as effective as antidepressant medication generally is but did not carry the drugs' risk for side effects.

Bright-light therapy also can successfully

treat a number of nonseasonal forms of depression, including chronic depression in women and men of various ages, bipolar disorder, and depression during pregnancy (offering a safe alternative to medications that might affect the fetus). There is also preliminary evidence of light therapy's positive effects for postpartum depression. Light therapy alone relieves mild, moderate, or even severe depression in some cases. In other cases, light therapy is used along with psychotherapy, medication, and/or other treatments.

Eyes must be open during light therapy, because it works through the eyes, not the skin. A simple neural pathway connects the retina to the area of the brain that houses the body's internal clock. This clock is vulnerable to getting out of kilter with respect to the local time of day, which can cause mood and energy to plummet and make it hard to get to sleep or to wake up feeling alert. Bright-light therapy sends a signal that resets the internal clock, shifting the circadian rhythm so it is in sync with the local day/night cycle, and this in turn has positive effects on mood. In addition, if melatonin activity is high at the time of the light signal, a reaction is triggered that reduces melatonin secretion, thus reinforcing the corrective effects on the internal clock. Light therapy also may increase the availability of the mood-boosting neurotransmitter serotonin by reducing activity of a "transporter" molecule that removes serotonin from active sites in the nervous system.

Light therapy works surprisingly quickly. Effects may be seen within a week of daily use and sometimes even faster.

HOW TO DO IT

You do not need a prescription to purchase a light box, and for people with mild depression, light therapy self-treatment generally is safe. However, certain people should use light therapy only under the supervision of a doctor. This includes anyone who:

+ **Suffers from moderate-to-severe depression,** whether or not they are being treated with medication and/or psychotherapy, because if used incorrectly (such as at the wrong time of day), light therapy could potentially worsen depression symptoms.

+ **Has bipolar disorder,** because if the condition is not being adequately treated with mood-stabilizing medication, light therapy could lead to mania, and because light therapy's timing may need to be adjusted to later in the day so as not to destabilize the circadian rhythm.

- **Takes medication that increases adverse reactions to sunlight,** such as drugs used to control irregular heartbeat, because bright light could damage the retina, which absorbs these drugs in its photoreceptors.
- **Has a degenerative eye problem,** such as macular degeneration, because bright white light could accelerate illness progression. (In such cases, a dimmer "dawn simulation" device, which also has an antidepressant effect, may be used instead.)

Using a light box at home: Buy a fluorescent light box that provides 10,000 lux of illumination, which is the type that has proven successful in clinical trials. (Lower lux levels can be effective but require more exposure time to get the same effect.) The light box should filter out ultraviolet rays that can damage eyes and skin and should give off white light, not colored light. Some insurance companies cover the cost if patients are using the light box under a physician's supervision.

Treatment typically involves sitting twelve inches from the light box for thirty minutes each day shortly after waking up. It's essentially a breakfast-time routine. You don't look directly into the light, but your eyes are open and bathed in light while you concentrate, for example, on your newspaper or laptop.

Important: The optimal time for and duration of treatment sessions varies among individuals.

People whose depression is not limited to winter can benefit from using a light box year-round. Most people experience no negative side effects from light therapy. A small number of users develop headaches, eyestrain, agitation, and/or mild nausea. These symptoms tend to subside after a few days, but if symptoms persist, reducing the duration of light treatment sessions or sitting farther from the light box often takes care of the problem.

> Michael Terman, PhD, psychologist and director of the Center for Light Treatment and Biological Rhythms at Columbia University Medical Center, and professor of clinical psychology, Columbia University College of Physicians and Surgeons, both in New York City. He is founder and president of the Center for Environmental Therapeutics (CET), New York City, and director of clinical chronobiology at the New York State Psychiatric Institute. A leading authority on the circadian clock and the role that light plays in regulating it, Dr. Terman is author of *Chronotherapy: Resetting Your Inner Clock to Boost Mood, Alertness, and Quality Sleep.* Columbia-Chronotherapy.org.

Music Therapy Helps Ease Anxiety and Depression

An *increasing body of evidence* shows that music therapy—whether it includes the listener's favorite Bach sonatas or Beach Boys' classics—can help improve symptoms associated with a wide variety of common health problems, including anxiety and depression.

ANXIETY

Anxiety can occur in response to a stressful situation such as public speaking or from chronic stress.

Important finding: A study in the journal *Heart* found that listening to relaxing music—such as sonatas by Bach or Mozart—reduced feelings of anxiety in patients about to undergo heart surgery even more than the antianxiety medication midazolam. Music therapy was found to help reduce patients' heart rates and their levels of the stress hormone cortisol.

What this means for you: Music can be used to reduce anxiety due to a stressful situation or chronic stressors. Prior to a speaking engagement or any other stressful event, listen to calming music or try singing your favorite song.

While Bach and Mozart were used in the study, look for music that you find soothing. Experiment with different types of music and test their impact on your mood. Then create your own playlist to elicit the desired feelings.

DEPRESSION

Americans who are depressed tend to rely mainly on prescription antidepressants. However, these drugs are notorious for side effects such as nausea, headaches, and sexual dysfunction.

Finding: After reviewing seventeen studies that tested whether listening to music could reduce depression symptoms in adults, a 2011 meta-analysis concluded that music can be used to help combat depression if listened to regularly for at least three weeks.

What this means for you: Using music to improve your mood can be a fun and cost-effective way to help ward off negative feelings caused by mild depression.

Important: Add music therapy to your daily life—not just when you are feeling blue. Play around with familiar songs and new pieces to find the music that makes you feel best.

....

› Suzanne B. Hanser, EdD, coauthor with Susan Mandel, PhD, of the book and CD *Manage Your Stress and Pain Through Music.* She is the founding chair of the music therapy department at Berklee College of Music in Boston and past president of the American Music Therapy Association and the World Federation of Music Therapy.

....

Beware Nighttime Exposure to Certain Colors of Light

W*hat color is the light* you sleep with? You may say that you don't sleep with any lights on. But if you take a closer look, you're likely to see some light coming from your alarm clock, cell-phone charger, computer, e-reader, night-light, and/or bedroom TV.

Problem: The color of the light you're exposed to at night, even while you're sleeping, may affect how you feel during the day, and not in a good way. In fact, certain colors are linked to signs of depression.

Good news: You can minimize your risk by making your room truly dark or, if you need a bit of illumination, by using the *right kind* of clock or night-light.

TESTING THE RED, WHITE, AND BLUE

It's thought that exposure to light at night interferes with the release of hormones that affect mood and various physiological functions. Researchers wanted to explore whether certain colors of light would be better or worse than others in this regard. The experiments were conducted on hamsters, but these mammals share enough physiological similarities with humans that the findings might well apply to us too.

For four weeks, all the hamsters were exposed to bright light (similar to normal daytime lighting) for sixteen hours each day. However, their nighttime light exposure differed. One group was exposed to no light at night, while three other groups were exposed to either dim white light, dim blue light, or dim red light. Then the hamsters were given various tests to assess depression-like symptoms. The tests were done during daytime, away from any immediate effects of nighttime light.

First, the hamsters were placed in tanks filled with room-temperature water for ten minutes. (From previous studies, the researchers knew that hamsters normally swim vigorously during this challenge, but those who demonstrate various depression-like behaviors are likely to just float passively.) In this study, hamsters that had slept in the dark spent almost all their time swimming (happy hamsters!), while those that had been exposed to white or blue light at night spent the least time swimming (not so happy). Most interesting of all, those that had been exposed to red light at night spent significantly more time swimming than the other light-exposed hamsters, indicating that red light did not affect mood nearly as negatively as white or blue light did.

Another measure of depression is anhedonia, the inability to derive pleasure from normally enjoyable activities. For hamsters, drinking sugar water is very pleasurable.

Findings: Hamsters not exposed to any light at night consumed the most sugar water, followed closely by those exposed to red light, whereas those exposed to white or blue light consumed only about half as much. So again, red did best among the colors of light, coming in second only to darkness.

Finally, the researchers looked at the hamsters' brains, particularly the neurons in the hippocampus, an area known to be involved in mood regulation. The hamsters that had spent their nights in blue or white light had significantly reduced density of dendritic spines (hairlike growths on brain cells that are used to send chemical messages between cells), another sign that has been linked to depression. The dark-night hamsters showed the highest density of these dendritic spines, with the red-light hamsters again coming in a close second.

WAVELENGTH INTERFERENCE

What explains these results? Researchers suspect that specialized light-sensitive cells of the retina, called ipRGCs, are responsible. These cells, which detect the unique wavelengths emitted by various colors, are most sensitive to blue wavelengths and least sensitive to red wavelengths. The ipRGCs also send messages to the part of the brain that helps regulate circadian rhythm. When circadian rhythm is disrupted—by nighttime light or some other factor—the body feels the effects physically and psychologically. In addition, ipRGCs send messages to the brain's limbic system, which controls mood and emotion. All these factors help explain why red light at night had fewer detrimental effects on mood than other colors of light.

Good-mood lighting at night: It's best if you can keep your bedroom totally dark, and to do that, besides having light-blocking shades or curtains on your windows, you'll need to turn off, cover, or remove all electronics and other light-emitting objects at night. (The one exception is your smoke alarm/carbon monoxide detector, for obvious reasons.) If you want to have a clock immediately readable at all times or if you need a small night-light (for instance, to illuminate the way to the bathroom), use a clock that emits red light, or use a red bulb in your night-light. It's a simple enough thing to try, and you might just start feeling better because of it!

› Tracy Bedrosian, PhD, postdoctoral researcher, Salk Institute, La Jolla, California. Her study was conducted while she was a graduate student at Ohio State University in Columbus and was published in the *Journal of Neuroscience*.

The Ten Very Best Foods to Prevent Depression and Build a Healthier Brain

H ere's a startling statistic—studies show that people who consume a healthy diet are 40 to 50 percent less likely to develop depression.

What are the absolutely best nutrients—and most nutrient-packed foods—to protect your brain from depression and other ailments?

What protects mood also protects against dementia and other brain-related conditions. The brain is the biggest asset we have, so we should be selecting foods that specifically nourish the brain.

Here's how to build the healthiest brain possible—starting in your kitchen.

NUTRIENTS BRAINS NEED MOST

These key nutrients as the most important:

+ **Long-chain omega-3 fatty acids.** There are two major ones. Docosahexaenoic acid (DHA) creates hormones called neuroprotectins and resolvins that combat brain inflammation, which is implicated in the development of depression (as well as dementia). Eicosapentaenoic acid (EPA) protects the cardiovascular system, important for a healthy brain.

+ **Zinc.** This mineral plays a major role in the development of new brain cells and can boost the efficacy of antidepressant medications.

+ **Folate.** Also known as vitamin B-9, folate is needed for good moods and a healthy brain. It helps produce defensin-1, a molecule that protects the brain and increases the concentration of acetylcholine, a neurotransmitter that's crucial to memory and cognition.

+ **Iron.** This essential element is a crucial cofactor in the synthesis of mood-regulating neurotransmitters including dopamine and serotonin.

+ **Magnesium.** This mineral is required to keep myelin—the insulation of brain cells—healthy. It also increases brain-derived neurotrophic factor (BDNF), which promotes the growth of new neurons and healthy connections among brain cells. A deficiency in magnesium can lead to depression, anxiety, symptoms of ADHD, insomnia, and fatigue.

- **Vitamin B-12.** This vitamin, which often is deficient as we age, helps makes neurotransmitters that are key to mood and memory.
- **Vitamin E.** This potent antioxidant vitamin protects polyunsaturated fatty acids in the brain, including DHA. Vitamin E–rich foods, but not supplements, are linked to the prevention of clinical depression as well as slower progression of Alzheimer's disease. One reason may be that most supplements contain only alpha-tocopherol, while other vitamin E compounds, particularly tocotrienols, play important roles in brain function.
- **Dietary fiber.** A high-fiber diet supports healthy gut bacteria (the gut microbiome), which growing evidence suggests is key for mental health.

BOOSTING YOUR MOOD AT THE SUPERMARKET

The best brain foods are mostly plant-based, but seafood, wild game, and even some organ meats make the top of the list too:

- Leafy greens such as kale, mustard greens, and collard greens
- Bell peppers such as red, green, and orange
- Cruciferous vegetables such as cauliflower, broccoli, and cabbage
- Berries such as strawberries, raspberries, and blueberries
- Nuts such as pecans, walnuts, almonds, and cashews
- Bivalves such as oysters, clams, and mussels
- Crustaceans such as crab, lobster, and shrimp
- Fish such as sardines, salmon, and fish roe
- Organ meats such as liver, poultry giblets, and heart
- Game and wild meat such as bison, elk, and duck

Eating these nutrient-dense foods is likely to help prevent and treat mental illness. When someone with depression is treated, the real goal is to prevent that person from ever getting depressed again.

EVERYDAY BRAIN FOODS

Not into eating beef heart? Having a little trouble stocking up on elk? When it comes to meat, wild game may not be widely available, but grass-fed beef, which is higher in omega-3 fatty acids than conventionally raised beef, is stocked in most supermarkets and may be independently associated with protection from depression.

Other foods that didn't make it to the top of the brain food scale but that still are very good for the brain include eggs (iron, zinc), beans (fiber, magnesium, iron), and fruits and vegetables of all colors (fiber, antioxidants), plus small quantities of dark chocolate, which gives you a little dopamine rush. Dopamine is a neurotransmitter that provides a feeling of reward.

....

› Drew Ramsey, MD, psychiatrist, Columbia University Medical Center, and assistant professor, Columbia University College of Physicians and Surgeons, both in New York City. His latest book is *Eat Complete: The 21 Nutrients That Fuel Brainpower, Boost Weight Loss, and Transform Your Health.* DrewRamseyMD.com.

....

Sexual Health

Natural Aphrodisiacs

Each spring, a young man's (and presumably young woman's) fancy turns to love, but what if you're no longer quite so young and ready? Age apparently matters. In a survey by Massachusetts General Hospital, four out of ten women expressed sexual concerns such as diminished libido (especially at middle age), while men reported a consistent trend toward more frequent sexual dysfunction with increasing age. But the truth is, you can have a healthy and fulfilling sex life at any age.

DON'T OVERMEDICALIZE AGING

A decrease in libido with age is commonly chalked up to declining hormone levels, but in reality, it's far more complicated. In addition to the hormonal effect of aging, your sex drive is also significantly influenced by what's going on in your life overall. The state of your health, relationship, job, mortgage, concerns about children, care for aging parents, the medications you take—all these and other factors come with you into the bedroom. Sexuality is a complicated equation, which is why you shouldn't believe that infamous "little blue pill" so relentlessly hawked on TV and the internet is the solution.

Menopause and andropause (its male equivalent) are life passages, not diseases. While treating low desire with pharmaceutical products may mask symptoms, it's important to recognize that these drugs have powerful and undesirable side effects. For example, in addition to sudden vision loss, sildenafil, tadalafil, and vardenafil have resulted in erections lasting four hours or more, which are dangerous and require a really embarrassing visit to the emergency room.

Testosterone (creams, gels, injections, pills) may help boost a woman's sex drive, but may also bring on baldness, a deep voice, liver damage, acne, and abnormal hair growth…not a pretty picture.

TROUBLE BREWING?

A *far better way to* address changes in libido is to provide gentle support to natural biological processes. Examine your day-to-day life. If you're driving yourself hard, eating poorly, or not getting enough sleep or exercise, it's not surprising you have trouble in the bedroom. Paying more attention to your health in general will soon pay off in a better sex life.

Sexual concerns may also be a sign of problems elsewhere in the body. For instance, erectile dysfunction is often one of the earliest signs of cardiovascular disease in men. And for both genders, problems in the large intestine or urinary tract may end up disturbing sexual function.

HOW TO GET A MORE SATISFYING SEX LIFE

Quell inflammation. Imbalances in the pelvic-abdominal region may be related to inflammatory disturbances that disrupt microbial colonies in the genital-urinary and lower gastrointestinal tracts. To correct this imbalance and restore digestive and immune health, which in turn support sexuality, I prescribe probiotics such as *Lactobacillus* and *Bifidobacterium*. Also helpful to this end is to cut back on sugar, white breads, dairy products, trans fats, and fried foods; eat protein at every meal; and two or three times a week, enjoy cold-water fish such as salmon or tuna, rich in omega-3 fatty acids.

Ease vaginal dryness or thinning. I prescribe a variety of topical low-dose bioidentical hormonal products, botanical extracts, and supplements.

Relax and take a deep breath—literally. Make a habit of consciously breathing deeply at every available opportunity—when waiting for the light to change, when you ride the elevator, each time you sit at your desk, whatever pattern works for you. Excess anxiety raises blood levels of the stress hormone cortisol and impedes the body's ability to manufacture the estrogen and testosterone that are vital to sexual response. My favorite breathing technique is the meditative deep breathing exercises of pranayama yoga, which fuel your natural balance, energy, and sexuality.

Exercise. Regular workouts not only clear your mind and improve your mood, they make you feel better about your body—often a libido boost. Aerobic activity such as brisk walking, biking, or dancing also increases blood flow to organs, including the sexual ones.

Practice Kegel exercises. To enhance pelvic muscle control and thus sexual satisfaction, I recommend daily Kegel exercises for both men and women. Learn to locate and isolate pubococcygeus (PC) muscles by interrupting urine flow next time you go to the bathroom. Next, three or four times a day, strengthen your PC muscles by alternately clenching and releasing them for five to ten seconds at a time.

Date your partner. Use novelty to break up humdrum routines. For instance, steal away for a romantic weekend or fashion your own "staycation" at home. Take a long walk together in the park or on the beach, buy lavender oil for a shared bath, light an aromatherapy candle, enjoy a leisurely dinner (make sure to go light on the sleep-inducing carbs), and see what happens.

Yohimbe bark extract. In cases of specific sexual dysfunction, I prescribe an extract of the botanical medicine yohimbe, derived from the bark of an evergreen tree in West Africa. This medicine can be taken by either men or women to stimulate desire. (**Note:** If you have high blood pressure, kidney problems, or a psychiatric disorder, do not use yohimbe.)

In the long run, making adjustments toward a healthier lifestyle—fitting in more exercise, eating healthier foods, spending more time with your partner and less time at the office—will do a lot more for your sex life than taking a pill. That way, when the moment is right, you'll be ready.

> › Andrew L. Rubman, ND, medical director of Southbury Clinic for Traditional Medicines in Southbury, Connecticut. He is a founding member of the American Association of Naturopathic Physicians. His blog, *Nature Doc's Patient Diary*, is published on BottomLineInc.com. SouthburyClinic.com.

Women: Revive Your Sex Drive

Diminished libido—little or no sexual desire—is the most common sexual complaint among women. But repeated attempts by the pharmaceutical industry to solve the problem with one or another form of "female Viagra" have failed.

My viewpoint: Reviving a mature woman's sex drive requires addressing multiple factors. These include:

+ **Balancing hormones,** which play a key role in both physical and mental aspects of arousal, particularly during the hormonal changes of perimenopause and menopause.
+ **Treating the pelvic problems of aging,** such as vaginal atrophy and dryness, which can cause painful sex.

Here are natural ways to boost libido that consistently work for the mature women in my medical practice. Choose one or two based on your particular needs. If you still have problems, consult a licensed naturopathic physician.

HORMONE HELP

Several herbs and herbal combinations can help balance a mature woman's hormones. Here are two of my favorites.

Maca. This powerful Peruvian herb is a good choice for women going through perimenopause or menopause because it is rich in plant sterols that balance and strengthen the entire hormonal system. The herb not only increases sex drive, but also improves perimenopausal and menopausal symptoms such as hot flashes, night sweats, and insomnia. Additionally, it supports the adrenal glands, reducing levels of energy-depleting stress hormones.

Typical dose: 1,000 mg, twice daily.

Two Immortals. This herbal formula from traditional Chinese medicine builds two types of chi, or life-energy—*yin* (feminine) chi and *yang* (masculine) chi—thereby boosting a woman's libido, which requires both nurturing (yin) and stimulation (yang). It also helps to balance hormones and control some symptoms of perimenopause (irregular menstrual bleeding and cramping) and menopause (hot flashes).

Many of my patients take it for six months to a year to rebuild their vitality.

Typical dose: Many companies manufacture the supplement, and dosages vary. Follow the dosage recommendation on the label.

SUPER SEX SUPPLEMENTS

Two nutritional supplements are particularly effective at stimulating sexuality.

L-arginine. This amino acid works by boosting nitric oxide, a compound that promotes blood flow—including blood flow to your genitals.

A study in the *Journal of Sex & Marital Therapy* showed that more than 70 percent of women who took a supplement containing L-arginine (ArginMax for Women) experienced increased sexual desire, more frequent sex and orgasm, enhanced clitoral stimulation, decreased vaginal dryness, and improved overall sexual satisfaction.

Typical dose: 3,000 mg daily.

Caution: Talk to your doctor before you take L-arginine, especially if you have low blood pressure, herpes, gastric ulcer, liver disease, or kidney disease.

PEA (phenylethylamine). Called the "love supplement," PEA boosts the neurotransmitter dopamine, enhancing feelings of well-being, joy, and pleasure.

Typical dose: 60 mg once a day.

(Higher doses can cause overstimulation, insomnia, or anxiety.)

Caution: Don't take PEA if you're nursing, pregnant, or take an MAOI antidepressant medication such as selegiline.

You also can boost PEA by exercising regularly, eating dark chocolate, and taking a blue-green algae called spirulina.

APHRODISIACS

Two aphrodisiacs are particularly effective for mature women because, by relaxing your body and improving your mood, they slowly and gently boost your libido.

Cordyceps. This mushroom is considered a potent sexual tonic in traditional Chinese medicine. It enhances both yin and yang chi, making it an ideal aphrodisiac for women.

Typical dose: 500 mg, twice daily.

What works best: Pills made by a hot-water extraction process that pulls out the herb's most active constituents, such as the cordyceps supplement from JHS Natural Products.

Ginkgo biloba. Often recommended for memory loss because it improves blood supply to the brain, ginkgo also promotes blood flow to the vulva and vagina. Studies show that it may help restore libido in women taking antidepressants, which can destroy sex drive.

Typical dose: 40 mg, three times a day. The label should read, "Standardized extract of 24 percent ginkgo flavonglycosides (or flavone glycosides)."

STATIN WARNINGS

Cholesterol-lowering statin drugs— taken by millions of older women— can lower libido, probably by damaging mitochondria, energy-generating structures inside cells. If you take a statin and notice a decrease in libido, talk to your doctor about your options.

VAGINAL WEIGHT TRAINING

The pubococcygeal (PC) muscle—a bowl-shaped "hammock" of pelvic muscle that contracts rhythmically when you have an orgasm and also supports your genital organs and bladder—is crucial to sexual pleasure. Using a vaginal weight (a small, round weight inside an oval tube that is inserted into the vagina like a tampon) is the best way to strengthen the PC muscle, enhancing erotic sensation and sexual response.

What to do: To start, insert the tube for one to five minutes, twice daily, squeezing your PC muscle repeatedly to hold the tube in place. You can do this standing or lying down. Gradually work up to twenty minutes, twice daily, using progressively heavier weights. Do this for three months.

Other benefits: Regular use of vaginal

weights can help prevent and treat urinary incontinence and prevent prolapse of the bladder or uterus.

VAGINAL DRYNESS AND PAINFUL INTERCOURSE

Enjoyable sex requires vaginal tissue that is healthy and well-hydrated. But the midlife drop in estrogen levels causes a decrease of blood flow to the vagina, which can lead to vaginal atrophy and dryness. This can be remedied as follows.

Vitamin E. The unique lubricating properties of vitamin E make it especially effective.

What to do: Pierce a soft 400 IU vitamin E gel capsule with a pin, squeeze the oil onto your finger, and apply it to the outside of the vagina and inside about an inch. Or use a vitamin E vaginal suppository. (I recommend the product from Earth's Botanical Harvest, available online.) Apply the gel or insert the suppository nightly at bedtime for at least two weeks. Taper use to three times a week.

> › Laurie Steelsmith, ND, LAc, a licensed naturopathic physician and acupuncturist and medical director of Steelsmith Natural Health Center, Honolulu. She is the coauthor of *Natural Choices for Women's Health* and *Great Sex, Naturally.* DrSteelsmith.com.

Everything You Always Wanted to Know about Personal Lubricants but Were Embarrassed to Ask

When vaginal dryness starts making sex uncomfortable, many midlife women (and seniors too) are delighted to discover how much enjoyment a little extra moisture provides. Personal lubricants can make sex more comfortable when any of these happen:

+ **Vaginal dryness** as a result of menopause, use of certain medications, such as antihistamines, antidepressants, or chemotherapy drugs, or stress (which raises adrenaline levels, in turn reducing blood flow to the internal organs and also reducing lubrication).

+ **Intercourse lasts a long time** as it often may, considering that older men typically take longer to climax.

+ **Using condoms,** which are advisable—even when pregnancy is no longer a concern—to protect against sexually transmitted diseases, unless you are in a long-term monogamous relationship.

What's available? The four basic types of products are:

- **Natural oils,** such as canola, corn, grapeseed, olive, peanut oil, and Yes oil-based brands.
- **Water-based lubricants,** such as Astroglide Liquid, Hydra-Smooth, ID Glide, K-Y Jelly, Liquid Silk, Probe, and Yes water-based brands.
- **Petroleum-based lubricants,** such as baby oil, mineral oil, petroleum jelly.
- **Silicone-based lubricants,** such as Astroglide X Premium Silicone Personal Lubricant, Eros Bodyglide, Passion Premium, and Wet Platinum.

Which type should you try? It depends on what is most important to you. If you want a product that:

- **Is inexpensive:** choose natural oils or water-based products.
- **Lasts a long time without being reapplied:** choose silicone-based, and avoid water-based products.
- **Carries no risk of staining sheets:** choose water-based products.
- **Has no taste:** choose petroleum-based products, and, of course, avoid products with added flavors.
- **Will not degrade latex condoms, diaphragms, or sex toys:** choose water-based, and avoid petroleum-based and some oil-based products.
- **Washes off easily with plain water:** choose water-based, and avoid natural oils, petroleum-based, or silicone-based products.

Why read the fine print? Most lubricant ingredients are what the FDA calls GRAS—"generally recognized as safe"—for consumers. Still, certain ingredients can cause problems for certain people, so check labels before you buy. If you:

- **Are prone to vaginal yeast infections:** avoid glycerin, a thickener, and look for a product labeled "pH neutral."
- **Often experience allergic skin reactions:** avoid propylene glycol (an emulsifier) and methylparaben (an antifungal preservative).

If you or your partner experience irritation or develop a rash after using a lubricant, stop using that product. Talk to your doctor about the need for treatment and ask for advice on products better suited to your needs.

What about those "warm" or "tingling" products? Some personal lubricants include capsaicin, menthol, and/or other ingredients designed to create a warm or tingling sensation on the skin. Such sensations enhance pleasure and intensify orgasm for some people, but other people find them irritating. The only way to tell how such a lubricant might feel to you is to give it a try.

....

> Irwin Goldstein, MD, director of sexual medicine at Alvarado Hospital in San Diego, clinical professor of surgery at the University of California, San Diego, editor in chief of the *Journal of Sexual Medicine*, and coauthor of *When Sex Hurts: A Woman's Guide to Banishing Sexual Pain*. SexualMed.org.

....

Intimacy after a Long Dry Spell

I f *you haven't been intimate* for a long time, intercourse is likely to be uncomfortable at first, because the vagina can atrophy from lack of activity. Vaginal tissues can become thin and dry after menopause due to the natural decline in estrogen and testosterone levels, exacerbating the discomfort of penetration. Fortunately, there is a lot you can do to prepare yourself so that intercourse will be enjoyable.

Try any or all of the following natural approaches:

+ **Start using a nonhormonal over-the-counter vaginal moisturizer,** which is a topical suppository, cream, or gel with long-lasting effects. Routinely applied two or three times per week,

it helps rejuvenate the vaginal tissues, making them more moist and resilient.

Good brand: Replens.

+ **Once daily, use a pin to pierce a vitamin E gel-cap supplement** (500 IU), squeeze the oil onto your fingertips, then rub it onto the labia and around the vaginal opening. This plumps up and strengthens the cells.

+ **Keep a water-based or silicone-based personal lubricant on hand** so you'll have it when you need it. Used during foreplay and intercourse, it helps minimize pain and heighten pleasure. Some lubricants contain ingredients that can irritate delicate tissues, particularly in menopausal women, so look for a product that is organic, hypoallergenic, and/or paraben-free. Excellent brands include Hathor Aphrodisia, Pink, and Sliquid.

+ **Do Kegel exercises,** aiming for twenty minutes or two hundred repetitions per day. Repeatedly squeezing and then releasing the muscles you use to start and stop the flow of urine can increase the flow of blood, oxygen, and nutrients to the pelvic floor, strengthening not only the muscles but also the tissues in that area.

Bonus: Kegels help prevent incontinence and may intensify orgasms.

+ **Masturbate on your own,** with a

vibrator if desired, to rediscover what makes you feel aroused. Sometimes getting back in the game takes practice.

- **Consider talking to your gynecologist about a vaginal dilator,** which is a set of smooth cylindrical probes in varying sizes. You use the dilator at home to gradually stretch the vagina, so that by the time you want to have intercourse, you are physically ready.

....

> Barbara Bartlik, MD, sex therapist and assistant clinical professor of psychiatry at Weill Cornell Medical College in New York City. She is the author of numerous scientific publications, and medical advisor for the book *Extraordinary Togetherness: A Woman's Guide to Love, Sex and Intimacy.* BarbaraBartlikMD.com.

....

Men: The Secret to Better Erections

If you're like most middle-aged and older men, you want better erections—erections that are reliable and hard. But better sex is only one of the benefits of better erections.

Surprising fact: A man's erection is an important barometer of his health. Erectile dysfunction (ED)—when a man can't get or keep an erection firm enough for sexual intercourse—often is an early warning sign of heart disease. An erection requires healthy blood vessels, nerves, and hormones.

Important scientific evidence: A seven-year study of more than four thousand middle-aged and older men, published in the *Journal of the American Medical Association,* showed that those who had ED at the beginning of the study or developed it during the study had a 45 percent higher risk of developing heart disease.

Unfortunately, ED affects roughly half of American men over age sixty (and many younger men), most of whom have cardiovascular disease or one or more risk factors for developing it, such as high cholesterol, high blood pressure, insulin resistance, diabetes, or obesity.

Of course, you can take an ED drug (such as sildenafil, tadalafil, and vardenafil) for the problem. But that won't take care of the underlying health issues. Plus, no man wants to be dependent on ED drugs—they're not without risk (blindness is a rare but possible side effect), and they don't always work.

Here's what you need to know to preserve or restore your erections—and the health of your body—naturally.

EXERCISE

Erections owe most of their hardness to nitric oxide, a molecule that signals blood vessels to relax, allowing blood to enter and pool in the penis. The body's most effective way of stimulating nitric oxide formation is exercise, even mild exercise, such as walking.

Scientific evidence: In a study of 180 men ages forty to seventy, published in the *International Journal of Impotence Research,* those who were sedentary were ten times more likely to develop ED than those who were physically active.

My recommendation: Ten thousand steps a day, which you can achieve through everyday physical activity (typically four to five thousand steps) and a brisk walk of four to six thousand steps (about two to three miles, or thirty to forty-five minutes).

Start with five thousand steps daily for one week. Increase to six thousand steps daily the second week and to seven thousand the third week until you reach ten thousand. Maintain that level. You can find an accurate pedometer—typically at a cost of twenty to thirty dollars—at your local sporting-goods store or on the internet at DigiWalker.com.

ERECTION-ENHANCING FOODS

Your sexual performance is greatly impacted by the foods you eat. Here are my recommendations.

Reduce the fats in your diet. Fatty foods lead to clogged arteries, which prevent blood flow from reaching the penis. Cut back on saturated fats such as egg yolks, butter, cream, fatty red meats, and palm oil.

Eat more fruits and vegetables. They reduce cholesterol and improve blood flow to the penis.

Eat whole grains, nuts, and seeds. They provide an important basis for cardiovascular and penile health.

Spice up your foods. Chili peppers stimulate the nervous system, helping with sexual arousal. Ginger has long been considered a sexual stimulant and an overall tonic for general health.

BEST SUPPLEMENTS

Several supplements can help restore erections.

L-arginine and **Pycnogenol.** The amino acid L-arginine (found in meat, whole grains, fish, nuts, and milk) is converted to nitric oxide in the body. But most men don't get enough in their diets, so I often recommend an L-arginine supplement.

Caution: Talk to your doctor before you take L-arginine, especially if you have low blood pressure, herpes, gastric ulcer, liver disease, or kidney disease.

L-arginine works best when combined with Pycnogenol, a patented amalgam of more than three dozen antioxidants extracted from the bark of the French pine tree. Together, the supplement allows for better nitric oxide production and utilization.

Scientific research: In a study of men with mild-to-moderate ED, published in *Phytotherapy Research*, taking a supplement with L-arginine and Pycnogenol for eight weeks improved erections and satisfaction with sex.

Typical dose: A daily dose of the supplement Prelox Blue, which contains a blend of Pycnogenol and L-arginine.

Omega-3 fatty acids (fish oil). Found in oily fish such as salmon and sardines, omega-3s can reduce plaque inside artery walls, decrease blood clotting, lower triglyceride (blood fat) levels, and decrease both blood pressure and blood vessel inflammation. Omega-3s are the nutritional building blocks of heart and penis health.

Typical dose: 2,000 mg daily, taken with a meal.

Horny goat weed (*Epimedium sagittatum*). This Chinese herb perks up sexual desire.

Scientific evidence: I conducted two studies on Exotica H-G-W, a brand of horny goat weed. The first study showed that the supplement enhanced sexual satisfaction in three out of five men. The second study—in which men took horny goat weed capsules one hour before sexual activity—resulted in a significant increase in hardness in two-thirds of the participants.

Typical dose: Two capsules daily, totaling 500 mg of horny goat weed. My patients take it for six weeks and then start to taper off. You can use it intermittently after that.

TESTOSTERONE SELF-CARE

Testosterone—the predominantly male hormone that helps drive sexual desire and performance—declines with age. But most of that decline is caused by lifestyle— poor sleep, relentless stress, and belly fat. Here are my recommendations to prevent that decline.

Sleep seven to eight hours a night. Going to bed at the same time every night (say, 11:00 p.m.) and getting up at the same time every morning (say, 6:30 a.m.) is one of the best habits for deep, refreshing sleep.

Add strength-training to your routine. Whether it's in the gym or at home with resistance bands, building and maintaining muscle are key to producing plenty of testosterone.

Breathe. Take a few slow, deep breaths a few times a day every single day—it does wonders for relieving tension and anxiety.

VISUALIZE FOR SEX SUCCESS

How do you prepare for an upcoming sexual encounter, especially if you didn't do so well in a previous effort and don't feel confident?

Sex is a physical act, and just as athletes practice visualization techniques so they can perform optimally, you can use the same techniques to build confidence in your bedroom "performance."

First, relax. Lie on your back on a mat or a rug with your arms at your sides and take a deep breath. Hold it for a moment, then exhale. Lie still, and continue breathing slowly.

Once you are relaxed, picture yourself about to have sex. Patiently go through the step-by-step sequence of events. Imagine every aspect of the session, including the sights, sounds, and smells associated with sex. Try to rehearse the action in your mind just as you would actually perform it. It's all about mental practice. When the time comes for the actual moment, your confidence will be higher.

....

› Steven Lamm, MD, practicing internist, faculty member at New York University School of Medicine, and director of men's health for NYU Langone Medical Center, both in New York City. He is author of several books, including *The Hardness Factor: How to Achieve Your Best Health and Fitness at Any Age.* DrStevenLamm.com.

....

Four Things That Can Ruin a Man's Sex Life

An erection is a manly miracle—a complex, coordinated effort of brain, blood vessels, nerves, muscles, and hormones that increases blood flow to the penis sixfold. But because so much has to go *right* for a man to have an erection, there's also a lot that can go wrong.

The problem is called erectile dysfunction (ED)—the inability to get or sustain an erection hard enough to have enjoyable and satisfying sex. And it's a very common problem. Nearly one in five men have ED, including 44 percent of men ages sixty to sixty-nine and 70 percent of men seventy and older.

A prescription ED drug such as sildenafil (Viagra), vardenafil (Levitra), or tadalafil (Cialis) can help. But this pharmaceutical solution isn't necessarily the best solution, because ED drugs don't address the underlying causes of ED, some of which can kill you.

What most men don't realize: An erection is the best barometer of a man's overall health, particularly the health of his circulatory system. The easier it is to achieve erections, the healthier the man. By identifying and correcting the factors that might be undermining erections, a man not only can restore his sex life—he might save his *life.*

Here are four factors that can ruin a man's sex life and what to do about them.

HEART DISEASE

An artery leads directly to the penis and subdivides into three more arteries, supplying the robust flow of blood on which an erection depends. If those arteries are narrowed or blocked, it's likely that there's a problem with all your arteries, including the arteries supplying blood to your heart.

Troubling finding: A decade-long study published in the *Journal of Sexual Medicine* shows that men over age fifty with ED are 2.5 times more likely to develop heart disease, and men under age fifty are 58 percent more likely. And a study of men with ED who were already diagnosed with heart disease shows that they are twice as likely to have a heart attack and 90 percent more likely to die of heart disease, compared with men who have heart disease but not ED.

What to do: Eat a Mediterranean diet, emphasizing vegetables, fruits, whole grains, beans, fish, and healthy fats (in olive oil, avocado, and nuts). It's a diet proven to prevent and treat heart disease, and several studies from Italy show that a Mediterranean diet also can prevent and cure ED.

Other conditions that increase the risk for ED: Type 2 diabetes, obesity, gout, and sleep apnea, and studies show that these conditions also are helped with a Mediterranean diet.

Important: If you have ED, make an appointment with your doctor, tell him/her about your problem, and ask for a complete workup to check for cardiovascular disease.

ALCOHOL

Alcohol is a central nervous system depressant, and despite what many people think, it dampens sexual arousal, and that's particularly true for older men.

What to do: Limit yourself to no more than one to two drinks per day. (A drink is one twelve-ounce beer, a five-ounce glass of wine, or 1.5 ounces of 80-proof spirits.)

What not to do: Washing down fried foods with beer (or any alcohol) is a double whammy. Eating fried food immediately spikes the level of blood fats such as triglycerides, impeding blood flow to the penis for several hours.

MEDICATIONS

ED can be a side effect of taking one or more prescription medicines. The most common offenders are drugs to treat high blood pressure, heart ailments, depression, and allergies.

Telltale sign: You start a new

medication, and you suddenly notice that you're having erectile difficulties.

What to do: Talk to your doctor about using a different medication to treat your health problem. For example, one class of antidepressants (selective serotonin reuptake inhibitors, or SSRIs) often leads to libido issues and ejaculation problems contributing to ED, but the antidepressant bupropion rarely does.

STRESS

Too much stress can undermine erections by slowing the production of hormones (including testosterone, the master male hormone) and by impeding blood flow to the penis.

What to do: The best way to reduce stress is to spend at least twenty to thirty minutes a day doing something you personally enjoy, whether it's watching your favorite comedian on Netflix, participating in a hobby such as woodworking, or going for a walk with your dog.

› Steven Lamm, MD, practicing internist, faculty member at New York University School of Medicine, and director of men's health for NYU Langone Medical Center, both in New York City. He is author of several books, including *The Hardness Factor: How to Achieve Your Best Health and Fitness at Any Age.* DrStevenLamm.com.

Blueberries Instead of Viagra?

Men, *if you like to* eat blueberries, you may beat the odds on developing erectile dysfunction (ED). It also helps if you eat strawberries, oranges, grapefruit, apples, and pears and drink red wine.

So suggests a recent study. But ED can be caused by some serious health issues. Could a handful of berries really be *that* powerful?

Nutrition expert and board-certified internist John La Puma, MD, reviewed the scientific literature on diet and men's sexual health and conducted original clinical research in preparation for his book, *Refuel: A 24-Day Eating Plan to Shed Fat, Boost Testosterone, and Pump Up Strength and Stamina.*

It turns out he's pretty positive about blueberries and other ways that diet and lifestyle changes can prevent—even *reverse*—ED.

THE FLAVONOID BOOST

In the study, Harvard researchers analyzed the diets and ED symptoms of twenty-five thousand men in the Health Professionals Follow-Up Study. In the period that this analysis focused on, the men were in their fifties, sixties, and seventies and older. The researchers focused on phytochemicals called flavonoids and the foods, mostly fruits, that are the biggest source of them in the American diet.

Results: Men whose diets were higher in these flavonoid-rich fruits were 14 percent less likely to develop ED over a ten-year period. Citrus fruits were a major flavonoid contributor. (Dark chocolate and soy foods, both of which are also flavonoid-rich, were not studied in this analysis.)

Blueberries stood out. In a separate analysis, men who ate them more than three times a week, on average, were *22 percent less likely to develop ED.*

What's so special about flavonoids? Berries here are acting in the same way as Viagra but they're a lot cheaper and they taste better. In animal studies, flavonoids inhibit a biological pathway that makes the penis flaccid and boost production of nitric oxide, which facilitates erections during sexual activity. In one study of rats with diabetes and ED, for example, adding a specific flavonoid (quercetin) to their chow actually reversed ED.

Medications such as sildenafil work through similar mechanisms, but unlike blueberries, they don't promote heart health, and they have side effects.

To be sure, no one is saying that you can pop a few blueberries in your mouth, wait a half hour, and jump into the sack.

The study unveiled not a quick fix but a long-term benefit of a flavonoid-rich diet.

Bonus: While you're saving your sexual function, you're likely saving your heart too.

BEYOND PREVENTION

The diet connection makes sense when you realize that erectile dysfunction often is a cardiovascular problem. The penile artery is about half the width of the coronary artery, so inflammation there creates symptoms first. Men with ED have cardiac disease until proven otherwise—it's an early warning sign.

That's why a heart-healthy diet is so important for prevention—and even treatment—of ED. In one study, men with ED who ate three ounces of heart-healthy flavonoid-rich pistachios for three weeks had improvement in their symptoms. Another study found that flavonoid-rich walnuts, like blueberries, boost nitric oxide production. A number of studies have shown that the dietary pattern, especially a Mediterranean diet—along with other interventions such as quitting smoking and increased physical activity—can be both preventive and therapeutic.

ANOTHER NOTCH IN THE BLUEBERRY BELT

On the other hand, if you're looking for just *one* food to add to your diet to improve your health and perhaps help preserve your sexual vitality, you can't go wrong with blueberries.

It's not just men who benefit. Blueberries are good for brain health in both men and women, improving cognitive function and memory in older adults.

And if any women are reading this article, there's a heart benefit for you too. The same Harvard group that discovered the ED connection reported a few years ago that women who consumed at least three servings of blueberries or strawberries a week were 34 percent less likely to get heart disease.

Blueberries—quite a sexy food indeed.

> Study titled "Dietary Flavonoid Intake and Incidence of Erectile Dysfunction" by researchers at Norwich Medical School, University of East Anglia, United Kingdom; Harvard T.H. Chan School of Public Health, Boston; Brigham and Women's Hospital, Boston; and Harvard Medical School, Boston, published in the *American Journal of Clinical Nutrition*.

> John La Puma, MD, board-certified specialist in internal medicine and trained chef with a private nutritional medical practice in Santa Barbara, California. He is the author of *ChefMD's Big Book of Culinary Medicine* and *Refuel: A 24-Day Eating Plan to Shed Fat, Boost Testosterone, and Pump Up Strength and Stamina*. DrJohnLaPuma.com.

A Health Problem Doesn't Have to End Your Love Life!

There are a multitude of reasons why some couples stop having sex as they age. But a chronic health problem is definitely a big one. Fortunately, it doesn't have to be that way.

Sexual satisfaction remains within reach for just about everyone who wants it, and most people still do want it. Not only that, sexual activity has its own health benefits. For example, it helps lower blood pressure, improves sleep, and relieves pain.

ADOPTING A NEW MIND-SET

If you're depriving yourself of sexual intimacy because of a health problem, the key is to start thinking about sex in a new way. Instead of viewing a sexual encounter as a pass/fail test that involves intercourse and mutual orgasm, it's time to think of it as an opportunity for sharing pleasure. How you achieve this is largely up to you. To get started, you'll want to talk to:

+ **Your doctor.** Schedule a single consultation for you and your partner to meet with your internist, cardiologist, oncologist, or other physician who is treating your health problem. Ask him/her to explain how your condition might affect your sexual intimacy and to give you any advice on what you can do medically to minimize those issues.

+ **Your partner.** It's crucial for you to be able to talk about sex with your partner. Don't wait until you're in bed or after a negative experience. Instead, bring up the subject (ideally on the day before a sexual encounter) while you're on a walk or having a glass of wine together. Avoid any blaming, and be clear that you're simply making sexual requests so that the experience is more comfortable and pleasurable.

In addition to what you learn by talking to your doctor and your partner, consider these specific steps to get your sex life back on track.

BACK PAIN

Take a man with lower back pain and have him engage in intercourse the way 70 percent of Americans do—with the man on top of his partner performing short, rapid thrusts—and you've got a perfect recipe for uncomfortable sex.

A better approach: The man with the bad back can invite his partner to go on top, and they can try a circular, thrusting motion. If a woman has back pain, the couple might try the side rear-entry position and long, slow thrusts. If your partner also has back problems, take lovemaking to the shower, where the warm water can loosen sore muscles.

Also helpful: If you're in chronic pain, such as that caused by arthritis, your doctor can refer you to a physical therapist, who can give you additional positioning tips.

Taking your favorite over-the-counter pain reliever or using a heating pad about thirty minutes before sex also helps. This approach often reduces back *and* joint pain for an hour or more.

Even if your pain is not entirely eliminated, you may get enough relief to enjoy yourself. And after orgasm, your pain will likely be less intense for a period of time.

CANCER

Cancer treatment, such as surgery, radiation, and medication, can create pain, fatigue, and all kinds of psychological and physical fallout.

With breast cancer, it's common for a woman to worry about her partner's reaction to her altered body and how her breasts will respond to touch, particularly if she has had reconstructive surgery, which reduces sensitivity.

What helps: When talking about these issues, don't be afraid to get specific. Some women will not want to be touched on the affected breast or breasts, at least for a while. Others will crave that touch. Some might feel uncomfortable about nipple stimulation but fine about touching on the underside of the breast.

Cancers that affect other parts of the body, such as cervical or testicular malignancies or even mouth cancer, can also interfere with intimacy. If a man has been treated for prostate cancer, for example, he may want to focus more on pleasure-oriented sexuality rather than the traditional approach of intercourse and orgasm. Whatever the situation, talk about these vulnerable feelings and enlist your partner's help as a sexual ally.

EXCESS BODY WEIGHT

Too much body weight can get in the way—both psychologically and physically.

It's common for a person who is overweight to think: *I don't feel sexy now, but I will when I lose some weight.* While weight loss is a healthy idea, putting your sexuality on ice until you reach some ideal state is not. Learn to love and care for the body you have.

What helps: Think beyond the missionary position, which can get pretty awkward and uncomfortable if one or both parties carry a lot of weight around the middle. Try lying on your sides instead. Or try a sitting and kneeling combination—a woman might sit on the edge of a sofa, supported by pillows behind her back, while her partner kneels before her.

HEART AND LUNG PROBLEMS

The fatigue often associated with heart and lung disease can douse your sexual flames. But a bigger issue is often the fear that a bit of sexually induced heavy breathing will prove dangerous or even fatal.

If this is a concern, ask your doctor whether you are healthy enough for sex. A good rule of thumb is to see if you can comfortably climb two flights of stairs. If the answer is yes, then almost certainly, you're healthy enough to have sex.

What helps: If you still feel nervous, you can gain some reassurance by pleasuring yourself. A bout of masturbation produces the same physiological arousal as partnered sex. And it gives you a no-pressure chance to see how that arousal affects your breathing and heart rate.

PARKINSON'S AND RELATED CONDITIONS

People with frequent tremors, muscle spasms, and other conditions in which a loss of control over the body occurs can still enjoy sex.

What helps: When talking to your partner about sex, decide between the two of you, in advance, on what you will say if, during lovemaking, your body becomes too uncooperative. It might be just a single word—"spasm," for instance—that tells your partner you need to pause.

Then agree on a "trust position" you will assume as you take a break to see if you want to return to sexual activity. For example, some people will cuddle or lie side by side.

> Barry McCarthy, PhD, psychologist, sex therapist, and marital therapist who is professor of psychology at American University in Washington, DC. He is coauthor, with Michael Metz, PhD, of *Enduring Desire: Your Guide to Lifelong Intimacy.*

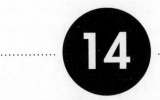

Sleep

How Sleep Sweeps Toxins from Your Brain

*I*t's tempting to shortchange ourselves on sleep. There's so much that needs to get done while we're awake, and science has never given us a good explanation for why we sleep away one-third of our lives, until now.

Using state-of-the-art imaging technology, researchers have made a startling discovery about the purpose of sleep. It turns out that, as our bodies rest, our brains are busy sweeping away a certain type of toxic detritus that collects during the day—the same type of detritus that's linked to Alzheimer's disease and other neurodegenerative disorders. This cleanup process involves changes in the actual cellular structure of the brain, changes we can liken, oddly enough, to a busy movie theater!

Here's the latest advice on how to keep your brain in top form, plus lots of tips on how to sleep better.

CLEANING A CROWDED SPACE

To understand this research, it helps to think of a movie theater. When a film is showing and the theater is packed, candy wrappers and popcorn and other garbage all fall to the floor. Moviegoers are making a mess, but it would be impossible to clean up while the people are still in their seats. The theater patrons wouldn't be able to concentrate on the movie, and there wouldn't be enough room for cleaners to maneuver.

Later though, after the movie, the people clear out and the seats fold up, and there is much more room. It's easier to get to the floor beneath to sweep away all the crud that the people left behind.

Researchers from the University of

Rochester Medical Center discovered that brains are like movie theaters. When we're awake, our brains are very active, guiding all our functions. As part of that process, our brains discard toxic proteins (such as the beta-amyloid that's linked to Alzheimer's) and other by-products, and there's little opportunity to clean up that debris. However, as the detritus builds up, our brains can't function as well.

Cool revelation: When we sleep, our brain cells literally shrink—similar to how theater seats fold up—thus enlarging the spaces around the cells. This allows brain fluids to flow more freely, doing their job of picking up the garbage that accumulated during the day and carrying it away.

HOW THIS DISCOVERY WAS MADE

In most of the human body, the lymphatic system is responsible for collecting and disposing of waste. But the lymphatic system doesn't make it past the protective blood-brain barrier that closely guards what enters the brain. Instead, cerebrospinal fluid circulates through the brain, picking up the interstitial fluid (fluid between the cells) along with the discarded proteins. This exchange of fluid was named the glymphatic system by the same Rochester researchers after they discovered the intricate network.

For the recent study, the researchers used a technique called two-photon imaging and different colored dyes to measure the rate of cerebrospinal fluid flowing through the brains of mice (the mouse brain is remarkably similar to the human brain) when the animals were awake, when they were sleeping naturally, and when they were under general anesthesia.

What the researchers found: The glymphatic system was nearly ten times more active when the mice were asleep or anesthetized than when they were awake, and the sleeping brains removed significantly more beta-amyloid and other debris. This occurred because, when the mice were asleep or anesthetized, their brain cells contracted by more than 60 percent, creating more space between the cells.

We already know that sufficient sleep helps us think more clearly, do better on tests, make smarter food choices, and perhaps keep blood sugar under control. Though it's too early to say that getting enough sleep helps prevent Alzheimer's and other neurodegenerative diseases, the recent study findings suggest that it might, giving us yet one more reason not to shortchange our slumber time.

....

› Maiken Nedergaard, MD, professor of neurosurgery, codirector, Center for Translational Neuromedicine, University of Rochester Medical Center, Rochester, New York. Her research was published in *Science*.

....

Eat Right to Sleep Tight

There's *nothing like a bad* case of indigestion to mess with a good night's sleep. But surprisingly, this is just one digestive factor that can keep you from sleeping well and feeling rested. What and how you eat impacts the absorption of critical nutrients and the flow of food through your digestive system.

SECRETS TO A GOOD NIGHT'S SLEEP

Well-nourished people sleep more soundly. Here are some secrets to getting a good night's sleep.

Get enough fiber. Doing so makes it less likely you'll awaken with stomach cramps and also helps with removal of wastes expelled by the liver. Adequate fiber—in foods such as steamed veggies, ripe fruits, whole grain bread, brown rice, and oats—is essential to efficient digestion, staving off problems such as constipation, irritability, and sleeplessness. Because Americans consume about half the fiber they should, I frequently prescribe the fiber supplement glucomannan to take thirty minutes before lunch and dinner and again before bedtime with a large glass of water.

Other helpful hints: Consume three square meals a day, chew food thoroughly, and limit beverages with meals to guarantee adequate stomach acid for digestion.

Avoid hard-to-digest foods. Excessive red meat, alcohol, white bread, fast foods, fatty or fried items, and sugary snacks and desserts require the stomach and liver to work overtime. Overwhelming the system interferes not only with digestion, but also with sleep.

Monitor your B vitamin levels, including B-6 and B-12. In order for the body to effectively convert dietary tryptophan—from foods such as turkey and other animal protein, dairy, eggs, and fish—into serotonin, the "good night moon" hormone, the body requires a sufficient supply of vitamin B-6.

Note: Remember that vitamins used for medicinal reasons require medical oversight.

Get enough calcium and magnesium. In addition to building strong bones, these vital nutrients relax the muscles of the digestive tract and decrease digestive irritability. I often prescribe the calcium supplement Butyrex (from T. E. Neesby in Fresno, California). It contains calcium, magnesium, and butyric acid, a fatty acid found in butter and milk. Butyrex is calcium and magnesium in their most easily absorbed forms.

Also beneficial: A warm, milky nightcap. My favorite is herbal tea with honey and a touch of heavy cream. If, like many people, you have trouble digesting cow's milk, consider goat's and sheep's milk, which are good alternatives.

Don't eat too close to bedtime. On average, the stomach takes between two and four hours to empty its contents after eating. A full stomach works best in an upright position.

Be careful about eating spicy foods that stimulate GI activity. These include dishes made with ingredients such as curry, cumin, cardamom, and hot peppers. Though these contain important nutrients, you'll do best to eat them many hours before retiring for the night.

These simple strategies will not only help you get a good night's sleep, they'll help your digestion overall, which will also make you feel and function better. If you continue to suffer from indigestion and/or sleep disturbances despite taking appropriate measures, be sure to consult your health-care professional.

› Andrew L. Rubman, ND, medical director of Southbury Clinic for Traditional Medicines in Southbury, Connecticut. He is a founding member of the American Association of Naturopathic Physicians. His blog, *Nature Doc's Patient Diary*, is published on BottomLineInc.com. SouthburyClinic.com.

Nutritional Deficiencies That Cause Insomnia

Every night, millions of Americans have trouble falling asleep or staying asleep. Quite often, this is caused by stress, anxiety, caffeine, or overstimulation before bed. But there is another common cause that few people even know to consider—a nutritional deficiency of one kind or another. If you have such a deficiency, once it is identified, you can easily correct it and start enjoying peaceful slumber once again.

CALCIUM: NATURE'S SEDATIVE

When you run short on calcium, you are apt to toss and turn and experience frequent awakenings in the night. This mineral has a natural calming effect on the nervous system. It works by helping your body convert tryptophan—an essential amino acid found in foods such as turkey and eggs—into the neurotransmitter serotonin, which modulates mood and sleep. Serotonin, in turn, is converted into melatonin, a hormone that helps regulate the sleep cycle.

It's always better to get the nutrients you need from food rather than supplements. Milk and dairy products are the most common dietary sources of calcium, but many people have trouble digesting cow's milk, especially as they grow older.

Excellent nondairy sources of calcium are leafy green vegetables such as kale and collard greens, canned sardines, sesame seeds, and almonds. The recommended dietary allowance (RDA) for adults over age eighteen is 1,000 to 1,200 mg/day. For those not getting enough from dietary sources, consider the calcium-magnesium supplement Butyrex from T. E. Neesby. Take it half an hour before going to bed.

RELIEVE LEG CRAMPS WITH MAGNESIUM

Nighttime leg cramps, often due to a magnesium deficiency, are a common cause of sleeplessness. Magnesium helps your body's cells absorb and use calcium, so this mineral pair works hand in hand to relax muscles, relieve painful cramps or spasms, and bring on restful slumber.

Leafy green vegetables are the best source of dietary magnesium, followed by artichokes, nuts, legumes, seeds, whole grains (especially buckwheat, cornmeal, and whole wheat), and soy products. The Butyrex I prescribe for calcium deficiency contains magnesium, so it helps solve this problem too. (The RDA for magnesium for adults is 400 mg/day for men and 310 mg/day for women.)

VITAMIN B-12 FOR SEROTONIN PRODUCTION

Vitamin B-12 supports the production of neurotransmitters that affect brain function and sleep, helping to metabolize calcium and magnesium and working with them to convert tryptophan into the neurotransmitter serotonin. Insufficient B-12 may be a factor if you have trouble falling or staying asleep.

Foods rich in vitamin B-12 include liver and other organ meats, eggs, fish, and, to a lesser degree, leafy green vegetables. For B-12 deficiency, I sometimes prescribe B-12 tablets taken sublingually (dissolved under the tongue) one hour before bedtime, but it's important to take a multivitamin that contains B vitamins twice daily as well, since it helps your body use the B-12 efficiently.

Note: Most B multivitamins contain B-12 but only a minimal dose, so further supplementation is usually necessary.

VITAMIN D MODULATES CIRCADIAN RHYTHMS

Again with the vitamin D! We can't hear enough about the importance of this vital nutrient, it seems, and indeed, vitamin D turns out to be essential to support your body's uptake and usage of calcium and magnesium. Its role in sleep involves modulating your circadian rhythm (the sleep/wake cycle that regulates your twenty-four-hour biological clock).

Most Americans have less than optimal levels of vitamin D, so I commonly prescribe daily supplements of D-3, the form most efficiently used by the body. Ten to twenty minutes of sunshine daily helps your body manufacture vitamin D, and foods such as fish and fortified milk are rich in this nutrient.

HERBS: SOME HELP, BUT SOME INTERFERE WITH SLEEP

Although they do not specifically address nutritional deficiencies, I also recommend relaxing herbal supplements such as chamomile, hops, or valerian to gently nudge you toward sleep. Try them in teas, capsules, or tinctures from reputable manufacturers, taken half an hour before retiring.

Though many people swear by melatonin, there is not enough scientific evidence yet to demonstrate that this popular sleep supplement works efficiently and without long-term ill effects. I do not prescribe it.

It's also important to be aware that a number of supplements are stimulating and may cause sleep irregularities in some individuals.

The biggest stimulators: Ginseng, ginkgo, St. John's wort, alpha-lipoic acid, and SAMe. If you take any of these, do so early in the day, take the lowest dose that seems effective for you, or discuss alternatives with your physician. These are all best used under professional guidance.

A SOOTHING BEDTIME SNACK

I generally advise against late-night snacking, which can disturb sleep, but if you must have something, keep it light. A high-protein, low-glycemic snack, such as a banana with peanut butter or half a turkey sandwich on whole-grain bread, can help encourage serotonin production...and sweet dreams.

> Andrew L. Rubman, ND, medical director of Southbury Clinic for Traditional Medicines in Southbury, Connecticut. He is a founding member of the American Association of Naturopathic Physicians. His blog, *Nature Doc's Patient Diary*, is published on BottomLineInc.com. SouthburyClinic.com.

Foods That Sabotage Sleep

You know that an evening coffee can leave you tossing and turning into the wee hours. But these other foods can hurt sleep too.

Premium ice cream. Brace yourself for a restless night if you indulge in Häagen-Dazs or Ben & Jerry's late at night. The richness of these wonderful treats comes mainly from fat—16 to 17 grams of fat in half a cup of vanilla, and who eats just half a cup?

Your body digests fat more slowly than it digests proteins or carbohydrates. When you eat a high-fat food within an hour or two of bedtime, your digestion will still be active when you lie down, and that can disturb sleep.

Also, the combination of stomach acid, stomach contractions, and a horizontal position increases the risk for reflux, the upsurge of digestive juices into the esophagus that causes heartburn, which can disturb sleep.

Chocolate. Some types of chocolate can jolt you awake almost as much as a cup of coffee. Dark chocolate, in particular, has shocking amounts of caffeine.

Example: Half a bar of Dagoba Eclipse Extra Dark has 41 mg of caffeine, close to what you'd get in a shot of mild espresso.

Chocolate also contains theobromine, another stimulant, which is never a good choice near bedtime.

Beans. Beans are one of the healthiest foods. But a helping or two of beans—or broccoli, cauliflower, cabbage, or other gas-producing foods—close to bedtime can make your night, well, a little noisier than usual. No one sleeps well when suffering from gas pains. You can reduce the "backtalk" by drinking a mug of chamomile or peppermint tea at bedtime. They're carminative herbs that aid digestion and help prevent gas.

Spicy foods. Spicy foods temporarily speed up your metabolism. They are associated with taking longer to fall asleep and with more time spent awake at night. This may be caused by the capsaicin found in chili peppers, which affects body temperature and disrupts sleep. Also, in some people, spicy foods can lead to sleep-disturbing gas, stomach cramps, and heartburn.

....

› Bonnie Taub-Dix, RDN, CDN, registered dietitian and director and owner of BTD Nutrition Consultants, LLC, on Long Island and in New York City. She is author of *Read It Before You Eat It: How to Decode Food Labels and Make the Healthiest Choice Every Time.* BonnieTaubDix.com.

....

Sleeping Pills Are Just Plain Dangerous

It's bad enough that people are so desperate for sleep that they resort to taking any of a long list of pharmaceuticals in an effort to help them get a good night's rest. Even worse is that these theoretical helpers come with a long list of associated dangers, including addiction.

Well, guess what? The list of dangers just got longer.

Research conducted by physicians at the Scripps Clinic Viterbi Family Sleep Center in San Diego and Jackson Hole Center for Preventive Medicine (JHCPM) in Wyoming has shown that use of sleeping pills has been associated with an increased risk for cancer and death.

The most troubling part is that this study found that it's not just daily users who are at risk. Those who use them less than twice a month may even be at risk. Robert Langer, MD, MPH, principal scientist and medical director at JHCPM, explained more about these frightening findings.

IT TAKES A WHILE FOR SIDE EFFECTS TO SURFACE

Most studies on the safety of sleeping pills last only six months or less. That's not enough time to examine the risk for many serious health consequences, such as cancer or death. Our research is more long-term, and we didn't just look at whether or not people were taking sleeping pills. We also looked at which type they were using and how often they were taking the pills.

The researchers looked at the electronic medical records of the population served by the Geisinger Health System (GHS) in Pennsylvania, the largest rural integrated health system in the United States. Subjects (mean age fifty-four years) were 10,529 male and female patients who received prescriptions of sleeping pills as sleep aids (on-label), and 23,676 matched controls with no prescriptions of sleeping pills. They were followed for an average of 2.5 years.

The researchers found that the more sleeping pills that subjects took, the greater their risk for death from all causes, and shockingly, even people who were taking them only sporadically were at higher risk for death. For example, compared with those who did not take sleeping pills, people who took…

- One to 18 sleeping pills a year were 3.6 times more likely to die within the 2.5-year follow-up period.
- 19 to 132 sleeping pills a year were 4.4 times more likely to die.
- 133 or more pills a year were 5.3 times more likely to die.

These results did not differ whether the subjects were using older sleeping pills, such as temazepam, or newer ones, such as zolpidem, eszopiclone, and zaleplon, which are marketed as being shorter-acting and safer.

Researchers also found an increased risk for all major cancers among moderate and heavy users of any sleeping pill. There was a 20 percent increased risk among any users who took 19 to 132 pills a year and a

35 percent increased risk among any users who took more than 132 pills a year.

It's important to note that none of these results prove cause and effect, but they certainly reveal an unsettling association.

UNDERSTANDING THE CONNECTION

Could the results simply be due to the fact that patients who take sleeping pills are usually in worse health? For example, perhaps they don't eat well or exercise as much as they should, or maybe they're more stressed. No. The study controlled for every possible variation, matching subjects and controls by age, gender, and health history, yet the results remained the same.

So why the increased risk for death and cancer? The study did not have adequate information to assess possible mechanisms. However, based on prior studies, potential mechanisms include increases in sleep apnea, accidents related to sleep walking/driving, aspiration pneumonia, and depression of respiratory function.

NOW WHAT?

This is a finding of major consequence, because nine million American adults took a prescription sleeping pill in 2013, according to a Centers for Disease Control and Prevention study. But the complicating factor is that sleeping pills do provide health benefits. In other words, not taking

a sleeping pill and potentially not getting enough sleep comes with its own set of risks. For instance, insomnia can raise the risk for heart disease, stroke, diabetes, obesity, depression, and other serious health conditions. So if you're taking sleeping pills, what do you do?

First, consult your prescribing physician. Don't stop cold turkey, because that can cause withdrawal symptoms and agitation, as well as sleepless nights. Figure out a plan with your doctor about how to taper off. And then ask your doctor about safer alternatives, such as melatonin or manipulating light exposure. You can also try cognitive behavioral therapy from an informed primary care doctor, behavioral therapist, or sleep medicine physician.

> Robert Langer, MD, MPH, principal scientist and medical director, Jackson Hole Center for Preventive Medicine, Wyoming.

What's Your Sleep Problem?

Most people assume that lack of sleep is more of an annoyance than a legitimate threat to their health. But that's a mistake. Lack of sleep—even if it's only occasional—is directly linked to poor health. If ignored, sleep problems can increase your risk for diabetes and heart disease.

About two out of every three Americans ages fifty-five to eighty-four have insomnia, but it is one of the most underdiagnosed health problems in the United States. Even when insomnia is diagnosed, many doctors recommend a one-size-fits-all treatment approach (often including long-term use of sleep medication) that does not correct the underlying problem.

Here are some ways to treat specific sleep problems.

IF YOU WAKE UP TOO EARLY IN THE MORNING

Early risers often have advanced sleep phase syndrome (ASPS), which is seen most commonly in older adults. With this condition, a person's internal body clock that regulates the sleep-wake cycle (circadian rhythm) is not functioning properly. ASPS sufferers sleep best from 8:00 p.m. to 4:00 a.m.

My solutions: To reset your circadian rhythm, try a light box (a device that uses lightbulbs to simulate natural light). Light boxes don't require a doctor's prescription and are available online or from retailers. Most people use a light box for thirty minutes to an hour daily at sundown. (Those with ASPS may need long-term light therapy.) If you have cataracts or glaucoma or a mood disorder (such as bipolar disorder), consult your doctor before trying light therapy. Patients with retinopathy (a disorder of the retina) should avoid light therapy.

Also helpful: To help regulate your internal clock so that you can go to bed (and get up) later, take a 3- to 5-mg melatonin supplement each day. A sleep specialist can advise you on when to use light therapy and melatonin for ASPS.*

IF YOU CAN'T STAY ASLEEP

Everyone wakes up several times a night, but most people fall back to sleep within seconds, so they don't remember waking up.

Trouble staying asleep is often related to sleep apnea, a breathing disorder that causes the sufferer to awaken repeatedly during the night and gasp for air. Another common problem among those who can't stay asleep is periodic limb movement disorder (PLMD), a neurological condition that causes frequent involuntary kicking or jerking movements during sleep. (Restless legs syndrome, which is

---

* To find a sleep center near you, consult the American Academy of Sleep Medicine (630-737-9700, sleepcenters. org).

similar to PLMD, causes an uncontrollable urge to move the legs and also can occur at night.)

My solutions: If you are unable to improve your sleep throughout the night by following the strategies already described, consult a sleep specialist to determine whether you have sleep apnea or PLMD.

Sleep apnea patients usually get relief by losing weight, if necessary, elevating the head of the bed to reduce snoring, using an oral device that positions the jaw so that the tongue cannot block the throat during sleep, or wearing a face mask that delivers oxygen to keep their airways open. PLMD is usually treated with medication.

IF YOU CAN'T GET TO SLEEP

Most people take about twenty minutes to fall asleep, but this varies with the individual. If your mind is racing due to stress (from marital strife or financial worries, for example) or if you've adopted bad habits (such as drinking caffeine late in the day), you may end up tossing and turning.

My solutions: Limit yourself to one cup of caffeinated coffee or tea daily, and do not consume any caffeine-containing beverage or food (such as chocolate) after 2:00 p.m. If you take a caffeine-containing drug, such as Excedrin or some cold

remedies, ask your doctor if it can be taken earlier in the day.

Helpful: If something is bothering you, write it down, and tell yourself that you will deal with it tomorrow. This way, you can stop worrying so you can get to sleep.

Also helpful: When you go to bed, turn the clock face away from you so you don't watch the minutes pass. If you can't sleep after twenty to thirty minutes, get up and do something relaxing, such as meditating, until you begin to feel drowsy.

IF YOU CAN'T GET UP IN THE MORNING

If you can't drag your head off the pillow, sleep apnea or a delayed sleep phase (DSP) disorder might be to blame. DSP disorder makes it hard to fall asleep early, so you stay up late at night and then struggle to get out of bed in the morning.

My solutions: To treat DSP disorder, progressively stay up for three hours later nightly for one week until you reach your desired bedtime. By staying up even later than is usual for you, you'll eventually shift your circadian rhythm. Once you find your ideal bedtime, stick to it. Also consider trying light-box therapy each morning upon arising. Light helps advance your body clock so that your bedtime should come earlier. Taking 3 to 5 mg of melatonin one hour before bedtime should also make you sleepy at an earlier hour.

IF YOU CAN'T STAY AWAKE DURING THE DAY

If you're getting ample rest—most people need seven and one-half to eight hours a night—and still are tired, you may have narcolepsy. This neurological disorder occurs when the brain sends out sleep-inducing signals at inappropriate times, causing you to fall asleep and even temporarily lose muscle function. Sleep apnea or periodic limb movements also can leave people feeling exhausted.

My solutions: Figure out how much sleep you need by sleeping as long as you can nightly (perhaps while on vacation) for one to two weeks. At the end of that period, you should be sleeping the number of hours you need. Give yourself that much sleep time nightly. If you remain sluggish, ask your doctor about tests for sleep apnea, PLMD, or narcolepsy, which is treated with stimulants, such as modafinil, that promote wakefulness.

....

› Lawrence J. Epstein, MD, instructor in medicine at Harvard Medical School in Boston, medical director of Sleep Health Centers, based in Brighton, Massachusetts, and author of *The Harvard Medical School Guide to a Good Night's Sleep.*

....

Insomnia Cure from Cherries

*C*an a glass of juice improve the quality of your sleep at night? Perhaps so.

Several years ago, scientists at a company called CherryPharm (now called Cheribundi) began studying the health benefits of juice made from fresh tart cherries, a type of cherry that is loaded with phytochemicals and antioxidants. Several company-sponsored studies indicated that this juice helps ease inflammation and sore muscles in marathoners and heavy exercisers. Coincidentally, some of the people in those studies mentioned that they also slept better after drinking the juice. This prompted the company to ask the University of Rochester Medical Center's sleep research lab to investigate whether the juice might ease insomnia in older adults.

Result: Drinking the tart cherry juice brought significant improvement in sleep continuity with study participants. In fact, the juice worked better than the popular herbal sleep aid valerian and at least as well as melatonin, which had been evaluated in similar sleep studies.

TWO THEORIES ON WHY IT WORKS

The cherry juice—simple, safe, and natural—did help. Tart cherries naturally contain melatonin, which is known to improve sleep in some people. The juice's anti-inflammatory properties may also explain the sleep improvements. It's known that inflammatory substances that naturally occur in the body are associated with the regulation of sleep and that poor sleep is associated with elevated levels of these substances. While this was just a small study and further investigation is needed, these preliminary findings suggest that tart cherry juice may provide some aid for insomnia.

The study used Montmorency tart cherries, available at specialty and high-end supermarkets. One eight-ounce bottle of tart cherry juice contains the juice from fifty tart cherries along with a bit of apple juice and has a fresh, slightly sour taste. Note that it packs quite a sugar wallop, with 28 grams of sugar. (You can buy tart cherry juice that is sweetened with stevia, which contains 17 g of sugar.) Another option is to take a cherry supplement that contains freeze-dried extract of tart cherries in capsule form. As always, check with your doctor first.

> Wilfred R. Pigeon, PhD, director, Sleep & Neurophysiology Research Lab, University of Rochester Medical Center, Rochester, New York. He is coauthor of *The Sleep Manual: Training Your Mind and Body to Achieve the Perfect Night's Sleep.*

Herbal Sleep Aids

The following sleep inducers may work as well as the popular pharmaceutical drugs but without their adverse side effects.

Valerian is a natural sleep aid and daytime sedative. Contrary to the popular myth, it is not related to the pharmaceutical drug Valium. Small doses of valerian can be used for calming during the day and higher doses as a sleep aid about a half hour before bedtime. Valerian can be taken in combination with lemon balm or other mildly sedative herbs (e.g., chamomile, hops, etc.), which makes it an even more powerful sleep aid.

Hops (*Humulus lupulus*) can also be helpful. Yes, this is the same ingredient used in making beer. It is a gentle sedative that promotes relaxation and is available in pills as well as in tincture and bulk flower form in health food stores. It can be taken together with valerian.

> Mark Blumenthal, founder and executive director, American Botanical Council, and editor, *HerbalGram.* ABC.HerbalGram.org.

Acupuncture Cure for Insomnia

Getting stuck all over with needles may seem the stuff of voodoo nightmares, but in fact, if you suffer from insomnia, it may be just the fix for your sleepless nights.

A meta-analysis of forty-six randomized trials found that acupuncture does ease insomnia. And a study published in the *Asian Journal of Psychiatry* found that acupuncture may be as effective as the sedative drug zolpidem in alleviating sleeplessness, particularly for women and older patients.

Big advantage: Acupuncture has no serious adverse effects, unlike sleeping pills, which can lead to breathing problems, pounding heartbeat, chest pain, blurred vision, and addiction.

I can confirm that acupuncture has helped many of my patients sleep. I use it on its own for mild insomnia. For chronic cases, I use it in combination with other natural modalities to address underlying conditions that can interfere with sleep.

How it works: From the perspective of Western medicine, acupuncture helps regulate various hormones and neurotransmitters—including melatonin, serotonin, endorphins, and many others—that play major roles in sleep regulation, according to a study from Emory University School of Medicine. In traditional Chinese medicine, the theory is that various symptoms develop when a patient's qi (vital energy) gets blocked, and acupuncture removes these blockages by stimulating specific acupoints that correspond to different parts of the body. Acupuncture helps strengthens the body's ability to heal itself. When tension and pain are removed, you eliminate much of what is causing the insomnia.

What to expect: While the course of treatment is tailored to an individual's needs, typically a patient receives ten to twenty hypoallergenic needles at a time in a treatment session that lasts about thirty to forty-five minutes. Placement of the needles depends on where the qi is blocked and on any underlying health problems that may be contributing to poor sleep. Discomfort is minimal—the needles are extremely thin and only go through the first layer of skin.

Insomnia patients typically go for treatment once per week for six to twelve weeks, then follow up once or twice a year for maintenance. Some feel a difference as soon as the third treatment, while others may take up to twelve sessions. If we are not seeing results by the eighth session, I start thinking about adding nutrients or herbs to the treatment plan.

Acupuncture generally is safe for everyone, there are no side effects except for rare cases of slight bruising, and some health insurance policies now cover it—all facts that may help you sleep better as you consider this treatment option.

To find a qualified acupuncturist: Visit the website of the American Association of Acupuncture and Oriental Medicine.

....

› Pina LoGiudice, ND, LAc, clinical director of Inner Source Health and Acupuncture, a center for integrative naturopathic care in New York City. She also is a contributing author of *Textbook of Natural Medicine* and a member of the adjunct faculty of the Natural Gourmet Institute for Food and Health in New York City. InnerSourceHealth.com.

....

Warm Hands and Feet to Bring On Sleep

Next time you have trouble falling asleep, do what Mom used to suggest—make yourself all cozy and warm—but perhaps not for the reasons you'd expect. In 1999, Swiss researchers found that temperature in the extremities relative to the core is the most important physiologic predictor of sleep onset, even more so than feeling sleepy. Researchers at Weill Cornell Medical College in New York City learned how these warm feelings—especially in your hands and feet—make you sleepy and why it's not as simple as wearing socks to bed.

WARM FUZZY THOUGHTS

What's at work here is not simply the temperature of your hands and feet but rather the physiological process involved in warming extremities. Prior to falling asleep, circulation increases to the periphery, including your hands and feet. Your body cools slightly, and sleep ensues.

HOW TO DO IT

Our research focused on the use of biofeedback to teach people how to bring warmth to their limbs. Currently used to treat several medical conditions, biofeedback involves using the mind to influence measurable physiologic aspects, such as lowering blood pressure or raising body temperature. Electrodes were attached to the hands and feet of subjects, all of whom suffered from insomnia. Temperature data fed into a computer, displaying the results so subjects could see how well their efforts worked. They were told to use whatever positive imagery they liked to try to increase the temperature of their hands and feet. Specific instructions were avoided, but general guidelines such as "think of the sun" or "imagine a beach" were suggested.

Most subjects quickly learned how to bring heat to their hands and feet. This is one technique you can safely try at home, and you don't even need a biofeedback device. Just paint a mental picture of the warm sun shining its rays on the paws of those sheep you've been counting…and counting…and off to dreamland you'll go.

. . . .

› Matthew Ebben, PhD, sleep expert, researcher, and psychologist at the Center for Sleep Medicine at New York-Presbyterian/Weill Cornell. Dr. Ebben is also an assistant professor of psychology in neurology at Weill Cornell Medical College.

. . . .

The Antisnoring Workout

*S*noring can be a nightmare, both for the sufferer and his/her bed partner. But until recently, the treatments have been limited. A snorer might be told to lose weight, for example, wear a mouth guard or a mask (part of a continuous positive airway pressure, or CPAP, system) that delivers a steady stream of air at night, change his sleeping position, or, in severe cases, get surgery.

Recent development: In a 2015 study of thirty-nine men who snored or had mild obstructive sleep apnea (OSA), a common cause of snoring, scientists found that performing mouth and tongue exercises reduced the frequency and intensity of snoring by up to 59 percent—a reduction on par with other therapies, including mouth guards or surgery.

And while snoring may seem like more of an annoyance than a health problem, that is simply not true. Snoring has been linked to medical conditions, including heart attack, stroke, and glaucoma. Here is how mouth and tongue exercises can help.

SIT-UPS FOR YOUR THROAT

If your bed partner has complained of your snoring or you have unexplained daytime sleepiness, consider trying the following exercises.

About half of my patients improve enough after doing these exercises (think of them as "throat sit-ups") for five minutes three times a day for six weeks to avoid surgery or other inconvenient therapies such as wearing a mouth guard or using CPAP. They also awaken feeling more refreshed and reduce their odds of developing OSA.

Here are the main exercises included in the recent study mentioned above (led by Geraldo Lorenzi-Filho, MD, PhD), along with some slight variations that I have found to be effective for my patients. The tongue positions for these exercises strengthen your tongue muscle and the sides of your throat. However, my variations give these muscles a more rigorous strength-training workout.

Tongue Push

What to do: Push the tip of your tongue forcefully behind your upper front teeth and move it all the way back along the roof of your mouth (palate) twenty times.

My variation: Say the vowel sounds "A, E, I, O, U" while doing the exercise.

Flat Tongue Press

What to do: Suck your tongue up against the roof of your mouth, pressing the entire tongue against your palate twenty times.

My variation: Repeat "A, E, I, O, U" while doing the exercise.

Say "Ahhh"

What to do: Focus on raising the back of the roof of the mouth and uvula (the fleshy appendage in the throat that's responsible for the rattling sound made by snorers) twenty times.

My variation: Say the vowel "A" (or "Ahhh") while doing the exercise.

OTHER HELPFUL THERAPIES

Colds, allergies, and sinus infections can cause nasal congestion and/or postnasal drip, two common conditions that can make your throat swell, increasing your risk for snoring. Here are some therapies that help:

+ **Nasal lavage** (using a saline solution to irrigate and cleanse the nasal cavity) helps clear nasal congestion and postnasal drip. Subjects in the study mentioned earlier performed nasal lavage three times a day. Based on my clinical experience, once a day does the job.
+ **Nose taping.** With age, the tip of one's nose naturally begins to droop some. This can obstruct the nasal valve, which impedes breathing and contributes to snoring.

  Try this simple test: Use your finger to press the tip of your nose up. If breathing feels easier when you do this, try taping your nose up before bedtime.

  What to do: Cut a three-inch strip of one-half-inch medical grade tape. Place it under the nose at the center, without blocking the airway. Gently lift the nose as you run the tape up the midline of the nose to the area between the eyes. The taping should be comfortable and is for use during sleep.

  Important: Commercial nasal strips, such as Breathe Right, spread the sides of the nose apart. Taping up the nose, as described above, also does this, with the additional advantage of opening the nasal valve.

› Murray Grossan, MD, board-certified otolaryn-gologist at Tower Ear, Nose & Throat, based at Cedars-Sinai Medical Center in Los Angeles. He is the author of *The Whole Body Approach to Allergy and Sinus Health*, founder of the Grossan Sinus & Health Institute (GrossanInstitute.com), and inventor of the Hydro Pulse (HydroMedonline.com).

Light Therapy: The Fifteen-Minute Secret to Sleeping Better

Many of us have trouble sleeping and experience times during the day when our energy or mood lags. This can be more pronounced in the fall and winter when the days are shorter and darker.

Well…you don't have to turn to medication to fix these problems. The way to restful sleep, increased energy, and a better mood may be as easy as exposing yourself to the right amount of light at the right time of day. Here's how to do it.

HOW LIGHT AFFECTS US
Many of us spend most of our days indoors. Even if our homes or offices seem to get a lot of natural light through windows, a light meter held in the room would show that the amount of light indoors registers much lower than just outside the window. In the evening, when our inner clock needs to wind down, we are inundated by artificial light from lamps, computer monitors, and television screens. In our bedrooms at night, a night-light, streetlights, bathroom light, etc., can disturb sleep timing and quality.

BRIGHT-LIGHT THERAPY
By changing the amount and patterns of your daily light exposure, remarkable changes in your mood, energy, and sleep can occur within days.

What to do: Buy a fluorescent light box that provides 10,000 lux of illumination (lux measures the light level reaching your eyes from the source). That is the equivalent of the amount of light that you would get while walking on the beach on a clear morning about forty minutes after sunrise. The lamp should have a screen that filters out ultraviolet (UV) rays, which can be harmful to the eyes and skin. It should give off only white light, not colored light, which has been hyped to be especially potent but is visually disturbing and no better than white. To be sure of a big enough field of illumination, the screen area should be about two hundred square inches (for example, twelve inches by sixteen inches) or larger.

Adjust the light box so that the light comes from above your line of sight and you feel comfortable and are not squinting. You should be positioned twelve to thirteen inches from the screen. You can get the benefits of the light while talking on the phone, using your computer, or enjoying breakfast. You sit facing forward, focused on the work surface, while the light shines down at your head from in front.

While side effects from light therapy are rare and relatively minor, they can occur. If you experience eyestrain, headache, queasiness, or agitation after beginning light therapy, reduce the light dose by sitting farther away from the light box, or shorten the duration of exposure.

SLEEP PROBLEMS

When do you prefer to go to sleep, and when do you like to wake up? Your answer indicates your chronotype, your individual inner clock. To determine your chronotype, take the chronotherapy quiz on the website of the Center for Environmental Therapeutics, the interdisciplinary research organization that I founded.

The quiz will tell you the amount

and timing of light therapy that will work best for you, but here are general recommendations.

You fall asleep too early. You find it hard to stay awake at night and typically wake up very early in the morning.

Prescription for light therapy: Use a bright-light therapy box for fifteen to thirty minutes about an hour before you typically get sleepy.

Other helpful strategies for staying awake and pushing your sleep cycle forward:

* **Make lunch your major meal of the day,** then eat only a light dinner.
* **Avoid napping,** especially in the afternoon and evening. Instead, distract yourself from your fatigue by moving around and doing stretches.
* **Turn up room lights** during the evening.

You fall asleep too late. You try to get to bed at a decent hour but can't fall asleep. Then you have trouble waking up for work or school.

Prescription for light therapy: Use a light box for fifteen to thirty minutes within ten minutes after your natural wake-up time. If this time is later than your work schedule allows, begin light therapy on a long weekend. Then begin shifting your wakeup time and light-therapy schedule earlier—in fifteen-minute increments—as soon as you feel comfortable waking up at the new time.

More strategies for shifting your inner clock earlier include:

- **Finish dinner at least three hours before bedtime.** Avoid alcohol after dinner.
- **Minimize napping,** especially in the second half of the day. Try to get outdoors, keep moving, and do some stretches instead.
- **Keep your bedroom dark until you wake up.** Early morning light seeping in through the windows actually can worsen a late-sleep pattern.

You sleep fitfully. You find it hard to stay asleep through the night, but you go back to sleep fairly quickly.

Prescription for light therapy: Take light therapy—or spend time in the sun—in the middle of the day. Enhancing midday light exposure often improves sleep quality at night.

Other strategies to help you sleep through the night include:

- **Do not drink alcohol after dinner.**
- **Keep your bedroom dark.**
- **Install amber-colored night-lights** in the bathroom and hallway so that if you tend to wake up at night to use the bathroom, you can use those instead of turning on bright lights, which can disrupt your sleep.

You are unable to fall back to sleep after waking in the middle of the night. There could be many causes for this type of sleep problem, such as anxiety, depression, and physical illness, so it is best to consult a doctor. However, using light therapy in the evening to push sleep onset later (see "fall asleep too early") may help some people sleep through the night.

ENERGY AND MOOD

You can use bright-light therapy at any time during the day to increase your energy and alertness. Some people can quickly recharge with a brief session of light therapy (as little as ten minutes) when they first feel an energy slump.

Caution: See a doctor if you are chronically lethargic. This can be a sign of depression, a medical sleep disorder (such as apnea), or other illness.

If you're feeling sad or mildly depressed, the light-therapy regimen is the same as the prescription for falling asleep too late.

Caution: It can be difficult for an individual to know the difference between mild depression and moderate or severe depression. If you are suffering from moderate or severe depression, a physician will need to monitor your progress with light therapy and consider other treatment options.

....

> Michael Terman, PhD, psychologist and director of the Center for Light Treatment and Biological Rhythms at Columbia University Medical Center, and professor of clinical psychology, Columbia University College of Physicians and Surgeons, both in New York City. He is founder and president of the Center for Environmental Therapeutics (CET), New York City, and director of clinical chronobiology at the New York State Psychiatric Institute. A leading authority on the circadian clock and the role that light plays in regulating it, Dr. Terman is author of *Chronotherapy: Resetting Your Inner Clock to Boost Mood, Alertness, and Quality Sleep*. Columbia-Chronotherapy.org.

....

For Better Sleep: Some Like It Chilly

Getting a good night's sleep is tough if your partner is a blanket hog or a relentless snorer. It's even harder when you can't find a happy compromise on the best bedroom temperature.

Temperature is one of the trickiest issues to resolve when it comes to sleep. Some people are polar bears—they get their best sleep when the bedroom is refrigerator-cold. Others are lizards—they're happiest when they can strip off their clothes and sleep in tropical warmth.

Problems arise when polar bears and lizards sleep in the same bed. No matter where you set the thermostat, it's likely that one of you won't be completely comfortable.

Sleep products, including temperature-regulating mattresses, that allow you to create the environment that's best for you and your partner. If you sleep alone, these products also may help by giving you the ability to control the temperature so that you can optimize the quality of your sleep.

COOLER USUALLY IS BETTER

Most people get their best sleep when the room temperature is in the 60 to 70°F range. Even though your body temperature is slightly lower at night than during the day, your bed is warmer than body temperature because it absorbs and traps your body heat.

The problem with heat: Studies have shown that people who sleep in a too-warm environment tend to have a longer sleep-onset latency (the time that it takes to fall asleep) and more arousals (awakenings) than those who are cooler.

For those who overheat, there's no easy solution. You can lower the thermostat, but your partner might suffer. You can sleep blanket-free, but the bed will still trap your body heat. You can take a cool shower before bed. Or if you like to take a warm bath to relax, your body temperature will cool once you're out of the tub. But for many people, these measures aren't real solutions to the problem.

Not just a gender issue: Many men and hot-flash-prone menopausal women are known for being "hot sleepers," but people who are overweight and those with fast metabolisms also tend to overheat, and it's often an undetected cause of poor sleep in these individuals.

FINDING YOUR PERSONAL CLIMATE ZONE

Manufacturers have introduced mattresses and other sleep products that are designed to keep the bed a few degrees—or, in some cases, many degrees—cooler than room temperature. If you and your partner cannot agree on the ideal temperature, you might want to look at products that control each side of the bed separately.

Important: Some temperature-controlled sleep products are quite expensive, and there's no conclusive scientific evidence that they'll improve the quality of your sleep. But they may be a good choice for people who can't cool or heat the room as much as they would like, especially if they are about to buy a new mattress.

Remember: Most mattresses should be replaced about every seven years or if

they begin to show signs of wear (sags or lumps) and/or you regularly awaken with stiffness and aches.

› Joseph M. Ojile, MD, clinical professor of medicine at St. Louis University School of Medicine. Dr. Ojile is also founder and CEO of Clayton Sleep Institute and president of the Clayton Sleep Research Foundation, www.ClaytonSleep.com, in St. Louis. Dr. Ojile serves on the board of directors of the National Sleep Foundation.

15

Urinary System

Keep Your Bladder Healthy

If you're age fifty or older and haven't had a bladder infection, count yourself lucky. The reality is that these infections are among the most common complaints of the AARP crowd.

Here's why: With age, women—and men—are at increased risk because tissues in the bladder weaken, making it more difficult for it to fully empty, so bacteria have more time to proliferate and cause a urinary tract infection (UTI). As we age, our immune systems also don't work as well.

Interestingly, the symptoms of bladder infection become less apparent with age. Instead of the burning, cramping pain and bloody urine that generally accompany a UTI in younger people, only a modest increase in urinary frequency and a dark urine color may indicate a bladder infection once you're middle-aged or older. After about age seventy, confusion, agitation, balance problems, and falling may be a physician's only clues of a bladder infection.

Fortunately, there are some highly effective natural approaches to help prevent UTIs.

Stay hydrated. You must drink a minimum of two quarts of plain water daily—no matter what other beverages you consume. If you take a prescription medication, you may need even more water. Diuretics and some other drugs will make you lose water, so you'll need to drink more than usual. Discuss this with your pharmacist.

Use good hygiene. OK, you might find this is a little embarrassing, but make sure that you wipe from front to back after a bowel movement, wash your genitals before and after sex, and change your undergarments regularly, particularly if you have incontinence or are sedentary (small amounts of stool on a person's underwear can increase infection risk).

Load up on cranberry. Everyone knows that cranberry is supposed to be good for the bladder, but recent research made some people doubt its effectiveness. One study found that cranberry may not be very effective at preventing UTIs. But don't write off cranberry. The same research showed that compounds in cranberry do prevent infections by making it difficult for bacteria to stick to the walls of the bladder. Because most brands of cranberry juice (perhaps the most convenient form of the fruit) have added sugar to make them less tart, I usually advise people who develop more than one bladder infection a year to take 600 mg of a freeze-dried cranberry extract daily.

Caution: People with a history of calcium oxalate kidney stones or who take warfarin or regularly use aspirin should avoid cranberry. It can increase stone risk and interact with these medications.

Get more probiotics. The beneficial bacteria found in yogurt and other cultured foods, such as kefir and miso, reduce risk for bladder infection. Eat one cup of plain yogurt, kefir, or miso soup daily or take a probiotic supplement.

Do Kegel exercises. Women—and men—listen up! Strong pelvic muscles

allow for more complete bladder emptying and reduce infection risk.

What to do: At least once daily, contract and release the muscles of your pelvic floor (the ones that stop urine flow) ten times while seated or standing.

....

› Jamison Starbuck, ND, naturopathic physician in family practice and a guest lecturer at the University of Montana, both in Missoula. She is past president of the American Association of Naturopathic Physicians. Starbuck is a columnist for the *Bottom Line Health Insider* and hosts *Dr. Starbuck's Health Tips for Kids* on Montana Public Radio. DrJamisonStarbuck.com.

....

Urinary Stress Incontinence: Causes and Treatments

I *laughed so hard, tears ran* down my legs."

When you can't hold back the tears—OK, what I really mean is *urine*—while coughing, exercising, sneezing, laughing, or lifting something heavy, it is called "urinary stress incontinence" and is a common phenomenon in postmenopausal women. The result is either a small little tinkle of urine or a complete flood and loss of control.

Remember, first things first! We need

to identify and treat the cause. This calamitous experience happens for a variety of reasons, and simply being aware of them can help you manage and "keep it inside."

After menopause, your estrogen levels are lower, and this can contribute to not only your pelvic muscles weakening, but the urethral tissue becoming thinner, less resilient, and less elastic, leading to reduced control over urination.

Other contributing factors to be aware of are certain medications such as diuretics or steroids, which can have urinary incontinence as a side effect. With my patients, I always go through the side effects listed of any medications that they are on. You would be surprised how many clinical complaints are actually due to them.

Chronic constipation can also weaken the pelvic floor muscles, making it harder to hold urine. Being overweight can put extra pressure on your bladder as well, worsening the situation.

Believe it or not, food sensitivities can also exacerbate the issue, causing irritation and inflammation to the bladder.

Here are some tips and tricks:

+ **Review and increase awareness of the side effects** of any medications you are taking.
+ **Rule out food sensitivities.** I often recommend the "Eat Right for Your Type" blood-type diet for a period of four weeks to effectively help rule out foods that might have become irritants. It is an inexpensive and effective modality.
+ **Reach and maintain an ideal weight** to reduce pressure on the bladder wall.
+ **Correct constipation.** Increase fiber, and by all means, stay hydrated, drinking at least half your body weight in ounces a day, and reduce caffeine and alcohol.
+ **Strengthen your pelvic floor muscles by using Kegel exercises.** Regular exercise can strengthen and build endurance in the group of muscles that control the opening and closing of your urethral sphincter (where the pee comes out). Kegel exercises are the standard and most effective treatment for incontinence caused by poor muscle tone, but *you have to do them!* The first step is to properly identify the correct muscle group. As you begin urinating, try to stop the flow of urine without tensing the muscles of your legs. It is very important not to use these other muscles, because only the pelvic floor muscles help with bladder control. When you are able stop the stream of urine, you have located the correct muscles. Feel the sensation of the muscles pulling inward and upward.

It feels like squeezing your buttocks so as to not pass gas. Consistency is the key when doing these exercises, so plan on ten minutes, two times each day. Morning and evening are good times for most people, but the important thing is to choose times that are convenient for you so you can develop a routine. No one will know what you are doing, so you can do these anywhere! Begin with tightening and relaxing the sphincter muscle as rapidly as you can for one minute. Take about a minute rest, and then contract the sphincter more slowly, holding for a count of three, gradually working to increase the count to ten. Then go back to the rapid contractions for a minute. Make sure to relax completely between contractions. If you stay consistent, you will start to see marked improvement within three to six weeks.

+ **Vaginal estrogen therapy** might be helpful, so see a qualified menopause practitioner, such as a licensed naturopathic doctor to assist in treatment options.

These simple and noninvasive interventions can not only lead you once more to crying tears of joy but can contribute to your overall well-being!

› Holly Lucille, ND, RN, naturopathic doctor whose private practice, Healing from Within Healthcare, is in West Hollywood, California. She is chair of the Natural Partners INC educational advisory board, vice chair of the Institute for Natural Medicine, and author of *Creating and Maintaining Balance: A Woman's Guide to Safe, Natural Hormone Health.* DrHollyLucille.com.

Don't Let Your Overactive Bladder Run Your Life!

People who scout out restrooms wherever they are may think that others don't have to worry so much about their bladders.

But that's not true.

Eye-opening statistic: One in every five adults over age forty has overactive bladder, and after the age of sixty-five, a whopping one in every three adults is affected. If you regularly have a strong and sudden urge to urinate and/or need to hit the john eight or more times a day (or more than once at night), chances are you have the condition too.

Postmenopausal women (due to their low estrogen levels) are at increased risk of having overactive bladder. Urinary tract infections, use of certain medications (such as antidepressants and drugs to treat high blood pressure and insomnia), and even constipation also can cause or worsen the condition.

But there is a bright side. Research is now uncovering several surprisingly simple natural approaches that are highly effective for many people with overactive bladder.

Most people don't connect a bladder problem to their diets. But there is a strong link. Here are some things to keep in mind.

Take a hard line with irritants. Alcohol, caffeine, and artificial sweeteners can exacerbate the feeling of urgency caused by overactive bladder. Cutting back on these items is a good first step, but they often creep back into one's diet over time.

What helps: Keep it simple. Completely avoid alcohol, caffeine (all forms, including coffee, tea, and caffeine-containing foods such as chocolate), and artificial sweeteners. Stick to decaffeinated coffee and herbal teas, and use agave and stevia as sweeteners.

Many individuals also are sensitive to certain foods, such as corn, wheat, dairy, eggs, and peanuts. They often trigger an immune reaction that contributes to overall inflammation in the body, including in the bladder. If your symptoms of urinary urgency and/or frequency increase after eating one of these (or any other) foods, your body may be having an inflammatory response that is also affecting your bladder. Eliminate these foods from your diet.

Keep your gut healthy. The scientific evidence is still in the early stages, but research now suggests that leaky gut syndrome, in which excess bacterial or fungal growth harms the mucosal membrane in the intestines, is at the root of several health problems, including overactive bladder.

The theory is that an imbalance of microbes, a condition known as dysbiosis, can irritate the walls of the bladder just as it does in the gut.

What helps: Probiotics and oregano oil capsules. Probiotics replenish good bacteria, and oregano oil has antibacterial properties that help cleanse bad bacteria and fungi from the gut.

Drink up! People with overactive bladder often cut way back on their fluid intake because they already make so many trips to the bathroom. But when you don't drink enough fluids, urine tends to have an irritating effect, because it becomes more concentrated. This increases urgency.

What helps: Drink half your body weight in ounces of water or herbal tea daily. Do not drink any fluids after 5:00 p.m. to help prevent bathroom runs during the night.

THE RIGHT SUPPLEMENTS

Cranberry supplements (*or unsweetened cranberry* juice) can be helpful for bladder infections, but they're usually not the best choice for overactive bladder. Here are some better options.

Try pumpkin seed extract. These capsules help tone and strengthen the tissue of your pelvic-floor muscles, which gives you better bladder control.

Typical dosage: 500 mg daily.

Consider *Angelica archangelica* **extract.** This herb has gotten positive reviews from researchers who have investigated it as a therapy for overactive bladder.

Research finding: When forty-three men with overactive bladder took 300 mg of the herb daily, they had increased bladder capacity and made fewer trips to the bathroom.

Typical dosage: 100 mg daily.

OTHER WAYS TO CURB AN OVERACTIVE BLADDER

Kegel exercises, *which help strengthen* the pelvic-floor muscles, are essential for getting control of overactive bladder symptoms. Unfortunately, most people who try doing Kegels end up doing them the wrong way.

How to do Kegels: Three to five times a day, contract your pelvic-floor muscles (the ones you use to stop and start the flow of urine), hold for a count of ten, then relax completely for a count of ten. Repeat ten times.

If you aren't sure you are contracting the right muscles, there is a possible solution. A medical device called Apex acts as an automatic Kegel exerciser. It is inserted into the vagina and electrically stimulates the correct muscles ($249 at www.pourmoi.com—cost may be covered by some insurance plans). Check with your doctor to see if this would be an appropriate aid for you.

Kegels can easily be part of anyone's daily routine—do them while waiting at a red light, after going to the bathroom, or while watching TV.

Try acupuncture. An increasing body of evidence shows that this therapy helps relieve overactive bladder symptoms. For example, in a study of seventy-four women with the condition, bladder capacity, urgency, and frequency of urination significantly improved after four weekly bladder-specific acupuncture sessions.

Go for biofeedback. Small electrodes are used to monitor the muscles involved in bladder control so that an individualized exercise program can be created. Biofeedback is noninvasive and is most effective when used along with other treatments. To find a board-certified provider, consult the Biofeedback Certification International Alliance, www.BCIA.org.

....

› Holly Lucille, ND, RN, naturopathic doctor whose private practice, Healing from Within Healthcare, is in West Hollywood, California. She is chair of the Natural Partners INC educational advisory board, vice chair of the Institute for Natural Medicine, and author of *Creating and Maintaining Balance: A Woman's Guide to Safe, Natural Hormone Health.* DrHollyLucille.com.

....

You Can Restore Your Pelvic Floor

If you're a woman who pees when you laugh or cough or sometimes feels overcome with a sudden nearly uncontrollable urge to pee—that is, if you have urinary incontinence—you've undoubtedly heard of Kegel exercises and maybe even tried them. The simple do-anywhere pelvic exercises often are recommended for this condition and a wide variety of other pelvic problems including fecal (bowel) incontinence, chronic pain, and pelvic organ prolapse, in which the bladder or uterus can bulge into the vagina.

But doing Kegels may be exactly the wrong thing for you. They actually could be making your problem *worse*. It's not that you're doing them wrong, although

many people do. In fact, it's *especially* an issue if you do Kegels right.

If you suffer from incontinence and have performed hundreds of Kegels with no improvement, or if you have chronic pelvic pain but think it can't be fixed, you are not alone—and there *is* help. Eventually, Kegels can be part of the solution, but there are steps you need to take *first*.

A PELVIC FLOOR PRIMER—THE MENOPAUSE CONNECTION

The pelvic floor is a network of muscles, ligaments, and tissue that acts like a sling to support a woman's pelvic organs—the uterus, vagina, bladder/urethra, and rectum. You control your bowel and bladder by contracting and relaxing these muscles and tissues. Twenty-seven percent of women ages forty to fifty-nine will experience pelvic floor dysfunction (PFD) in their lifetime.

There's a strong menopause link: The estrogen drop that typically begins some time in your forties during perimenopause and is typically complete when you enter menopause (usually by your early fifties) can cause the pelvic floor to thin out, making prolapse more likely. Plus age, obesity, repeated heavy lifting, traumatic injury—such as may happen during childbirth or from a hip or back injury—can cause pelvic muscles and connective tissues to become sensitive, strained, and weak. Over time, the likelihood of a pelvic floor disorder increases.

WHAT MOST WOMEN GET WRONG ABOUT KEGELS

Women with PFD often think their internal muscles are too weak and do Kegels in an effort to strengthen them. While that often is true, it's not the biggest problem. For 99 percent of my patients, the real problem is muscles that are *too tight.*

These too-tight muscles often get stuck in a contracted position, unable to control the flow of urine or to fully relax and contract in a pleasurable way during intercourse. For these women, Kegels can worsen the situation by strengthening already too-tight muscles. What they really need is to *relax* them.

The first step: Bring up your symptoms with your internist, ob-gyn, urogynecologist, or urologist. He/she can rule out any concerns that are not musculoskeletal, and if physical therapy is the next best course of treatment, he can refer you to a women's health physical therapist (WHPT). WHPTs partner with ob-gyns, urologists, and other specialists to diagnose and treat not just the pelvic floor but the body as a whole. Three to six months of weekly or biweekly manual therapy sessions,

combined with homework, can typically ease symptoms of urinary incontinence, painful intercourse, and/or pelvic pain.

A WHPT will perform an internal exam to assess your areas of strength and weakness and design a plan to retrain your muscles. You can find a WHPT with the locator on the website of the American Physical Therapy Association. Insurance typically covers these services.

Note: Some chiropractors, occupational therapists, and naturopaths may also perform similar treatments, but I am not familiar enough with their exact practices to recommend them. Midwives are typically not trained in these techniques.

TONING THE PELVIC FLOOR — THE RIGHT WAY

A crucial component of treatment with a WHPT is manual therapy. It may take some getting used to, but it's the gold standard of practice. In manual therapy, a WHPT uses her hands to gently massage, stretch, and release spasms and trigger points within the deep and soft tissues of the vagina. This helps reduce tightness and tension and can even break up scar tissue that's further restricting tissues, allowing the pelvic floor muscles to fully relax and contract. Though manual therapy can feel uncomfortable initially, any pain quickly recedes as the muscles and tissues relax.

Manual therapy is a prime opportunity to assess how you do Kegels. Many women do it so that it only strengthens, never relaxes. During such therapy, I will insert one finger into the vagina and then ask my patient to perform a Kegel by imagining she is stopping the flow of urine midstream. (Once a woman learns how to do this correctly, she can do it herself.) Two out of three women do this incorrectly, tightening their pelvic floor muscles *but not releasing them all the way back down*, or not tightening their pelvic floor at all, recruiting their abs or glutes instead. The goal is to teach them how to relax their muscles all the way down to starting position. Here are some ways to teach this technique.

Reverse Kegels. In a conventional Kegel, you tighten your pelvic floor muscles, hold the contraction for ten seconds, then fully relax back down, maintaining the relaxed position for ten seconds. (Sometimes I tell patients to imagine they are controlling an elevator with their vagina and send it to the top floor, hold it there, then send it down to the basement.) In a reverse Kegel, you begin "in the basement," so to speak, relaxing the muscles as you do when you've just sat down on the toilet with a full bladder and are able to urinate. You should feel your anus relax as well. After relaxing for ten seconds, send the elevator back up to the top and hold ten seconds, then release again.

This pain-free, nonsurgical technique allows patients to see their pelvic muscles at rest and while contracted and improves their ability to retrain the pelvic floor. A sensor or small weight is inserted into the vagina, while a nearby computer provides visual feedback. More than 75 percent of PFD patients who try biofeedback benefit from it.

Home biofeedback. The apps Elvie ($199, Apple/Android) and PeriCoach ($249, Apple/Android) use intravaginal devices to assess the strength and endurance of vaginal contractions and then send data to your smartphone via Bluetooth. I only recommend them for women who've had a professional pelvic floor assessment, because if you're not performing Kegels correctly, a product like this could contribute to further tightness/tension. But if you've learned to do Kegels so that you relax as well as strengthen, they can be helpful.

LIFESTYLE SOLUTIONS

Shallow chest breathing also can contribute to pelvic floor disorders. The diaphragm, a sheet of muscle that separates the chest cavity from the abdomen, gets stuck in a contracted position, causing pelvic muscles to contract too.

Solution: Learn diaphragmatic (belly) breathing. Lying down, pretend your belly is a balloon, and fill it with air, keeping your chest still (you may need to start with shallow breaths). Now exhale, deflating the balloon. Try this once an hour for five breaths and again for five minutes before bed. In two to three weeks, you should notice a change in the way you breathe.

In general, chronic stress can make urinary incontinence worse, so mind-body relaxation methods, such as meditation and yoga, also help.

One final tip: Sit-ups can put even asymptomatic women at risk of developing incontinence, prolapse, or other PFD issues.

A better way to strengthen your abs: Plank.

....

› Lesli Lo, DPT, women's health physical therapist, Northwestern Medical Group, and instructor of obstetrics and gynecology at Northwestern University Feinberg School of Medicine, both in Chicago.

....

Do You Pee in Your Pants after You Pee? There's a Cure for That

Have you heard of *postmicturition dribble (PMD)?* The term might not be familiar, but the sight of it probably is—a wet spot smack on the front of a man's pants. It happens when the last few drops of urine leak out after a gent thinks he's done using the bathroom. It can happen to women too.

But you can fix it.

The first thing to know is that postmicturition dribble—which we will refer to as urinary dribble here—is not a sign of a dangerous health problem. It sure is annoying and embarrassing, though, a major cause of stress, not at all surprisingly.

How many people have urinary dribble is not exactly clear, but it's not rare. A Finnish study, for example, asked people about it and found that 6 percent of adults between the ages of eighteen and seventy-nine have it—more men than women. In an American study, 11.8 percent of men and 8.5 percent of women between the ages of thirty and seventy-nine said they have it.

But those percentages are probably low, because urinary dribble is the sort of problem that many people, especially men, are too embarrassed to admit having.

PMD is not caused by poor hygiene or problems with the bladder or, for men, the prostate. It differs from stress incontinence (involuntary urination caused by weakness of the pelvic floor muscles) or urge incontinence (urination caused by involuntary contraction of the bladder muscles). Although weakened muscle tone does cause urinary dribble in men—and we'll explore the solution for that below—in women, it is not muscle weakness but rather anatomical glitches that are generally responsible for urinary dribble.

WHY WOMEN DRIBBLE AFTER THEY PEE

Urinary dribble is occasionally found in women who have anatomic abnormalities that prevent complete emptying of the bladder. Abnormalities include:

+ **A tiny pouch, called a diverticulum, on the wall of the urethra** (the tube that carries urine out of the body). Urine can become temporarily trapped in this pouch, only to trickle out later. Most women adapt to having a diverticulum and wear a pad to catch moisture. Another option is to have the diverticulum surgically removed.

+ **An abnormal opening between either the vagina and bladder or vagina and ureter** (a tube that connects the kidney to the bladder) through which urine can leak. This kind of abnormality is corrected by surgically sealing off the opening.

WHY MEN DRIBBLE

For men, gravity and muscle weakness are responsible for urinary dribble. The male urethra doesn't run in a straight downhill line. It has a little dip in the middle of it, creating a pool where urine can collect. Normally, a muscle called the bulbocavernosus that fits around the urethra will automatically squeeze to force the urine out, but this muscle can lose its tone, especially in men older than fifty. Instead, movement and gravity will cause the last few drops of urine that pool up in the dip of the urethra to involuntarily spill out of the body at an unpredictable time, leading to those embarrassing wet spots.

STRENGTH TRAINING FOR MEN WITH URINARY DRIBBLE

The problem is correctable. Like any other muscle, the bulbocavernosus will be strengthened only by working it out. The muscle is part of the pelvic floor, the area between the scrotum and the anus. To work the pelvic floor muscles, sit or lie down. Then tighten your muscles as if you were trying to hold in your urine (and trying not to pass gas). Don't hold your breath or squeeze muscles in your abdomen or buttocks, as some men tend to do, because the extra effort will make focus on the pelvic floor muscles more challenging.

Hold those muscles tight for ten

seconds and then relax for ten seconds. Repeat this exercise six to ten times for one set, and complete two or three sets each day. You may have guessed it—this is the male version of the Kegel exercise, an exercise that many women do to strengthen their pelvic floors.

A biofeedback session or two for a man will most effectively help him learn how to work his pelvic floor muscles. Here's how it works. Band-Aid-like stick-on sensors are placed around the pelvic area, and a small rectal sensor is inserted a little way into the anus. Sensors are also placed on the abdomen. How does all that go over with patients—especially the rectal sensor? The sensors are small and do not cause discomfort. All together, they help the biofeedback therapist see which pelvic muscles are being used. The therapist can then guide the patient to contract only the muscles that need strengthening to prevent urinary dribble.

Urinary dribble is usually cured within three months in about 60 percent of male patients. The remaining 40 percent achieve partial cure and adapt to living with some dribble, although a few may need surgery to correct the problem. The key to cure is to be very regular and disciplined about doing the exercises.

And as a big bonus, exercising the bulbocavernosus muscle can help sexual performance, because that same muscle also helps create and maintain erections. You get a two-for-one!

> Geo Espinosa, ND, LAc, CNS, naturopathic physician, director of integrative urology, New York University Langone Medical Center, New York City.

Kegel Exercises for Men

Just about every woman who has experienced childbirth or gone through menopause has heard of Kegels. These simple exercises are widely used to treat and prevent urinary leaks.

What you may not realize: Kegels, named after the American gynecologist Arnold Henry Kegel, are also useful for men, not just for reducing urinary and bowel incontinence, but also for easing prostate discomfort and relieving premature ejaculation.

Bonus: Many men report that these exercises enhance sexual pleasure as well.

You don't have to set aside a specific time to do these exercises. Because no one can see what you're doing, you can exercise the muscles almost any time—when you're standing in line, driving your car, or watching TV.

But even people who have heard of Kegels—or perhaps tried them—may not be getting all the possible benefits if they're making some common mistakes while performing the exercises.

WHAT GOES WRONG

The goal of Kegel exercises is to strengthen the pelvic floor, a group of muscles that control urination and defecation and help support pelvic organs, such as the bladder.

In men, urinary incontinence is usually due to prostate enlargement or prostate surgery. Prostate enlargement causes the bladder muscle to become overactive, resulting in urinary incontinence. Prostate surgery can damage the sphincter or nerves that control the sphincter.

HOW TO DO KEGELS PROPERLY

Kegels are simple—they involve contracting and relaxing your pelvic-floor muscles. Yet many make these mistakes when performing the exercises.

Mistake #1: **Not identifying the pelvic-floor muscles.** Some people simply can't feel these muscles. When contracting them, there should be no movement of the abdominal muscles and minimal movement of the buttocks. Men can see a shortening of the base of the penis.

Solution: The next time you urinate, try to stop the flow in midstream. If you can do this, you're contracting all the right muscles. You can also tighten the muscles

that prevent you from passing intestinal gas. (Once the proper muscles have been located, do *not* do Kegels while urinating or defecating.)

If you still can't locate the muscles: A man can place a finger in his anus and tighten the muscles to squeeze his finger. If he is tightening the correct muscles, he will feel a contraction on his finger.

A physical therapist trained in pelvic-floor rehabilitation can also teach you where the muscles are. He/she may use biofeedback, which involves placing electrodes on the abdomen or in the vagina or anus. A machine can then monitor the contraction/relaxation of the appropriate muscles and alert patients when they're doing it right. This procedure is painless.

Mistake #2: **Stopping too soon.** It's common to do a few Kegels then stop.

Solution: Make sure you know how to correctly count your repetitions. To begin, squeeze the muscles as hard as you can for three to five seconds. Then relax for five seconds. This is one Kegel. Start with five or ten repetitions. As your muscles get stronger, you'll easily be able to do twenty in a row and hold each Kegel for about ten seconds.

Mistake #3: **Not doing the exercises often enough.** Until you've incorporated Kegels into your daily schedule, it's easy to try the exercises a few times, then forget about them for several days.

Solution: As with any exercise, Kegels are more effective when you do them regularly. To get the most benefit, do ten or twenty Kegels, relax for a minute, then do ten or twenty more. Repeat this three times daily. Be patient. It may take six to twelve weeks to see any benefits, but many people report beneficial effects earlier.

For improved sexual function: Men who experience premature ejaculation can learn to delay their orgasms by squeezing the muscles, hard, during masturbation or intercourse.

Important: Avoid devices sold online that claim to strengthen pelvic-floor muscles. They aren't necessary and often don't work.

....

› Jonathan M. Vapnek, MD, urologist and associate clinical professor of urology, Mount Sinai School of Medicine, New York City. A member of the American Urological Association, he's been named by *New York Magazine* as one of New York City's best urologists.

....

Solution to Nocturia— Get Moving

Are you a man who has a buddy who is sleep-deprived, not because he's living the high life but because he admits to visiting the john to pee several times a night? Or does that describe *you*?

Having to urinate repeatedly during the night is called nocturia, and it's a common symptom of benign prostatic hyperplasia (BPH), the medical term for enlarged prostate. It starts showing up in middle age, and by the time a man hits eighty, the likelihood that he has nocturia is more than 90 percent. But even if you can't avoid BPH, you can avoid nocturia if you get serious about one thing, says a study that analyzed data from a huge, ongoing program called the Prostate, Lung, Colorectal, and Ovarian Cancer Screening Trial (PLCO, for short).

It's exercise. Although being physically active does not necessarily prevent BPH, studies show that exercise can delay its development and help keep symptoms— especially nocturia—to a minimum if BPH does set in.

The study looked at 28,404 men who had long-term BPH and 4,710 participants with newly diagnosed BPH. The men ranged in age from fifty-five to seventy-four at the start of the study. All kinds of information related to prostate health, outcomes related to BPH (whether a man had surgery for it, for example), exercise habits, and other lifestyle habits were analyzed to better understand the role of exercise in preventing nocturia and other symptoms of BPH. Exercise included activities such as walking, jogging, and bike riding.

A TRUE BATTLE OF THE BULGE

The study findings were an eye-opener about BPH, exercise habits, and nocturia. Although exercise had little impact on other symptoms and issues related to BPH, it did make a difference in whether nocturia developed and the degree of severity if it did. For example, men who had long-time BPH and nocturia but got at least one hour of exercise per week were 35 percent less likely, on average, to need to urinate more than twice per night (severe nocturia) than men who got less than one hour of exercise per week.

Among those in whom BPH developed during the study, those who exercised at least one hour per week were an average 13 percent less likely to report nocturia than were inactive men, and that rate didn't much differ whether men got in one hour or more than four. And among those men who did have nocturia, those who exercised at least one hour per week were an average 34 percent less likely to need to make a bathroom run more than twice per night compared with men who were inactive—in other words, their nocturia was far less disruptive to their sleep. In this case, men who got more rather than less exercise were better off. For example, compared with men who didn't exercise, men who got one hour of exercise were 25 percent less likely to need more than two bathroom runs, whereas men who got three hours of exercise were 43 percent less likely.

Researchers recorded exercise levels going back to when each participant was forty years old. Men who had stayed physically active at least since their forties were (no surprise) better protected against nocturia than men who only recently started exercising or never exercised. But don't think that it's ever too late to get some control over nocturia. Men who were currently exercising—even if they hadn't in the past—were better protected than men who were once physically active but stopped.

HOW IT WORKS

Physical activity gives you a triple whammy of goodness—it promotes weight loss in those who are too heavy, works off stress, and reduces inflammation, which all have an impact on nocturia, according to the researchers. They also noted that exercise probably has a stronger effect on nocturia and even BPH than what was seen in their study, because it is likely that many of the participants exaggerated when reporting the amount of exercise they actually got. Studies show that most American men are sedentary, and this fact should have been more strongly represented in the study population, considering that the large majority of participants were overweight. Still, the take-home message is, if you are more active by day—if you make a habit of brisk walks or jogs, bicycling, or gym workouts—you can help your bladder be less active at night when you want to sleep. It's easy and powerful.

›   Study titled "Physical Activity and Benign Hyperplasia-Related Outcomes and Nocturia," published in *Medicine & Science in Sports & Exercise.*

The Right Selenium Supplement for Prostate Health

I f you are a health news junkie, you've probably found yourself frustrated by what seems like completely contradictory information. For example, one day, a perfectly sound study will show that a certain supplement does something great, and the next day, another study will show that it's no better than a sugar pill. Results that don't agree make it hard to know what to believe. But we can find the truth if we really know how to look. And that's the case right now with the mineral selenium. If you are interested in preventing cancer—particularly prostate cancer—you'll want to see exactly how some conflicting studies about selenium supplements can be unraveled to get to the truth.

THE *RIGHT* RIGHT STUFF

Selenium has strong antioxidant properties, and many studies have shown that cancer is less likely to develop in people who have more selenium in their diets. But there has been a lot of controversy about how effective it is in preventing prostate cancer. One large study showed selenium supplementation cut risk of prostate cancer by up to two-thirds, while another large study showed that it was no better than a placebo.

Where does the truth lie? In the not-so-fine print, actually, because some recent research has brought to light what may be obvious but easily missed. It turns out that the particular *type* of selenium supplement used may make it a hit or miss when it comes to protection against prostate cancer.

The study that showed a drastic reduction in prostate cancer used a supplement made of selenium yeast, which is yeast that has been enriched with selenium. The study that showed no effect used a supplement made of selenomethionine, which is the amino acid that contains selenium. To find out why one type of a selenium supplement was effective and another not in terms of prostate cancer protection, a research team recruited sixty-nine healthy men between the ages of twenty-three and seventy-eight to participate in a year-long study. The men were divided into four groups. One group received a placebo, one group received the maximum daily recommended dosage of selenium (200 micrograms per day) in the form of selenomethionine, another group received the maximum daily dosage in the form of selenium yeast, and, because higher doses of selenium yeast are currently being studied as therapy for prostate cancer, the last group received a higher dosage (285 micrograms per day) of selenium yeast.

Before starting the study and at three, nine, and twelve months, all the men had blood and urine tests to evaluate levels of selenium and prostate-specific antigen (PSA, a marker for prostate cancer) as well as signs of oxidative stress related to prostate cancer development.

The results: Although blood levels of selenium increased in all the men taking any form or dose of selenium, they substantially increased in the men taking selenomethionine (by 93 percent) and high-dose selenium yeast (86 percent).

You would think that the higher the blood level, the higher the prostate cancer protection, but the study findings hinted that this may not be the case. The only form of selenium that had an impact on oxidative stress in this particular study was high-dose selenium yeast. The researchers theorized that, although selenomethionine may be able to get more selenium into the blood than selenium yeast, it may be missing the compounds that reduce oxidative stress in the prostate gland or allow sufficient absorption of selenium into prostate gland tissue.

Selenium is naturally found in seafood, meats, grains, and eggs. Adults should get at least 55 micrograms per day, according to the National Institutes of Health. Most people in the United States who maintain well-balanced diets get enough selenium, although studies show that selenium levels are commonly low in men with prostate cancer. But if you are a man concerned about prostate health, get your selenium level checked first to find out whether taking a selenium yeast supplement is right for you. Getting too much selenium, such as from going overboard with supplement use, can cause gastrointestinal, cardiovascular, and kidney problems.

....

› Study titled "Comparative Effects of Two Different Forms of Selenium on Oxidative Stress Biomarkers in Healthy Men: A Randomized Clinical Trial," published in *Cancer Prevention Research.*

....

Foods and Supplements That Relieve Prostate Pain

When it comes to men's health, we hear a lot about enlarged prostate and prostate cancer. But there is another prostate ailment that gets much less attention yet affects many men. Prostatitis, a very painful condition, is inflammation of the prostate gland. It can be difficult to diagnose because its symptoms (persistent pain in the pelvis or rectum; discomfort in the abdomen, lower back, penis, or testicles; difficult, painful, or frequent urination or painful ejaculation) are similar to those of other conditions such as an enlarged prostate or a urinary tract infection.

It is estimated that almost half of all men will be affected by prostatitis at some point in their lives. If the condition lasts for three months or longer, it's considered to be chronic prostatitis.

Mainstream medicine often is unsuccessful in treating chronic prostatitis, leaving men in pain and without hope of feeling better. In my practice, I have had lots of success treating chronic prostatitis as both an inflammatory condition (which it always is) and as a possible fungal infection.

REASONS BEHIND PROSTATITIS

For a long time, it was thought that prostatitis could be caused only by bacterial infection. That view was dispelled when several studies found that the bacteria in the prostates of both healthy men and men with prostatitis were essentially identical. It's now understood that most prostatitis cases are not caused by bacteria. Still, most mainstream physicians routinely prescribe antibiotics for it, a treatment that is appropriate only if your case is one of a very small number actually caused by bacteria.

Although prostate inflammation is not well understood, the inflammation could be the result of inadequate fluid drainage into the prostatic ducts, an abnormal immune response, or a fungal infection.

PROSTATITIS TREATMENT PLAN

If you experience any of the symptoms of prostatitis mentioned earlier, see your doctor. Your visit should include a rectal exam to check for swelling or tenderness in the prostate and a laboratory test of prostatic fluid to check for bacterial infection. (Fluid is released during prostate gland massage.) I also recommend that you have your doctor order a urine culture to test for fungal infection (most medical doctors don't test for this).

In a small number of cases, the lab

test does reveal a bacterial infection, and an antibiotic is appropriately prescribed. But if there is no bacterial infection, then I recommend that men with this condition follow an anti-inflammatory, antifungal treatment plan for two months. If symptoms subside but don't disappear, continue for another two months. Even if you don't have a test for fungal infection, I often advise following the antifungal portion of the program (along with the inflammation portion) to see if it helps to relieve symptoms.

FOODS THAT BATTLE PROSTATITIS

Anti-inflammatory diet. *If you are thinking, Why is Dr. Stengler telling me again about an anti-inflammatory diet?* I'm telling you because it works. Eating a diet of whole foods and cutting out packaged and processed foods go a long way to reducing inflammation in general and prostate inflammation in particular.

Eat: A variety of plant products to maximize your intake of antioxidants, which are natural anti-inflammatories; cold-water fish such as salmon, trout, and sardines, which are high in omega-3 fatty acids; and pumpkin seeds, which are high in zinc, a mineral that helps reduce prostate swelling.

Don't eat: Foods that are high in saturated fat, such as red meat and dairy, which can make inflammation worse. Avoid alcohol, caffeine, refined sugar, and trans fats, all of which tend to contribute to inflammation.

Antifungal diet. If you already are following the anti-inflammatory diet described earlier, then you have eliminated refined sugar from your diet. (Fungi thrive on sugar!) Also try eliminating all grains (including whole grains and rice) from your diet. Fungi thrive on these foods.

PROSTATE-PROTECTIVE SUPPLEMENTS

The following supplements have targeted benefits for prostate inflammation. They are safe to take together, and there are no side effects. Many men feel much better within two weeks of taking these supplements.

Rye pollen extract. Studies show that rye pollen extract can relieve the pain of chronic prostatitis. In one study published in the *British Journal of Urology*, men with chronic prostatitis took three tablets of rye pollen extract daily. After six months, 36 percent had no more symptoms, and 42 percent reported symptom improvement. Follow label instructions. The pollen component in rye pollen does not contain gluten, but if you have celiac disease or a severe allergy to gluten, look for a certified gluten-free product.

Quercetin. This powerful flavonoid helps reduce prostate inflammation.

Dose: 1,000 mg twice daily.

Fish oil. In addition to eating anti-inflammatory foods, these supplements are a rich source of inflammation-fighting omega-3 fatty acids.

Dose: 2,000 mg daily of combined EPA and DHA.

ANTIFUNGAL SUPPLEMENTS

Many patients benefit from taking one or more antifungal remedies. Several herbs—such as oregano, pau d'arco, garlic, and grapefruit seed extract—have potent antifungal properties. They are available in capsule and liquid form. For doses, follow label instructions. Most patients feel better within two to four weeks of taking antifungal supplements.

....

› Mark A. Stengler, NMD, naturopathic doctor and founder of the Stengler Center for Integrative Medicine in Encinitas, California. He is author and coauthor of numerous books, including *The Natural Physician's Healing Therapies* and *Bottom Line's Prescription for Natural Cures*, and is the author of the newsletter *Health Revelations*. MarkStengler.com.

....

Surprising Ways to Avoid Kidney Stones

Plenty of people who develop kidney stones are shocked when this common condition occurs. How do these extremely painful stones take hold, and what can be done to prevent them?

Before you tell yourself that kidney stones are something that you'd never suffer, consider this—one of every ten people is destined to develop at least one of these excruciating stones in his/her life. Each year, more than one million people see their doctors because of kidney stones. Already had a kidney stone? You're not off the hook—about half of kidney stone sufferers will develop another stone in five to seven years. Read on for how to stay in the stone-free zone.

HOW STONES FORM

Kidney stones can usually be prevented by making the right changes to your diet and lifestyle. The problem is that many of the prevention strategies are counter-intuitive and involve some surprising approaches, such as cutting back on foods that are widely considered to be healthful.

The majority of kidney stones are made of calcium and oxalate. During normal digestion, oxalate (found in many healthful foods, such as spinach and beets) combines with calcium (another generally healthful nutrient) and makes its way through the digestive system before being excreted.

If there is excess oxalate, however, it gets absorbed into the bloodstream and carried to the kidneys, where urine is produced. Most of the time, oxalate is removed in the urine, but if the urine becomes saturated with oxalate, stones can develop. Here are some surprising ways to stop stones from forming.

Add just two daily servings of fruit and vegetables to your diet. When researchers at the University of Washington analyzed the diets of more than eighty thousand postmenopausal women, they found that women who consumed the most fiber, fruits, and vegetables had a 6 to 26 percent lower risk of developing kidney stones than women who ate the least.

Just two additional servings a day were enough to make a big difference.

Simple way to get two more fruit/ veggie servings daily: Have an extra apple and a handful of carrot sticks.

Consume calcium. You might be wondering why foods that contain calcium—a main constituent of kidney stones—would help *reduce* your risk of developing the stones. Calcium gives the oxalate something to latch on to in the stomach. Otherwise, the oxalate ends up in the urine, where stones are more likely to form.

Good sources of calcium: Yogurt, kale, bok choy, and calcium-fortified foods.

Exception: People who use calcium supplements may face a higher risk for kidney stones. If you use calcium supplements, take them with meals. That way, the calcium can bind with any oxalate that may be in the food.

Go easy on oxalates. Eating oxalate-rich foods in moderation usually doesn't promote kidney stones. But if you start getting large amounts of these foods—for example, by regularly using lots of spinach or beets in homemade juices—you might have a problem.

If you have had kidney stones or your doctor believes that you may be at increased risk for them due to such factors as a strong family history of the condition, talk to your doctor about limiting your intake of oxalate-rich foods such as spinach, Swiss chard, rhubarb, beets, all nuts (including almond milk), chocolate (especially dark), and soy/tofu products.

Eat less fish and other animal protein. Wait a minute—isn't fish good for you? Fatty, omega-3-rich fish usually is healthful, but people at increased risk for kidney stones (including anyone with a history of stones) should limit their intake of fish and any type of meat to six ounces a day.

Here's why: Protein is made up of amino acids and gets broken down into uric acid. Eating lots of animal protein acidifies the urine and can increase uric acid levels in the blood, leading to gout, or in the urine, leading to calcium-based or uric acid kidney stones.

Drink the right beverages. Staying well hydrated is crucial—drink enough water and other fluids so that your urine is clear or light yellow. But pay attention to *what* you drink. One very large study showed that drinking sugar-sweetened sodas and punches increased risk for kidney stones by a whopping 33 percent. However, orange juice, coffee (both decaf and caffeinated), and tea decreased risk by varying amounts, beer cut risk by 41 percent, and wine reduced risk by 33 percent. Even so, these fluids should be consumed in moderate amounts.

Make lemonade: About one-third of stone formers are low in citrate (your doctor can test your levels), which is a known stone inhibitor. Since lemons have more citrate than any other citrus fruit, low-citrate patients may benefit from drinking a mixture of one-half cup of fresh or bottled lemon juice and seven and one-half cups of water (sweetened to taste). Consume the entire batch throughout the day to keep a steady stream of citrate flowing through the kidneys.

Watch your salt intake. Sodium causes the kidneys to excrete more calcium into the urine, and many studies show that increased salt consumption raises the likelihood of kidney stones. Don't get more than 2,000 mg of sodium per day.

Get moving! You might not think that exercise would affect your risk for kidney stones, but it does. A recent study showed that even a small amount of physical activity reduced risk for kidney stones in women with no history of stones by 16 percent. Moderate activity (four hours of gardening or three hours of walking a week) reduced risk by 31 percent. There's no added benefit to very strenuous exercise.

Physical activity, especially weight-bearing exercise, may increase calcium absorption into bones, which means less calcium is excreted in the urine.

› Mathew D. Sorensen, MD, assistant professor of urology at the University of Washington School of Medicine in Seattle and director of the Comprehensive Metabolic Stone Clinic at the Puget Sound VA. His specialties include the treatment and prevention of kidney stones.

Best and Worst Drinks for Preventing Kidney Stones

Mention kidney stones and everyone within earshot winces, because we've all heard how painful these stones can be. So if you want to be stone-free, you're probably following the common advice to drink lots of liquids. But instead of focusing on how *much* you drink, the crucial question is *what* you drink. Certain beverages—including some very surprising ones, such as beer!—are particularly helpful in protecting against stones, while other drinks do more harm than good.

Unfortunately, kidney stones are common, plaguing 19 percent of men and 9 percent of women in the United States at least once in their lifetimes, and recurrences are quite common. Drinking plenty of water helps prevent stones from forming, but actually, there are other fluids that can be even more effective.

DRINK THIS, NOT THAT

Using data from three large studies, researchers followed 194,095 people, none of whom had a history of kidney stones, for more than eight years. Participants periodically completed questionnaires about their diet and overall health. During the course of the study, there were 4,462 cases of kidney stones.

Researchers adjusted for health factors (age, body mass index, diabetes, medications, blood pressure) as well as various dietary factors (including intake of meat, calcium, and potassium) known to affect kidney stone risk. Then they calculated the stone risk associated with various types of beverages.

How the comparison was done: For each analysis, the effects of drinking an average of *one or more servings per day* were compared with drinking *less than one serving per week*. Because data from three different studies were used, serving sizes were not necessarily alike across the board. But in general, a serving was considered to be twelve ounces of soda or beer; eight ounces of coffee, tea, milk, or fruit punch; five ounces of wine; and four to six ounces of juice. The researchers' findings were eye-opening.

Kidney stone risk boosters:

- Sugar-sweetened noncola sodas increased kidney stone risk by 33 percent.
- Sugar-sweetened colas increased risk by 23 percent.
- Fruit punch increased risk by 18 percent.
- Diet noncola sodas (but surprisingly, not diet colas) increased risk by 17 percent.

Kidney stone risk reducers:

+ Beer reduced kidney stone risk by 41 percent.
+ White wine reduced risk by 33 percent.
+ Red wine reduced risk by 31 percent.
+ Caffeinated coffee reduced kidney stone risk by 26 percent.
+ Decaf coffee reduced risk by 16 percent.
+ Orange juice reduced risk by 12 percent.
+ Tea reduced risk by 11 percent.

Consumption of milk and juices other than orange juice did not significantly affect the likelihood of developing kidney stones.

Theories behind the findings: Because sugar-sweetened sodas and fruit punch are associated with higher risk, researchers suspect that their high fructose concentration may increase the amount of calcium, oxalate, and uric acid in the urine, and those substances contribute to kidney stone formation. So how to explain the beneficial effects of orange juice, which is also high in fructose? Perhaps orange juice's high concentration of potassium citrate offsets the fructose and favorably changes the composition of urine.

Regarding the beneficial effects of coffee and tea, it could be that their caffeine acts as a diuretic that promotes urine production and thus helps prevent stones.

Tea and coffee, including decaf, also contain antioxidants that may help combat stone formation. Alcohol too is a diuretic, and wine and beer contain antioxidants as well, though of course, with any type of alcoholic beverage, moderation is important.

› Pietro Manuel Ferraro, MD, physician, department of internal medicine and medical specialties, Catholic University of the Sacred Heart, Rome, Italy. His study was published in *Clinical Journal of the American Society of Nephrology.*

Resources

American Association of Acupuncture
and Oriental Medicine
866-455-7999
www.aaaomonline.org

American Board of Integrative Holistic
Medicine
www.abihm.org

American Massage Therapy
Association
877-905-0577
www.AMTAmassage.org

American Physical Therapy Association
800-999-2782
www.apta.org

American Podiatric Medical
Association
301-581-9200
www.apma.org

Association of Acupuncture and
Oriental Medicine
www.aaaomOnline.org

Bonnie Prudden Myotheraphy
800-221-4634
www.BonniePrudden.com

Center for Environmental Therapeutics
646-395-8241
https://www.cet.org/

Clayton Sleep Institute
314-645-5855
www.ClaytonSleep.com

Earth, Inc. Shoes
877-372-2814
www.earthfootwear.com

Glaucoma Research Foundation
800-826-6693
www.glaucoma.org

International Association of Yoga Therapists
928-541-0004
www.iayt.org

National Certification Commission for Acupuncture and Oriental Medicine
904-598-1005
www.nccaom.org

National Parkinson Foundation's Helpline
800-4PD-INFO (473-4636)

Pilates Method Alliance
866-573-4945
www.PilatesMethodAlliance.org

USDA Farmer's Market Database
www.usdalocalfooddirectories.com

USDA Food Database
www.nal.usda.gov/fnic/foodcomp/
search

Yoga Point
www.yogapoint.com

Index

About Bottom Line Inc.

For more than forty years, Bottom Line Inc. (formerly Boardroom Inc.) has provided consumer health and financial insights to more than twenty million readers worldwide. Our vast array of expert-sourced content is published in both subscription-based newsletters and books.

Our mission is to provide the help people need to take on the challenges they face in their lives—how to stay healthy and how to heal when sick, how to make more money, and how to spend it wisely. Simply, how to be happier with their lives.

To empower your life with expert advice, please visit us at BottomLineInc.com.

Don't miss these other titles from Bottom Line books and newsletters

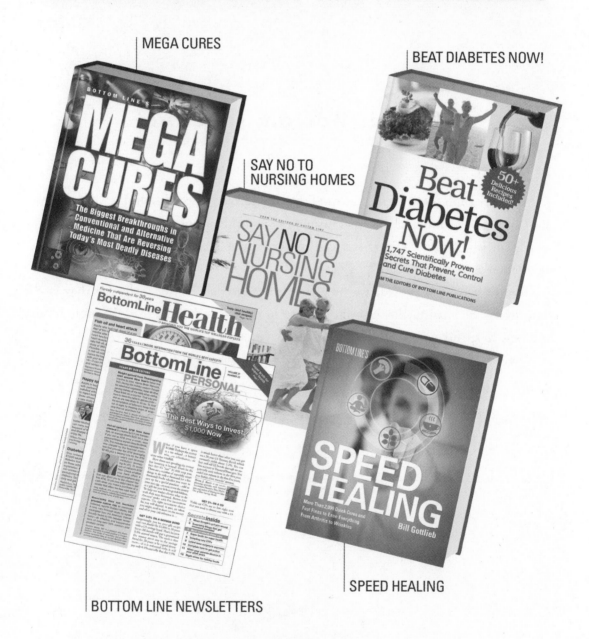